Disability Studies and the Classical Body

By triangulating the Greco-Roman world, classical reception, and disability studies, this book presents a range of approaches that reassess and reimagine traditional themes, from the narrative voice to sensory studies.

It argues that disability and disabled people are the 'forgotten other' of not just Classics, but also the Humanities more widely. Beyond the moral merits of rectifying this neglect, this book also provides a series of approaches and case studies that demonstrate the intellectual value of engaging with disability studies as classicists and exploring the classical legacy in the medical humanities. The book is presented in four parts: 'Communicating and controlling impairment, illness and pain'; 'Using, creating and showcasing disability supports and services'; 'Real bodies and retrieving senses: disability in the ritual record'; and 'Classical reception as the gateway between Classics and disability studies'. Chapters by scholars from different academic backgrounds are carefully paired in these sections in order to draw out further contrasts and nuances and produce a sum that is more than the parts. The volume also explores how the ancient world and its reception have influenced medical and disability literature, and how engagements with disabled people might lead to reinterpretations of familiar case studies, such as the Parthenon.

This book is primarily intended for classicists interested in disabled people in the Greco-Roman past and in how modern disability studies may offer insights into and reinterpretations of historic case studies. It will also be of interest to those working in medical humanities, sensory studies, and museum studies, and those exploring the wider tension between representation and reality in ancient contexts. As such, it will appeal to people in the wider Humanities who, notwithstanding any interest in how disabled people are represented in literature, art, and cinema, have had less engagement with disability studies and the lived experience of people with impairments.

Ellen Adams is Senior Lecturer in Classical Art and Archaeology at King's College London, UK. She has published extensively on Minoan Crete, including a book entitled *Cultural Identity in Minoan Crete: Social Dynamics in the Neopalatial Period* (2017, CUP). For many years, she has also investigated how a dialogue between disability studies and Classics might enhance both disciplines.

Routledge Studies in Ancient Disabilities

Routledge Studies in Ancient Disabilities is a series dedicated to the investigation of new perspectives, the application of new approaches, and the promotion of period-based and cross-cultural investigations of disability throughout antiquity. Extending beyond the core disciplines of ancient history, archaeology and classical studies, the series aims to provide a forum for scholars with diverse backgrounds, including bioarchaeology, biblical studies and contemporary disability studies, to explore the evidence for disabilities within communities extending from the Bronze Age to late Antiquity. Encouraging cross-disciplinary studies, the series aims to bring questions of disability and impairment into dialogue with those concerning status, gender, sexuality, ethnicity, and other lived experiences, as well as to consider how successive generations have received, appropriated, or reworked these forms of identity. Ultimately, the series seeks to expand the geographical, cultural, and chronological scope of work on ancient disabilities and broaden our understandings of physical impairment and mental and intellectual disabilities (and related conditions).

For further information about contributing to the series, please contact Dr Emma-Jayne Graham at emma-jayne.graham@open.ac.uk

Disability Studies and the Classical Body
The Forgotten Other
Edited by Ellen Adams

For more information on this series, visit: https://www.routledge.com/Routledge-Studies-in-Ancient-Disabilities/book-series/ANCDIS

Disability Studies and the Classical Body

The Forgotten Other

Edited by
Ellen Adams

Routledge
Taylor & Francis Group
LONDON AND NEW YORK

First published 2021
by Routledge
2 Park Square, Milton Park, Abingdon, Oxon OX14 4RN

and by Routledge
52 Vanderbilt Avenue, New York, NY 10017

Routledge is an imprint of the Taylor & Francis Group, an informa business

British Library Cataloguing-in-Publication Data
A catalogue record for this book is available from the British Library

Library of Congress Cataloging-in-Publication Data
Names: Adams, Ellen, 1975- editor.
Title: Disability studies and the classical body : the forgotten other / edited by Ellen Adams.
Description: Milton Park, Abingdon, Oxon ; New York, NY : Routledge, 2021. | Series: Routledge studies in ancient disabilities | Includes bibliographical references and index. |
Identifiers: LCCN 2020050910 (print) | LCCN 2020050911 (ebook) | ISBN 9780367221959 (hardback) | ISBN 9780367765965 (paperback) | ISBN 9780429273711 (ebook)
Subjects: LCSH: People with disabilities--History--to 1500. | Disabilities--History--To 1500. | Sociology of disability. | Civilization, Classical. | Disability studies.
Classification: LCC HV1552 .D58 2021 (print) | LCC HV1552 (ebook) | DDC 305.9/080938--dc23
LC record available at https://lccn.loc.gov/2020050910
LC ebook record available at https://lccn.loc.gov/2020050911

ISBN: 978-0-367-22195-9 (hbk)
ISBN: 978-0-367-76596-5 (pbk)
ISBN: 978-0-429-27371-1 (ebk)

Typeset in Sabon
by Taylor & Francis Books

This volume is dedicated to the activists and allies from all political persuasions who demanded the disability rights that I now enjoy and don't dare take for granted.

Contents

Illustrations

Figures

Tables

Contributors

Ellen Adams is Senior Lecturer in Classical Art and Archaeology at King's College London, UK. She has published extensively on Minoan Crete, including a book entitled *Cultural Identity in Minoan Crete: Social Dynamics in the Neopalatial Period* (2017, CUP). For many years, she has also investigated how a dialogue between disability studies and Classics might enhance both disciplines. She has established MANSIL (Museum Access Network for Sensory Impairments, London: www.mansil.uk), which supports access staff, and has run several events in museums (the British Museum, Courtauld Gallery, and Whitechapel Gallery) to explore the extended use of audio description, touch tours, and British Sign Language (BSL) tours for mainstream visitors. These were mainly funded by the Wellcome Trust and King's College London. She has also learned BSL to an advanced level (as congenitally deaf) and has a keen interest in signed art tours and the relationship between this visual-spatial language and visual culture.

Patricia Baker is currently an Affiliated Scholar in the Department of History at Virginia Tech, Blacksburg, Virginia, where she was Visiting Associate Professor in 2014. She is also an honorary academic at the University of Kent, where she was formally a Senior Lecturer. She has a wide range of publications on ancient medicine, including two monographs. Her most recent (2013) is *The Archaeology of Medicine in the Greco-Roman World*. She has also published two edited volumes dedicated to the subject – Patricia Baker, Han Nijdam, and Karine van't Land (eds) (2012) *Medicine and Space: Body, Surroundings and Borders in Antiquity and The Middle Ages* (Leiden: Brill) and Patricia Baker and Gillian Carr (eds) (2002) *Practitioners, Practices and Patients New Approaches to Medical Archaeology and Anthropology* – and more than 30 papers. She is currently working on aspects of healthy environments, considering what we might learn from the Greeks and Romans to help with environmental sustainability today (www.paxinnature.com). Her interest in ancient disability studies stems from being congenitally deaf from microtia of her right ear and conversations she had with her co-author, Dr Sarah Francis, about exploring the subject from an interdisciplinary perspective. They organized a joint conference on the subject at the University of Leeds in 2009.

Lennard J. Davis is Distinguished Professor of Liberal Arts and Science at the University of Illinois, Chicago, USA. He is the author and editor of numerous books on disability and Deafness, including *Enforcing Normalcy* (1995), *The Disability Studies Reader* (2021, 6th ed.), and *The End of Normal* (2014).

Jane Draycott is Lecturer in Ancient History at the University of Glasgow, UK. Her research investigates science, technology, and medicine in the ancient world. She has published extensively on the history and archaeology of medicine, impairment, and disability in the ancient world. Her publications include the monographs *Roman Domestic Medical Practice in Central Italy from the Middle Republic to the Early Empire* (2019) and *Approaches to Healing in Roman Egypt* (2012) and the edited volumes *Prostheses in Antiquity* (2019) and *Bodies of Evidence: Ancient Anatomical Votives Past, Present and Future* (2017, co-edited with Emma-Jayne Graham). Her current research project, which has been funded by the Wellcome Trust and the Royal Society of Edinburgh, focuses on prostheses and assistive technology in the ancient world. A monograph is in preparation, and several articles on this subject have been published in *History Today* and *Argo*.

Michael J. Flexer is a publicly engaged research fellow on the Wellcome-funded Waiting Times project at the University of Exeter, UK. His work involves co-creating storytelling and story-sharing interventions with different publics to explore and articulate their experiences of waiting and temporality. Prior to this, he worked at Imperial College London, teaching medical humanities to medicine and biomedical science undergraduates, and at Sheffield Hallam, teaching psycholinguistics. His PhD from the University of Leeds was in the semiotics of 'schizophrenia', and his contribution to this collection developed out of post-doctorate studies at King's College London with Professor Hurwitz, looking at published medical case reports since 1945. They intend to publish further on this. He has recently published on viral time and the revolutionary potential of the Covid-19 conjuncture; Peircean semiotics, abduction, and reasoning with cases; psychosis and mental time travel. Before his career in academia, Michael worked for 10 years as a semiotician and ran a small theatre company.

Sarah Francis (now known as Sarah Smart) is an independent scholar who previously held posts at the Universities of Newcastle, Leeds, and Liverpool (all in the UK), starting at Newcastle as Research Assistant on the Wellcome Trust-funded project Aristotelianism and the Development of Medical Science. She has researched the influence of the ancient philosophy on ancient medicine (and vice versa) and has published on the interaction between physiological and psychological processes in Aristotle's ethical works. She has collaborated on work investigating attitudes to disability in the ancient world, with particular regard to mental health, and how discussions of this in ancient philosophy relate to wider attitudes in ancient society.

Sophie Goggins is the Senior Curator of Biomedical Science at National Museums Scotland, UK. She is responsible for the medical and veterinary collections, including her specialism, contemporary biomedicine. Sophie's research interests include contemporary collecting in biomedicine, patient experience, and prosthetics.

Emma-Jayne Graham is Senior Lecturer in Classical Studies at the Open University, UK. Her research focuses on aspects of material religion, votive offerings, mortuary practices, and ancient disability, primarily in Roman Italy. She is General Editor for the Routledge *Studies in Ancient Disabilities* series and co-founder of the Votives Project (thevotivesproject.org). Recent publications include *Reassembling Religion in Roman Italy* (Routledge, 2021), which draws on assemblage theory, posthuman perspectives, and new materialism to explore the ways in which lived religion was produced and experienced in Roman Italy. Other relevant work includes *Bodies of Evidence: Ancient Anatomical Votives Past, Present and Future* (edited with Jane Draycott, Routledge, 2017) and a series of chapters exploring experiences of mobility impairment in the ancient world.

Edith Hall is Professor of Classics at King's College London, UK. She has published more than 30 books on ancient Greek and Roman culture and their reception since the Renaissance. Her latest book, co-authored with Henry Stead, is *A People's History of Classics: Class and Greco-Roman Antiquity in Britain and Ireland 1689–1939* (Routledge, 2020). She is the winner of the Erasmus Medal of the European Academy 2015 and was awarded an honorary doctorate from the University of Athens (2017).

Brian Hurwitz trained in general practice in central London and worked for 30 years as an inner-city GP. Since 2002, he has been Professor of Medicine and the Arts at King's College London, UK, where he co-directs the Centre for the Humanities and Health, a multidisciplinary research unit offering education at PhD and postdoctoral levels for both humanities scholars and clinical professionals, and seminars for the public (https://humanitiesandhealth.wordpress.com/). Based in the English Department at King's, his research interests include narrative studies in relation to medical practice, ethics, law, and the logic and literary form of clinical case reports and anecdotes. He has published in humanities, medical, and interdisciplinary journals and has held honorary chairs at: the Centre for Value Ethics & Law, Faculty of Medicine, University of Sydney, Australia; the Institute of Neurology (Motor Disorders Group) Queen Square, UCL, UK; the School of Humanities, Hong Kong University; and the Faculty of Medicine, Hong Kong University. Prior to his current position, he was Professor and Head of the Department of Primary Care and General Practice at Imperial College London, UK.

Helen King is a historian of medicine and the body and is Professor Emerita at the Open University, UK, from which she retired in 2017. Since then, she has held a 1-year post at Gustavus Adolphus College, USA, promoting interdisciplinary approaches to history. Originally trained in ancient history and social anthropology, her career began with fellowships at Newnham College, Cambridge, and at Newcastle University, before she worked at Liverpool Hope University College and Reading University (all in the UK). She has also held visiting roles at the Peninsula Medical School, UK, and the universities of Vienna, Austria; Texas, USA; Notre Dame, USA; and British Columbia, Canada. She has published on many aspects of medicine, particularly gynaecology and obstetrics, from classical Greece to the nineteenth century. Her most recent book, *Hippocrates Now*, was published in 2019. She is currently working on a history of the female body.

Georgia Petridou is Senior Lecturer in Ancient Greek History at the University of Liverpool, UK. She works on Greek literature, history of Greek and Roman religion, and ancient medicine in its sociocultural context. Her work on Greek and Roman religion has focused on the areas of divine epiphany, mystery cults, lived religion, religious professionals, religious innovation, and appropriation. In the field of the social history of medicine, she has a special interest in the lived experience of pain, patient history, and cultural framings of health and disease. She is the author of *Divine Epiphany in Greek Literature and Culture* (2015) and the editor of a special issue of the journal *Religion in the Roman Empire* (3.2, 2017): 'Embodying Religion: Lived Ancient Religion and the Body'. She has also co-edited *Homo Patiens. Approaches on the Patient in the Ancient World* (2016, with Chiara Thumiger) and *Beyond Priesthood. Religious Entrepreneurs and Innovators in the Imperial Era* (2017, with Richard L. Gordon and Jörg Rüpke).

Foreword

Lennard J. Davis

History is a creaky, gnomic time machine that would, if it could, take us back to the past and try to raise shadows and figures from runes and tracings. It is a clunky device with elegant aims. If scholarship seeks to be a light shone retrospectively on the darkness of the past, it is often one whose light falls off dramatically by the square of the distance. Historians know this misprision well, but common readers hope for clarity among the ruins. Tell us the story, let us imagine, let us feel the experience of those who came before, these readers ask the scholars. Some of these scholars comply and write books with absolute assertions and crystal-clear visions. Many readers like that clarity, as much of an illusion and a story as it may be.

But if it takes so much effort to actually pull a single moment in a single life from the abyss of the past, how much more effort does it take to animate (or reanimate) multifarious lives? And the inevitable paradox—the angel of history's face, as Walter Benjamin (1969, 249) wrote about Paul Klee's etching *Angelus Novus*—is turned to the past as its body is hurled into the future. Benjamin wrote:

> A Klee painting named *Angelus Novus* shows an angel looking as though he is about to move away from something he is fixedly contemplating. His eyes are staring, his mouth is open, his wings are spread. This is how one pictures the angel of history. His face is turned toward the past. Where we perceive a chain of events, he sees one single catastrophe which keeps piling wreckage upon wreckage and hurls it in front of his feet. The angel would like to stay, awaken the dead, and make whole what has been smashed. But a storm is blowing from Paradise; it has got caught in his wings with such violence that the angel can no longer close them. The storm irresistibly propels him into the future to which his back is turned, while the pile of debris before him grows skyward. This storm is what we call progress.

It looks back so that it can go forward. The farther forward it aims, the farther back it must look. When it comes to the ancient world, this misprision must be multiplied by the layers of translational fog and the continual possibility of errors piling on errors. Careening toward the future, we must (must we not?) look back. Simply saying that we can't be sure of what we recount isn't really enough to avoid leading the writer and reader down a winding path of fake truth. Instead, we must honor, as this collection does, the dialectic between future and past.

This book posits a forgotten other who is much harder to find than a remembered self. The big names of the ancient world are hardly forgotten, carved in stone as they are, remembered in British and European history, which claims an ideological descent from the ancient world, even adapting that conquering history to its own imperialist culture. We have been told that democracy began in ancient Greece, not in the foothills of South Dakota—although both ancient cultures had what we might call democracies. Philosophy began, again we are told, in ancient Greece, not perhaps in Africa or India whose thinkers either committed their philosophies to the ears alone, not the papyrus, or daubed them on wet clay temple walls. Dialectic began in the agora, not in the synagogues of arguing rabbis. We have been conditioned to believe this all too well, I am afraid.

People in the West live in an age now when, unlike earlier societies, we strive, when we are at our best, to make the other into the self. (Well, of course, not all of us do, as our daily political struggles show us—but it is a political and cultural goal for many.) We seek, successfully or aspirationally, to find that other in the present and the past, in the ashes of conquered cultures and burned libraries. We find the other in the fragilely preserved DNA of bones and the carbon of burial sites. We seek the other in asides in texts, between the numbers in economic data, within the descriptions of textiles or ores in trade transactions. We seek humanity in fragments of papyrus, shards of pottery, discarded materials and the bodies of servants entombed (and probably sacrificed) alongside their owners and rulers. That research is a dodgy game of hide and seek, and only the lonely devote their lives and livelihoods to play the long game instead of the quick bet.

And when that other is the disabled person, how much more difficult is it to find even the first foothold down the wormhole that links two spaces of time? The popular imagination, structured by the cultural surround of available images and prejudices, imagines the Greeks and Romans as marmoreal presences aglow in health and vitality. Muscular, wise, warlike, and rational, with Barthean classical fringes, elite accents, sybaritic lifestyles, they populate an imagined community drinking wine and debating the finer points of love. True, they are pedophiles, oppress women, keep slaves, only let property owners vote, and occasionally murder democratically elected leaders—but no one is perfect. But what of the disabled Greeks and Romans? They don't fit so easily into the popular imaginations taking their place in museums next to the muscular gods. True, there is Hephaestus, Polyphemus, and Philoctetes—these the exception rather than the rule. But how to find the ordinary blind woman, deaf man, mobility-impaired child?

Robert Garland (2010, xi) has written that there were 'no memoires written by the disabled in classical antiquity—the classical world was anything but confessional and there would have been no market for such revelations'. As we look for the confessional amidst the remnants of the ancient world, we are unlikely to find any written whispers to the self. One of the revelations of this book is that there are at least some confessional writings around illness and disease that begin to open the disabilities hidden by time and tide. People did write about their health, a perennial topic of discussion amongst humans. And when those notations concern pain and longstanding illness, we might get a fleeting glimpse into the disabled person.

But there is a larger paradox considered in these essays. Was the other in the ancient world actually an other? In a warrior culture, disability would be routine. In a world of incident and accident, or disease and chronic conditions, would there not be a multitude of people who were disabled? In the modern world, it is routinely estimated that between 15 and 20 per cent of the population is disabled. Would that number not be exponentially higher in the past? So might the 'other' actually be less othered than now? Would it be the case that there is not so much a forgotten other as there was a self that was only later othered as disability became less common? In that case, it is not so much the case of the forgotten other (since how could a self be other?), and more a case of an erasure of those selves by later historians? In reality, we may be talking about a forgotten 'forgotten self' that had become, only later, othered.

Without being precious about this point, I might focus more on the issue of memory. When a culture finds something unusual, it remembers it in art, writing, tabulations, and the like. But if disability, for example, would have been very common, then in some ways it would have gone unnoticed and would not be remembered or memorialized. Would we remark that our citizens all have noses, when noses are pretty common? Or, to put the point the way Marshall McLuhan once did: 'We don't know who discovered water, but we're pretty sure it wasn't a fish'. As the essays in this collection show, disability may have been more like the hard-to-see water than the more obvious iceberg or land mass—ubiquitous rather than unique.

Indeed, the larger issue comes up of the applicability of current linguistic usage to the past. Disability has a longish history in English, but, as a concept related to the social, cultural, and political implications of physical impairment and mental variation, would it seamlessly apply to other cultures? Helen Meekosha (2011) has written about the way that disability studies has followed a pattern of other 'northern' ideologies in terms of being (mis)applied to the global south. Shilpaa Anand (2013) has shown us that the term does not map easily onto Indian culture and history. And some of the authors in this collection ponder the relevance of the term for the past. In a warrior culture, for example, would disabilities related to war be seen as a negative or as a 'red badge of courage'? Would disabilities related to old age be seen as a sign of weakness and fallibility or would they be seen as markers of respect and accumulated wisdom? These are the subtle nuances that any historical approach would have to consider and about which, perhaps, hesitate to make large, definitive claims.

To return to Benjamin's angel of history, the bi-directionality of history—its backward stare versus its being hurled forward—takes us to the bi-directionality of trying to grasp disability in the past through the consciousness of the present. The editor of this volume has taken into account this stance in a mindful way. By having contemporary physicians oscillate their diagnostics between the poles of past and present, we get a better understanding of the complexities of the Hippocratic legacy bequeathed to those operating in the postmodern moment.

Likewise, focusing on museums—the living embodiment of the angel of history's dilemma—this book wakes us up to the fact that, for most people, memory of the past will be embodied in objects in the present and in the way those objects are made comprehensible to today's observers. That dialectic is particularly complex when the observers themselves are people with disabilities who may have trouble directly interacting with museum objects. Hinduism has the concept of *darshan*, or 'viewing', in which the beholding of a deity, particularly in an image form, creates a reciprocal type of experience between the person and the object. It is important, therefore, to travel, if possible, to holy sites to see and touch the carved image or painting of a god. The being-in-the-presence of that deity is crucial to the experience, perhaps similar to Benjamin's idea of 'aura' or Adorno and Horkheimer's notion of 'manna' (2002, 10–1). Likewise, much of Renaissance religious art, particularly paintings and sculptures of Madonnas, now mostly in museums, had this same aura and were seen as possessing powers to heal, forgive, and encourage devotion. These museum objects are much the same, requiring *darshan* or presence of the observer (they never do the same thing to the observer when they are reproduced in print or photography), and they act as intermediaries between the viewers who want the past to speak to them and the somewhat reticent history itself.

The essence of the angel of history's paradox perhaps might be best embodied in the face-to-face encounter between the disabled museum visitor and the mute classical object. We recall Keats's attempt to make the urn speak when it is itself the 'foster-child of silence and slow time' (*Ode on a Grecian Urn*). Attention paid to the disabled people of ancient Greece must, of course, bring attention to the disabled or Deaf citizen who stands before these valuable, if stolen (because stolen?), artifacts. Like the reader of history, the museum visitor must engage in the complex Hegelian dialectic between subject and object. But that interaction can only happen if the object is sensorily available to the viewer. It is imperative that our forgotten other not be a forgotten viewer if we are to get the fullest view of disability in the past through the present. As the disability activist's slogan goes: 'Nothing about us without us!' Disability can no longer be the thing we forget to mention about the past or the work done by non-disabled scholars and curators about an unknown other. Ideally, the story of disability in the past will be told and remembered by those who remembered not to forget in the first place.

References

Adorno, Teodor and Max Horkheimer (2002) *Dialectic of Enlightenment: Philosophical Fragments*. Edited by Gunzelin S.Noerr and translated by Edmund Jephcott. Stanford: Stanford University Press.

Anand, Shilpaa (2013) 'Historicising disability in India: Questions of subject and method.' In Renu Addlakha (ed.) *Disability Studies in India: Global Discourses, Local Realities*. New Delhi, Routledge, 35–60.

Benjamin, Walter (1969) 'Theses on the philosophy of history.' In his *Illuminations: Essays and Reflections*. Translated by Harry Zohn. New York: Schocken Books, 196–209.

Garland, Robert (2010) *The Eye of the Beholder: Deformity and Disability in the Graeco-Roman* World. Bristol: Bristol Classics Press.

Meekosha, Helen (2011) 'Decolonising disability: thinking and acting globally.' *Disability & Society* 26:6, 667–82.

Acknowledgements

This volume originated in an international 2-day conference held in June 2018 at King's College London, organized by Emma-Jayne Graham (Open University) and myself. It was generously funded by the Wellcome Trust (Small Grant for the Humanities and Social Science 208724/Z/17/Z) and the Open University, with further conference support from King's College London. Special thanks are owed to Richard Ashcroft, Lennard Davis, Rosemarie Garland-Thomson, Christian Laes, Michiel Meeusen, Aleksander Musiał, Alexia Petsalis-Diomidis, Tom Shakespeare, Michael Squire, Hannah Thompson, and Stephanie Evelyn Wright who made lively contributions to the conference, but whose papers do not appear here. Further thanks are owed to the chairs who lent fantastic support: Brian Hurwitz, Jessica Hughes, Kate Nichols, John Pearce, Alexia Petsalis-Diomidis, and Will Wootton. I am further grateful to Jessica Hughes for producing a podcast based on the workshop, as part of the Classics Confidential series (classicsconfidential.co.uk). Many thanks to Routledge (Taylor & Francis), Amy Davis-Poynter and Lizzie Risch, Emma-Jayne Graham as Series Editor, and the production team for great support.

This volume was finalised during the Covid-19 pandemic. Personal safety was jeopardized, the dread of isolation crept into every aspect of daily life, authorities made very invasive decisions regarding personal freedoms 'in your best interest', feelings of helplessness, frustration, and self-doubt surged. Overnight, the world got a taste of what it can mean to be disabled. This was a heartbreaking and economically crippling crisis, the impact of which will be felt for many years to come. Perhaps, from this chaotic crisis, we may take the opportunity to finally incorporate disabled people and disability studies into all areas of academic thought, including Classics, that most traditional stronghold. In this endeavour, I am particularly grateful to all contributors to this volume for their fantastic insights, support, and good cheer.

Chapter 1

Disability studies and the classical body: the forgotten other

Introduction

Ellen Adams

Abstract

This chapter argues that an awareness of disability studies is essential in Classics and the Humanities more widely. Studying historic disabled people requires an engagement with this relevant if seemingly anachronistic field, as we would expect with other identities, such as gender, sexuality, and ethnicity. Dialogue between past and present will help combat the ableism of our scholarly work, which is not only morally dubious, but also intellectually blinkered. This introduction sets out many of the key background issues, such as how to define disability and categorize impairments in both Western modernity and classical antiquity, and the construction of bodily aspirations and aesthetics, particularly around 'the norm' and 'the ideal'. It introduces the standard medical and social models of disability studies, but argues that we need to move beyond them, for example, considering a ritual model involving divine intervention. Unusually for a work on a disadvantaged minority, it investigates modern (British) equality and human rights law as a transparent, practical framework for exploring the complexities and tensions that the disabled body holds to the light.

Introduction

The title of this volume makes a bold claim that disability is the forgotten 'other' or minority in Classics and cognate disciplines, despite intermittent attempts to address this (e.g. Snyder, Brueggemann and Garland-Thomson 2002).[1] Many identities and statuses might lay a claim to this label, and perhaps it cheapens a serious issue if this is made into a competition. But impairment and illness are not particularly unusual, and for a proportion of society such conditions are a life-long norm. Neither are they mundane and boring, especially when the ingenuity behind substitution strategies is brought into account. Although *representations* of disabled people have long been a fascination in classical studies, especially if they can stand as metaphors or be 'good to think with', it is true that scholars have been much warier of engaging with disabled people themselves. This may partly be owing to the fact that a disproportionally low number of academics in the Humanities appear to be disabled (although the environment is increasingly inclusive), leading to such people being very much considered the 'other'. But 'other' also carries connotations of abnormality, and, historically, disabled people have been considered to be freaks. Activists for civil rights for other identities have 'bristled' with being associated with disability (Kudlick 2003, 766). This denies a stark reality: unless you die reasonably young after a healthy life, it is normal to experience impairment and debilitating conditions at some point, whether physical or mental. So why is this considered outside the realms of normal experience? There is a moral case for correcting this omission, as recently argued by Silverblank and Ward (2020), but there are also many intellectual reasons for engaging with these issues.

The 'classical body' of the title serves three purposes. First, it is a reference to the body's lived experience, rooted in empirical knowledge rather than imagined empathy. Second, it nods towards the ideal classical form, particularly as preserved in iconic marble sculptures. But these sculptures are so often broken and impaired – such as the *Venus de Milo* and her absent arms. Why, in our mind's eye, do we substitute phantom arms and ignore the damage? Why do we venerate the shattered Venus, but belittle those born with this form (e.g. Adams 2017, 206–9)? Third, 'classical body' refers to the large corpus of scholarship and sources, handed down over millennia, that has shaped modern Western thought and culture. This influence extends to the very ideas about disabilities and attitudes towards people with impairments that disability studies was established to assess and challenge.

A certain triangulation occurs across this volume. One point of reference is the Greco-Roman world itself, and the acknowledgement of the impaired or different bodies that breathed and moved within it. Another is the modern field of disability studies, very much an anachronism in terms of antiquity; it is unlikely they had the same concept of 'disability', and they certainly did not explicitly study it. Classical reception is the third point of reference that links these two contrasting worlds – the classical legacy as preserved and (mis)remembered over the centuries, and the process by which modernity has shaped, reused, and manipulated this ancient familiar/exotic/ideal world for its own agenda. It is this dialogue that ultimately justifies the juxtaposition of Classics and disability studies.

Why disability studies?

> Although the so-called reflective disciplines, such as philosophy, literature … rhetoric, art, and history, evoke disability everywhere, they seem unable to reflect on it. It appears in treatises on the ravages of war, aesthetic theories that expound on perfect form, metaphors dripping with disability imagery, modernist notions of progress, and artistic representation of anomalous bodies. Yet, outside the disability studies literature, it is barely 'unpacked'. Disability has become, then, like a guest invited to a party but never introduced.
>
> Linton (1998: 87–8)

This introduction argues that Classics and cognate Humanities disciplines need to break free from the traditional shackles of ableism and engage closely with disability studies. The absence of impairment and the failure to acknowledge physical, sensory, and mental difference permeate these fields. Take, for example, an auditory reader that includes a chapter on 'hearing loss' to explore the 'silence of the past', while excluding a consideration of actual impaired hearing and deafness (Bull and Back 2003). Much bodily research is *about* the body, as externally studied and observed (etic), rather than *from* the body as experienced (emic), and this is particularly true in studies of the disabled body (Kosut and Moore 2010, 2). Kosut and Moore's *The Body Reader* is unusual in that it focuses on the body's workings and non-workings rather than its social construction, and it also draws from disability studies (see also Breckenridge and Vogler 2001). As Shakespeare (2014, 67) states: 'academics who want to make comments about the impact of impairment, might do well to base their analysis on empirical evidence about how disabled people feel about their embodiment'. So why is this so rare in the Humanities?

Mainstream awareness of disability rights and issues are lagging at least a generation behind those of gender, sexuality, and ethnicity. The term 'disablism' does not have the same traction in identity studies or the world at large as its equivalents – various common software or social media sites (such as Microsoft Word, used for this chapter, and Facebook) mark the term 'disablism' as a misspelling, with that red, wiggly underscore (excitingly, this has now changed with the latest 2020 update of Word – progress!).[2] 'Racialism' and 'racism' are the earliest negative '-ism' terms known, used from the early twentieth century. 'Sexism' is first cited in the *OED* in 1965, 'ageism' in 1970 ('feminist', as a progressive '-ism' word is, however, first cited in the 1890s: Nagle, Fain and Sanders 2000, 267). All of these behaviours existed earlier: 'before there was *racism*, there was racism; before the word there was the practice' (Bauman 2008, 13, original italics). These terms were coined in order to fight *against* these attitudes; similarly, 'Islamophobia' was popularized by the 1997 British Runnymede Trust Report, which raised concerns about prejudice against British Muslims. The widespread lack of recognition that 'disablism' is a word and a problem is partly due to the lack of disabled people's agency and voice: this group needs to be decolonialized.

Colonialism is a form of dominance that occurs through various means, such as military or psychological, and is primarily used to refer to one country or people asserting control over another. It can also be used in a wider sense, such as the call to 'decolonise the curriculum' by challenging all structured inequalities. Colonialism is practised externally through aggressive culture contact, and a similar process can occur within societies, whereby certain groups are 'othered' (even if they are not a minority, such as women). Although this form of manipulation is a human universal, in recent centuries, upper-class, White, heterosexual, able-bodied, Western males have celebrated particular triumphs. Modern progressive societies are tasked with deconstructing this artificial, normative default in order to encourage the active participation of under-represented groups. Disability studies not only supports activism in attaining rights and adjustments for disabled people, but also challenges fundamental concepts of 'the norm', while celebrating bodily differences.

Framing this discussion in terms of colonialism can be useful in other ways. Both disabled and racial minorities are under-represented in Western academia. As 'whiteness' assumes the guise of neutrality, and therefore normality (McCoskey 2012, 26), so does being able-bodied. For example, Genie Gertz (2008, 219) has taken Joyce King's work on dysconscious racism – which implicitly accepts dominant White norms and privileges – and introduced the idea of dysconscious audism, a particular form of ableism that Deaf people who use sign language (rather than speech) encounter.[3] These assumptions are reflected in the choice of research questions and the parameters of projects.

A consideration of colonialism is a reminder that modern disability studies is a particularly Western phenomenon, so the 'us' versus 'them' narrative does not just run through time. The global south and developing countries are keen to assert *their* voice on how to promote the rights of disabled people (e.g. Anand 2013). Readers will note that there is a strong focus on the British context in this volume. This is deliberate, to a point, as claims of universality so often just uphold Western values and assumptions and impose them on others. In other words, a more local focus responds to the particular histories that constitute the structured ableism of that environment – it is unrealistic to assume that this will be the same across the world. And, if this assumption is made, all too often it is the Western template that is applied (Anand 2013).

Although we should not expect only disabled people to research these issues within each society (the insufficient representation in academia means that this would lead to their continued neglect, and we should not feel obliged to take a professional interest in this topic if we tick that box), there needs to be a grassroots-based approach, and this requires close engagement with disability studies. There is a long way to go in this, both in Classics and in the Humanities more generally. For example, in body studies (e.g. Borić and Robb 2008) and sensory studies (e.g. auditory archaeology: Scarre and Lawson 2006; Boivin et al. 2007; Mills 2014), there are few references to sensory impairments (but see Blackman 2012, 3–4; Mladenov 2015). The recent Routledge series on *The Senses in Antiquity* pays little attention to impairments or disability studies (see Graham, Chapter 7, this volume). One relevant topic this series could have explored is the plasticity of the brain – for example, how a blind person may rely more on hearing, redeploying cognitive function to this (Rodaway 1994, 101–3). The series includes a volume on ancient synaesthesia (Butler and Purves 2013), but little consideration of sensory impairment.

Rather than being a strategic decision or deliberate slight, this does seem to be a genuine and common oversight. One groundbreaking contribution to sensory archaeology includes a self-declaration statement that plants numerous flags of identity and education, without mentioning any impairment, sensory or otherwise. This 'excavation of the researcher's own sensorial prehistory, the ways by which our sensory realms and biographies define our engagement with the world' leaves us to assume that there is no such disability (Hamilakis 2013, 10). As someone with a significant sensory (hearing) impairment, I noticed this lack of comment immediately. However, reviewers of this work have not picked up on this omission, including one that referred to this page of self-analysis (Tringham 2015, 708; see also Rojas 2015; Sørensen 2015). This reflects the dominant ideology of able-bodied normality, or ableism. Furthermore, whereas other disciplines are drawn upon, such as anthropology, art history, and film studies, there seems to be no engagement with disability issues in Hamilakis's approach. Scholars engaging with sensory studies usually do so in interdisciplinary terms; for example, Day (2013, 2) invokes an impressive range, including history, sociology, ethnography, sociocultural anthropology, food studies, human geography, art and cinema, and archaeology – but again not disability studies. Although both volumes have much to contribute in terms of the archaeology of the senses, this absence presents a missed opportunity.

Within Classics, important work on disabled people in antiquity has been conducted (e.g. Garland 2010; Rose 2003; Laes, Goodey and Rose 2013; Laes 2018; Laes 2020a), but engagement with disability studies has been much more uneven. This chapter argues that disability issues are *particularly* relevant to Classics. 'Disability studies teaches that an assumed able body is crucial to the smooth operation of traditional theories of democracy, citizenship, subjectivity, beauty, and capital' (Breckenridge and Vogler 2001, 350). As Classics has done so much to define these terms in the modern Western context, it provides an appropriate and exciting starting point for renegotiating them in the light of a wider appreciation of Being Human, disabilities and all. Returning to sensory studies, we find that Greco-Roman antiquity has substantially influenced modern thought. As late as the seventeenth century, Aristotle's theory of taste perception was followed (Jütte 2005, 41). The ocularcentrism of the modern West is thought to stem ultimately from Aristotle, who also split the senses into our familiar five (*De Sensu* and *De Anima II*, 424b: Jütte 2005, 61–2; Skeates 2010; Day 2013, 4).[4] In order to widen our understanding, we need to unpack this legacy, while simultaneously surveying unexplored territories. For example, other senses may be considered, such as using sound studies and deaf studies to explore the experience of low-frequency vibrations (Friedner and Helmreich 2012). Here, engagement with a particular disability group contributes towards our wider understanding of the human senses.

The field that deals with the impaired body and the social impact of disability can take us beyond the aesthetics of the beautiful body, that most classic motif of Classics. Furthermore, in a two-way, dynamic dialogue with the past, we may explore how modern interpretations of ancient attitudes have shaped the perceptions and expectations of disabled people today (e.g. Adams 2020 on deafness). The challenge lies not only on the general level of reconstructing how (disabled) bodies act and are integrated socially, but also with retrieving them from a silent, specific past. There is a moral case for turning attention to disability, but this volume seeks to persuade the reader that there is an intellectual one as well. As bridges have already been built between Classics and other identity studies, such as gender, ethnicity, and sexuality studies, we may look sideways to them when considering how best to incorporate disability studies, and it is to these potential guides that we now turn.

Disability studies and classics: integrating the 'others'

Disability studies emerged in the UK and America as a distinctive discipline in the 1980s. In the following decade, it 'developed a new disability history, focused on concepts of otherness' (Laes, Goodey and Rose 2013, 4). The concept of the 'other' has been very influential in Classics, while assumptions about 'normality' are perpetuated. Perhaps as a result of being relatively new, disability studies is also an interdisciplinary area of research, requiring expertise from psychology, sociology, linguistics, economics, anthropology, politics, history, and media studies (Swain, French and Cameron 2003, 5). On the one hand, the very presence of this field of study sets the modern West apart from antiquity – it is a 'quite obvious statement that Greco-Roman writers could not and did not share our concept of disability' (Laes 2020b, 1). On the other hand, an explicit discipline on disabilities opens up our understanding in ways that can benefit the field of Classics. For example, disability studies challenges assumptions not only about the individual body, but also about the relationship between the individual and society. But the concept of 'disability' is culturally specific – as are all identities. So how can we open a dialogue between past and present?

A start may be to make retrospective diagnoses by deploying current medical knowledge, but this is a limited approach (Goodey and Rose 2013, 19–20). Part of the problem is that medical terminology and categorisation have changed beyond recognition (see next section). Furthermore, our 'modern' views have changed greatly over the decades, and medical opinions can be highly contested (just as the Greco-Roman world was not itself a static, homogeneous entity). However, rough retrospective diagnoses can provide a loose analytical framework for reconstructing past experiences (e.g. Baker and Francis, Chapter 8, this volume) and interpreting representations (e.g. Hall, Chapter 9, this volume). Broad identity labels, such as 'ethnicity', 'class', and 'disability', mask very striking variations within them that need to be qualified, even before bringing in intersectionality.[5] In the case of disability, I would argue that such qualification necessitates some kind of diagnosis. This approach enables a link between medical humanities and disability studies (e.g. Flexer and Hurwitz, Chapter 2, this volume; Petridou, Chapter 3, this volume; King, Chapter 10, this volume), the line between which is perhaps arbitrary. Some grasp of the specific impairment is required to build convincing bridges between past and present, in terms of experiencing the condition or representations of the condition.

Evidence for disabled people in antiquity is extremely limited, particularly concerning their experience rather than how they were viewed. This is the case for other minorities (or perceived minorities), so at least we can turn to other areas for guidance on how to proceed (e.g. see Davis 2017 on depictions of/by disabled people in film, in contrast with other minorities). Women and disabled people are comparable, as both are 'defined in opposition to a norm that is assumed to possess natural physical superiority' (Garland-Thomson 1997, 19). Indeed, Aristotle (*Generation of Animals* 737a 26–30) defined the female as being 'as it were, a deformed male'.[6] Feminist studies have wrestled with the fact that past cultures and traditional studies are inherently misogynous, or at least patriarchal (Grosz 1994). Women in antiquity lacked a voice, so how can they be written into the past, given the absence of surviving evidence and the expectations of modern sensitivities (e.g. Meskell and Joyce 2003)? One way is to explore how men *represented* women in literature and art, and this can also be applied to disabled people.

Considerations of ancient disability have focused on mythological cases and philosophical literature (e.g. Coo 2016 refers to Homer, Oedipus, and Teiresias and focuses on Thampris on the Athenian tragic stage; see also Ebenstein 2006; Kelly 2007; MacFarlane 2010). Studies have also considered how disabled people are represented in art, and how they were externally viewed (e.g. Trentin 2015). This is a practical response to the nature of the evidence, but it may also encourage a certain kind of objectification. Arguably, writing *about* disabled people is not the same as listening to the disabled voice, although there is some evidence for patient agency and voice (e.g. Letts 2016). However, Quayson (2007, 36) has argued that:

> [it] is important to bear in mind that attitudes to people with disabilities at any historical conjuncture are often multifarious, even in contexts that appear more enlightened and progressive. It is literature more than anything else that helps refract these multivalent attitudes towards disability.

Whereas women may be objects of the male gaze, the disabled body is the object of the (sometimes medical) stare (Garland-Thomson 2009; see also Foucault 1973; Garland-Thomson 2002). This stare conveys a detached, clinical response to the disabled individual, rather than providing insights into their experiences. A recent study of the body language of 'grotesques' in the ancient world includes a section on 'cripples', a term that, 'while vague and unsympathetic … has the virtue of being widely used and understood in scholarship' (Masséglia 2015, 279, fn. 44). This use of such an outmoded term is surprising and reflects the lack of engagement with disability studies and those affected by such conditions today (notwithstanding the ownership of 'Crip Pride' in some activist corners, which is not universally endorsed and is divisive). It is also a consequence of the focus on the etic *portrayal* of these figures. American scholars of disability studies are usually located within Humanities, with a tendency towards cultural representations (e.g. cinema), whereas British experts are generally placed in the Social Sciences – dealing with empirical evidence, lived experience, and policy (Shakespeare 2014, 52–3). One consequence of this split has been the lack of any engagement with lived disability issues in the British Humanities.

Although we are dealing with ancient societies for which 'disability studies' would have been inconceivable, the same could be said about gender, sexuality, class, and ethnicity studies, and classicists have engaged with them. On the one hand, anachronistic ideas should not be projected back – such as the Western distinction between sex (nature) and gender (culture) that emerged during the late 1950s (which the ancient world helped to shape: Holmes 2012; Foxhall 2013). On the other hand, we should avoid the 'add [minority] and stir' approach that does not engage with modern theory, as was applied to women in antiquity during the early 1970s (Skinner 2013). An investigation into ancient women would appear odd without some awareness and engagement with feminist literature. For example, Judith Butler's views concerning how gender is produced, performed, and regulated through social and cultural practices is of relevance even in prehistoric contexts (Butler 1990; 1993; Perry and Joyce 2005; Brady and Schirato 2011, 3). Butler's ideas of performance and femininity (rather than being a female) have been picked up in disability studies (e.g. Davis 2008).

The application of modern ideologies on to past worlds is complicated. The title *Making Silence Speak* (Lardinois and McClure 2001) indicates the role and (lack of) voice women had in the Greek world, as opposed to the present situation. Or is it so contrasting? The silencing of women remains deeply rooted, as their absence in so much modern data collection indicates (Criado Perez 2019). Our relationship with the ancient past rests on shifting sands, as both cultures are continually re-evaluated. In terms of sexuality, Orrells (2011) has wrestled with the tension between current sensitivities – with liberal attitudes to homosexuality that may more readily be mapped over ancient views – and the suffocating intolerance that existed in the earlier, Victorian period, when Classics was, ironically, more influential than it is today. We can expect similar changing tensions when considering disability. Furthermore, it is not the case that only elite, Western males engaged with antiquity, as Hall and Stead's (2020) work on class indicates. Reception studies also needs to attend to how disadvantaged groups engage with Classics, including disabled people (e.g. Adams, Chapter 6, this volume).

Unlike the identities of gender, ethnicity, and sexuality, which are perceived to be socially constructed, disability is understood to have 'real' limitations (Mitchell and Snyder 2000, 2; Shakespeare 2014, 29–30). Modern Western culture, so tolerant in other regards, remains essentially ableist – 'disability studies reminds us that feminism, sexuality and gender studies, and critical race theory meet at a point of incomprehension when faced with the corporeality of the disabled body' (Breckenridge and Vogler 2001, 350–1). There are clear advantages to being able-bodied; what is less palatable is the further assumption that all disabled people should strive for a 'normal' body, rather than accepting impairments as a natural and normal part of human life. Disability differs from other minorities in that there is strong support for the use of medical technology and aids to normalize the individual. The nearest equivalent perhaps is the attempt to 'cure' homosexuality (Conrad 2007, Chapter 5), although an equivalent comparison has been made concerning the use of melanin, hair straighteners, and dyeing products by Black people (Dunn 2008). Modern medical developments have ventured into areas well beyond the capabilities of ancient medicine, which poses difficulties in terms of bridging the cultures: the medical and ethical parameters are worlds apart. However, the main social issues are broadly comparable – and here we may again return to the Greco-Roman world.

Antiquity has influenced our attitudes towards disabled people in two contrasting, apparently contradictory ways, united only in othering them. The first is based on disgust and stigma, whereby impairments mirror character weaknesses and faults, so that the individual is to blame, monstered, and rendered subhuman (Oliver and Barnes 2012, 56; Vlahogiannis 1998, 14; 2005). Such thinking can be seen in the form of modern fictional villains, where a scar or hunchback signals inner inadequacies (e.g. Allan 2013 for representations of disabilities in science fiction). The second is the elevation of the inspiring souls who achieve goals against all the odds. Archaic tyrants and oikists were often depicted as deformed or disabled – for example, lame, blind, or with speech impediments. Ogden (1997) argues that the impairment served to demonstrate the extraordinary power of the ruler, as they were able to overcome it. Likewise, Demosthenes 'beat' his speech impediment by practising speaking with pebbles in his mouth (Rose 2003, 50, 65). The god Hephaestus's impairment becomes his strength, or *mētis*, and 'his disability is his ability' (Dolmage 2006, 122), although, in mythology, the god was often ridiculed. Today, the Paralympians similarly represent heroic achievement. These examples – subhuman and superhuman – remain as stereotypes, and, in both cases, disabled people are not 'normal'. A dialogue with the Greco-Roman world is therefore a crucial part to understanding, unpacking, and challenging such attitudes.

Antiquity has also influenced modern medicine and disability rights discourse to a (perhaps surprisingly) significant extent. Scientific medical discourse has drawn from key historical figures, such as Hippocrates, Aristotle, and Galen (King, Chapter 10, this volume). Occasionally, classical work targets this market specifically – for example, aiming to provide 'stimulating comparative perspectives for medical students and practitioners interested in the experience of the patient' (Petridou and Thumiger 2016, 6). King (2019) has explored in detail Hippocrates's role in modern medical confirmation bias and his adoption as a role model. This classical legacy has not always been positive. 'Negative reception' is detectable in two ways: first, how antiquity has influenced adverse attitudes regarding disabilities (see above), and, second, in terms of how the reception has been flawed, with mistranslations flourishing through Chinese whispers that misrepresent the original meaning (e.g. on deafness: Adams 2020, 89–90; see also Silverblank and Ward 2020).[7]

To summarize: Classics and disability studies may seem to be unlikely bedfellows, but there is much moral justification for such cross-fertilization, and the intellectual potential is far greater than simply adding disabled people to the status quo.

> Just as gender and race have had an impact well beyond women and people of color, disability is so vast in its economic, social, political, cultural, religious, legal, philosophical, artistic, moral, and medical import that it can force historians to reconsider virtually every concept, every event, every 'given' we have taken for granted.
>
> Kudlick (2003, 767)

The challenges are considerable, not least because 'disability' is a modern word and concept, although bodily impairments existed in the Greco-Roman world just the same. It is to this issue that we now turn.

Defining disability, categorizing impairments

Around 15% of people are in some way disabled, according to the 2011 WHO *World Report on Disability* (framed within Western views of 'disability' and 'normality').[8] It is clear that this group comprises a significant minority in all societies, even if 'disability' has just been used since the sixteenth century (Adams, Reiss and Serlin 2015, 6). But what does it mean to be disabled? In modern media, there is a tendency to speak of 'disability', 'disabled people', or even 'the disabled' as a single demographic category, without making even simple distinctions between different types of impairment and illness. However, 'disability is an overarching and in some ways artificial category', and polysemy is a problem (Garland-Thomson 1997, 13; see also Leshinskaya and Caramazza 2014; Altman 2001). As '*disability* itself covers a multitude of heterogeneous axes of difference' (Breckenridge and Vogler 2001, 352, original italics), it may be preferable to italicize the term – thereby signalling the need to qualify it further.[9] Dictionaries' definitions of 'disability' include 'incapacity, a disadvantage, deficiency, especially a physical or mental impairment that restricts normal achievement; something that hinders or incapacitates, something that incapacitates or disqualifies' (Linton 1998, 11). The UK Equality Act 2010 defines disability as 'a physical or mental impairment which has a substantial and long-term adverse effect on [your] ability to carry out normal day-to-day activities'.[10] This definition is necessarily vague, in order to cover a wide range of conditions and illnesses, meaning that 'the question of how the protected class is identified arises more acutely in relation to disability than it does for any of the other strands' (Hepple 2014, 43).

In social policy (such as the British 1978 Warnock Report), the different types of impairment and required need are considered separately. Today, our medical terminology has achieved a level of specificity well beyond that of the ancient world.[11] There are different types of impairment – mobility, learning, sensory, communication, mental, cosmetic disfigurements, chronic illness (including pain) – and many different grades. Some impairments are more visible than others. These different impairments (or combinations of them) demand different responses. One might, for example, distinguish between impairments (e.g.

deafness) and disease and/or pain (e.g. earache, a pain and symptom). There are also significant implications for one's identity if the condition is congenital or occurs later on in life (so that one feels a loss). Furthermore, it matters whether the problem is temporary or permanent; in the latter case, the compensatory strategies adopted are likely to have a long-term impact on personality and behaviour.

The only conditions that automatically confer on an individual the status of 'disabled' in Britain are HIV, multiple sclerosis, cancer, or being registered blind or partially sighted. For this reason, this volume welcomes discussions of serious illness and pain as well as disability based on motor/mobility, sensory, or mental impairments. This flexibility also renders disability 'not as a given entity or fact, but describes it as a discourse or as a process, experience, situation, or event' (Waldschmidt 2017, 25). In other words, disability is framed within the real-life presence of an impairment, but focused on the *consequences* of it, sociopolitical, personal, legal, economic, and so on.

It is possible to be a high-functioning person with significant impairments, and 'disabled' does not necessarily mean *un*able. India favours the term 'inconvenience' rather than 'impairment' (Bolt 2014, 4), but there are clearly many cases where this term is too mild in terms of lived experience (and it is debatable whether these terms, as understood in English, can be applied to other countries: see Anand 2013). Disability categorizations are usually set within the framework of modern Western medicine and are always in flux: the history of the diagnosis of autism illustrates this well (Silberman 2015).[12] Terminology is important in not only reflecting but also shaping attitudes. For example, there is much more acceptance of 'learning difficulties' and those who have them than previous labels such as 'retard'. The stigma of being mentally ill is reflected in the widespread use of derogatory terms such as 'nutter' and 'looney'. These are not innocent labels, and the public acceptance of vast differences in funding for mental health in comparison with other illnesses (notably cancer) stems partly from this framing: words structure attitudes, attitudes shape social policies.

Only with clear terminology and analysis can disability rights be pursued (Riddle 2013a) – even if many groups within the wider field, such as blind people or people with restricted growth, reject or deny the label 'disabled' (Shakespeare, Thompson and Wright 2010). Furthermore, some Deaf people do not consider themselves to be disabled, as sign language facilitates communication as complex as spoken English. This is an interesting argument, but not without its problems (Brueggemann 2009, 12–3; Leigh 2009). Many will feel uneasy about the relish with which the term 'disabled' is cast aside, which increases the stigma for those stuck with it. This rejection of the term can also occur among non-signing, oral deaf people. Mabel Bell (wife of Alexander Graham Bell) was a 'disability-denier': 'I shrink from any reference to my disability, and won't be seen in public with another deaf person' (quoted in Lane 1992, 98). Is it not more productive and progressive to be accepting of the label 'disabled'? Stating that Deaf people have a culture based on sign language does not in itself refute the fact that there is also a medical impairment (Baynton 2008, 300). In more practical terms, this identification is necessary in order to receive certain types of support, such as Britain's Access to Work programme (Scully 2012, 115), of which D/deaf people comprise the largest group of users. Such rights are recognized on the grounds of disability, not ethnicity or culture, and this box needs to be ticked.

How does all this compare with the vocabulary deployed in the Greco-Roman world? It has been argued that there was no single and general ancient Greek word for 'disabled', although they did have terms for specific impairments (Rose 2003, 11; this has been cited in many works since, e.g. Horn 2013, 116; see also Bien 1997; Cuny-Le Callet 2005; Laes 2008; Laes, Goodey and Rose 2013, 7). However, Laes (2020b, 3) explores the use of *anaperoi* for permanent impairments, notably the root *peros*. *Debilis* in Latin is rather vague, and can simply mean weak (Stahl 2011, 715), but Laes (2020b, 5) has pointed out that Latin distinguishes between illnesses or temporary afflictions (*morbus*) and more permanent impairments (*imbecillitas*, *infirmitas*, or *vitium*). Although this category of people clearly existed, there was apparently no need for a single collective noun for them. However, this category was recognized at some level, as disabled people were unable to draw lots for political office (Lysias, Speech 24.13–4; Dillon 1995, 38), and 'abnormal' bodies could be separated in death (Graham 2013; Southwell-Wright 2013).

One concern raised about integrating disability studies with Classics has been that there is no ancient equivalent to the term and concept of 'disability', and so we are doomed to applying inappropriate anachronisms. However, classical reception offers the space to engage with the clash of values between modernity and antiquity. There has been a recent interest in antiquity and anachronism (e.g. Rood, Atack and Phillips 2020; Umachandran and Rood 2020), which focuses on the development of the term and how it was applied in antiquity. But there is also great scope to consider how to navigate a path between 'us' and 'them', and to consider how the apparent barrier of anachronism might actually become a fruitful way of reviewing and reinventing antiquity (e.g. the consideration of 'queer temporality' in Plato: Atack 2020). This revision of antiquity opens it up to numerous more people and identities than the staid traditional elite White male, and is important – or essential – for the sustainable relevance and survival of Classics (Hall, Chapter 9, this volume).

I end this section by pointing out again that our modern term is highly problematic in itself. As stated above, 'disability' needs to be qualified, although it rarely is, itself indicating how disability rights are less developed than other minorities. The United Nations City Group concerned with this (the Washington Group on Disability Statistics) deliberately rejects the use of 'disability' in its recommended questionnaire, partly because of the potential stigma attached to the term.[13] And how do we assess whether a person is disabled or merely inconvenienced by a mild condition? The Washington Group system relies on the self-reported assessment of functioning and, in the case of sensory impairments, asks the respondent to judge their difficulty in seeing or hearing while using auxiliary aids (namely glasses and hearing aids). This, therefore, differs from the British definition (following the 2010 Equality Act), whereby the individual is assessed *without* the use of any aid. Both systems possess an internal logic (whether aids are incorporated in the assessment or not), but they contradict one another. A deaf person using hearing aids could be considered disabled in one method, but not in the other (although it is widely understood that hearing aids do not 'correct' the impairment as glasses usually do).

Furthermore, let us consider standard equal opportunities monitoring forms, such as the template provided by Britain's Advisory, Conciliation and Arbitration Service (ACAS 2020). The category of gender includes 'man', 'woman', 'intersex', 'non-binary', 'prefer not to say', and a space for 'own term'. Ethnicity contains 27 boxes, and other identities, such as sexual orientation, religion or belief, and marriage status are considered sensitively with many options. In contrast, age is set in restricted bands, and so there is a clear expectation that there is a single, factual right answer here. With disability, the options are 'yes', 'no', or 'prefer not to say', with a limited amount of space to address the question: 'What is the effect or impact of your disability or health condition on your ability to give your best at work? Please write in here: …'. In contrast to the other sections and protected characteristics, 'disability' is not broken down into a choice of categories, although further information is still required on the impact (which one might be unwilling to disclose as part of a job application). Disabled people are expected to out themselves as different from the norm, rather than just select from a diverse range of 'normal' options. This is not an unproblematic situation, and modern definitions are not straightforward. Indeed, disability studies offers a very productive starting point for exploring 'the norm' in both contemporary society and historically.

The normal body, the ideal body

How is 'normalcy' used as a synonym for 'able-bodied'? Since the early nineteenth century, the word normal 'has been used to describe how things are, as well as to prescribe how they ought to be – often both at once' (Baynton 1996, 141). Although both ancient and modern societies have bodily ideals, the scientific, statistical approach to current medical practice has brought about a focus on the *typical* body (Davis 1995; Crawford 2014; 2015; Adams 2019). Governments have increasingly managed populations in this way, with an impact on social attitudes – for example, regarding sex and gender (Orrells 2015, 4). Covid-19 brought the role of data management, state oversight, and citizen tracking in public health to global headlines. Scientific discourse valorized uniformity – 'statistics quantified the body, evolution provided a new heritage; eugenics and teratology policed its boundaries; prosthetics normalized it; and asylums cordoned off deviance' (Garland-Thomson 1996, 12). The atypical was pathological, and the normal becomes the model to aspire to.

But is this aspiration realistic? 'The body is up against an abstraction with which it cannot compete because the norm is an idealized quantitative and qualitative measure that is divorced from (rather than derived from) the observation of bodies, which are inherently variable' (Mitchell and Snyder 2000, 7). By this twist, the norm is an ideal, but one that disabled people are expected to become, rather than society catering for normal diversity (Stiker 1997). A disabled person's life is their norm, and so suggesting that normality should be a sought-after ideal can exert a great strain in terms of self-acceptance and personal identity. The contrast between congenital and introduced impairment presents a further challenge to ideas of normality. For example, we can compare the experience of war amputees, who have to adjust to a new reality, with people such as the quadrilateral amputee Diane DeVries, 'who has refused, seemingly since birth, to accept the notion that she is disabled, or, indeed, 'abnormal' (Messinger 2008, 110; Adams 2019). Here we loop back to the 'disability-deniers' referred to above, although my preference would be to state that it is perfectly normal to have a disability.

The desire for conformity or normality is not uniquely modern. There was, likewise, a drive to conform to a standard in various aspects of ancient Greco-Roman life, illustrated, for example, by the practice of Greek hoplite warfare or the Roman military tortoise. But the most celebrated aspect of the body in the ancient world is that of the Body Beautiful, as demonstrated by the 2015 British Museum exhibition, *Defining Beauty: The Body in Ancient Greek Art.*[14] Reactions against this notion include Beth Cohen's *Not the Classical Ideal* (2000), although this book focuses on ethnicity and gender, not disability. There has also been a shift towards thinking about fragmented, broken, and disabled bodies in ancient Greece and Rome (e.g. Draycott and Graham 2017).[15]

William J.T. Mitchell (1994, 1–2) observed how the political position of academic research falls into either the narrative of 'truth, beauty and excellence' as exposed by the right, or the drive to expose and address the 'political horrors' of inequality and structured discrimination. This tension may be seen in this volume. For example, Chapter 6 (Adams) addresses art appreciation, with its traditional engagement with beauty, in the context of access provision for blind and partially sighted people. Hall (Chapter 9, this volume) offers a rousing espousal of the power of representations to promote equality.

The need to take a more flexible approach to 'normality' is increasingly recognized, particularly in institutions that engage with the general public and disability access issues, such as museums (e.g. Sandell, Dodd and Garland-Thomson 2010). For example, the ivory statuette of a hunchback from the British Museum (museum number 1814,0704.277) was accredited in 1907 to an artist able to show 'an unsparing realism and the most minute observation of an abnormal' (Yeames 1907, 279). Updated, the British Museum website, on 1 November 2015, noted the melancholic pose of the piece, and focused on the artist's 'interest in the characterization of the individual' (quoted in Trentin 2015, front matter; British Museum Hunchback Catalogue, British Museum n.

d.). As of 12 December 2019, the British Museum's catalogue entry simply stated: 'Carved ivory figure of a hunchback displaying the symptoms of Pott's disease'.[16] No comment is offered on the aesthetics of the figure; instead, the label is limited to a clinical assessment of its medical status – this seems to be felt to be the most politically correct, objective framing.

In the 2008–9 British Museum *Statuephilia* exhibition, Mark Quinn raised further questions regarding the classical ideal (Fig. 1.1). The *Lely (Crouching) Venus* peers behind her towards the brash, golden statue of Kate Moss (*Siren*), posed in a yoga position well beyond the abilities of most people.[17] This juxtaposition highlights how 'ideal' equals 'unachievable', whether deity or knotted supermodel. These are different cultures, with different ideals of female body shape, roles, and attitudes – in contrast to the unsuccessful attempt by the curvy Venus to protect her modesty, tiny Moss stares straight out, defiant, at the viewer. The *Lely Venus* is a relatively unusual classical sculpture in that she is complete, which reminds us of the conceptual link between being able-bodied, normalcy, and completeness. The ideal built upon fragmentary classical sculpture contrasts with modern attitudes towards 'incomplete' disabled bodies (Adams 2017; see also Hughes 2017). For example, Mary Duffy deliberately sets her own, armless body against the 'amputated' *Venus de Milo*, but it is Duffy's body that is 'whole, complete and self-bounded' (Nead 1992, 79; see also Davis 2005). Duffy is not 'less' of a person owing to these missing parts: her claim to emic normality is as valid as anyone else's.

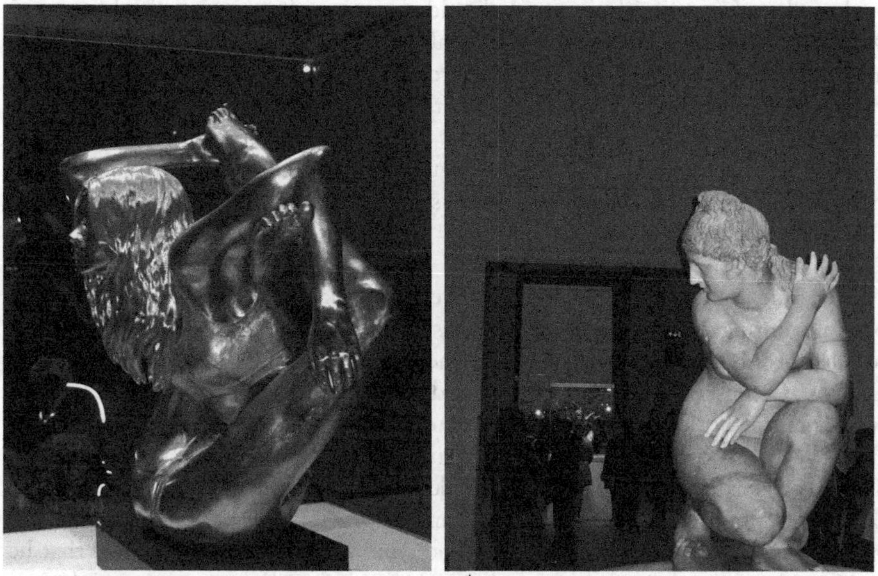

a b

Figure 1.1 1.1a *Siren* by Mark Quinn; 1.1b: The *Lely Venus* (photographs by author)

Likewise, the presence of double-amputee Aimee Mullins on the cover of *Dazed and Confused* (September 1998), topless, but wearing tracksuit bottoms and her Cheetah feet, is a direct challenge to the viewer to reconsider their ideas of completeness and beauty (Sobchack 2006; see also Goggins, Chapter 5, this volume; Draycott, Chapter 4, this volume). Alexander McQueen designed ash wood prostheses for her, carved with vines and leaves, which she modelled in his 13th fashion show in 1999 (Victoria and Albert 1999). Classicists will appreciate a comparison with the Roman tree-trunk props (or prostheses?) of marble sculpture, which offered support for these stone copies of more robust bronze originals. At one point, Cinderella glass (or clear polyethylene) slippers/legs were made for her, a nod to an imaginary, fairy-tale world. In her 2009 TED talk, Mullins asks the questions: 'what does a beautiful woman have to look like?' and 'what does it mean to have a disability?' She did not *feel* disabled and was genuinely startled to be described as such – instead, 'my legs might be wearable sculpture' (Mullins 2009). The point, in her talk, is not to normalize her body, but to improve and inspire our idea of humanity. These are ideals, perceptions and aesthetic categories. We now shift to how states and individuals respond to impairment in a rather more functional way, and the support mechanisms and practices put in place to mitigate the impact of disabilities.

Dealing with disabilities: ancient and modern approaches

A society may be judged on how it treats disabled people. Are they able to work and perform life duties, and should the state offer personalized support? Does being disabled mean you are unable to work? State support has been enshrined in wealthier countries' laws from the late twentieth century, but has the modern world created problems of its own? Clocking-in culture, stemming from the Industrial Revolution, requires a level of standardization that leaves less flexibility to absorb and accommodate diversity. The rise of capitalism and industrialism brought with it increasing segregation of the 'defectives', as there was little apparent room for disabled people in this new way of working (Oliver and Barnes 2012).

Over time, modern societies have intervened to enable such people to work. For example, during 2013–4, the British Access to Work programme supported 35,540 disabled people to retain or find employment, spending £108m (DWP 2015, 4). In contrast, Gellius (*Noctes Atticae* 4.2) understood 'able-bodied' as being literally functional for work (Laes, Goodey and Rose 2013, 7). To understand ancient attitudes towards those unable to work, we invariably turn to Lysias's Speech 24 on classical Athens (Dillon 1995). Here, the defendant is facing the accusation that he has been claiming the Athenian pension undeservedly. Rose (2003, 95) has argued that *adunatos* here does not mean 'disabled', and that this plaintiff argued that he was 'unable' to work (and therefore in need of aid) for other reasons, mainly personal circumstances and the ability to partake in a trade to only a limited extent (likewise, we have varied reasons for being 'unable' to work, including parental leave and acting as a carer). The existence of such a pension suggests a degree of social responsibility – even if this grant was not necessarily made for altruistic reasons, despite the claims of Lysias's defendant (Dillon 1995). If you were unable to work, you might seek a rich patron for survival, and then be at their command politically – which would be undemocratic. Notably, the plaintiff in Lysias (24.10) states that, if you have a misfortune, you will find the means and strategies to combat or circumnavigate it if possible – the onus initially being on the individual.

In this section, we explore sociological models developed in disability studies, which consider the relationship between the disabled individual and their society, and then turn to modern equality and human rights law (focusing on British and, by extension, European law). We will consider how appropriate such models are for the Greco-Roman world, and what insights modern legislation may give us into the practical consequences of having an impairment, as this is the area where the challenges have been considered in most depth.

Moving beyond the medical versus social models

Modern medicine is one of the great successes of contemporary times. Some diseases have been eradicated, the body can be repaired to an extraordinary extent, and everyday prevention measures, from hygiene to lifestyle practices, are well understood (if not always followed). The individual body, or patient, looks to the professional doctor to deploy all available resources to save and improve lives. In increasingly secular times, the doctor plays god, with the vital proviso that life must not be deliberately shortened. Medical advances have understandably increased doctors' authority, while the abnormal individual becomes a patient to be fixed. Furthermore, this authority is shifting to powerful pharmaceutical companies, who are 'now marketing diseases, not just drugs' (Conrad 2007, 19).

There are a variety of ways in which the body may be clinically fixed, or 'normalised' – surgery, prostheses, and drugs are just some. Biomedical enhancements (such as human growth hormone) and performance-enhancing drugs may be used to achieve normal or extraordinary ability. In some cases, the line between 'treatment', 'normalization', and 'enhancement' is not always clear (Conrad 2007). Furthermore, cosmetic (or 'aesthetic') surgery serves to help individuals 'pass' as categories or ideals that they want to belong to (Gilman 1999, 144–56). Minor cosmetic, or 'remedial', surgery is mentioned by Celsus (Jackson 2005, 23: quoting *De medicina* 7.8.3, 7.9, 7.25). The process of focusing on the physiological or biological feature deemed to be at fault, fixing the body, and rendering it normal (whatever that means) is known as the 'medical model'.[18]

If the medical model describes the fixing of individuals so they can fully rejoin society (or 'integration'), the social model calls for adjustments to social and environmental 'norms' in order to remove the disadvantage (or 'inclusion'). In other words, it is society that needs to be fixed, not the individual, with the removal of any social and environmental constraints that prevent the person from overcoming the consequences of their impairment (Anderson and Carden-Coyne 2007; Thomas 2007; Schillmeier 2010). A paradigm shift has occurred whereby the responsibility of dealing with the issue has passed from the impaired individual to the disabling society (Swain, French and Cameron 2003, 1). Structured support, such as reasonable adjustments (see below), is designed to circumnavigate any hurdles. Disability rights groups make a distinction between 'impairment' – namely, the physiological and biological missing part or defective element – and 'disability', which refers to the disadvantages that arise from this impairment and the consequent social segregation. The American Union of Physically Impaired Against Segregation argued that society had to take responsibility for the fact that its 'normal' includes a significant impaired minority, who are entitled to full access (UPIAS 1976).

Tom Shakespeare argued that a disservice is done if one neglects the predicament of bodily limitation and difference, and the role of the individual in responding to it (Shakespeare 2006, 2, 31; see Riddle 2013b for strong support of this interactionalist model, which seeks practical and realistic advances). An uncompromising social model has little room for the impact of pain in certain disabilities, which can only be managed, rather than wished away as if it were a case of mind over matter (see Zurhake 2020 for pain as a cultural phenomenon – but this does disregard the neurology of pain). On a personal level, I do not believe there is a magic wand that can alleviate all the environmental implications of having an impairment, as dedicated advocates of the social model seem to believe. Medical advances have been remarkable and do not deserve to be undervalued – and, indeed, often form part of the levelling-up process. Furthermore, some social interventions intended to support one disabled group have had unintended negative consequences for another. For example, in Canada, curbs were removed as they served as a barrier to wheelchair users, thus making it more problematic for blind walkers to traverse roads (Shakespeare 2006, 43). The modern medical and social models should be applied with caution to the ancient world, where a further ritual or moral model seems appropriate.

Martha Edwards (M. Lynn Rose) has argued that all pre-modern societies follow the social model (or community model, as she terms it), whereas the medical model is purely modern: 'the medical model did not exist in Greece' (Edwards 1997, 44). However, from the evidence of medical tools and literature, it is clear that great attempts were made to fix the body. Foucault emphasized the specifically modern nature of the clinical gaze, but he still recognized that the basic tools of medicine went back to the Greeks (Foucault 1973, xviii). Ancient medicine (as recognized by the terms of modern Western practice, focusing on human intervention to heal the patient) is a well-studied phenomenon (e.g. Draycott 2011; Hughes 2008; Nutton 2012). For example, Plato refers to amputation (*Symposium* 205e, quoted in Rose 2003, 20), and Celsus (7.33.1–2) describes the technique in some detail (quoted in Garland 2010, 134–5). Holmes points out that it is part of the Greek legacy that 'we believe there is a concept of a physical body whose nature (*physis*) must be known by the physician (*iatros*)' (Holmes 2010, 84). Ancient authors, such as Pliny in his *Natural History*, offer great insights into the variety of ancient practice. Although the humours formed an important part of ancient belief (eventually having much influence on early modern Western practice), medics also focused on particular parts of the body, such as the eyes, head, teeth or stomach (Herodotus, *Histories* 2.84; see also Horstmanshoff 2012). We have plenty of evidence for ancient medicine; it was just not as successful as modern practice.

The social model in the ancient world has been overstated. For example, it has been argued that the lack of information about disabled people is because they were integral to Greek society – blending in so seamlessly that they were not worthy of note: 'the notion of physical disability as a classification was foreign to the Greeks' (Rose 2003, 95, 98; see Dean-Jones 2005 for further criticisms of this stance). Rose rightly observes that attitudes towards disabled people are culturally specific, but the fact remains that the ancient world *did* apply medical methods to 'fix' the body. Classical scholars have pointed out that medical definitions of 'abnormalities' as a starting point for a study do not necessarily exclude sociocultural factors and nuances (e.g. Laes, Goodey and Rose 2013, 7; Graham 2013, 252). Graham (2020; Chapter 7, this volume) has advocated using the interactional perspective, which focuses on the emic experiences of impairment (see also Flexer and Hurwitz, Chapter 2, this volume; Petridou, Chapter 3, this volume). This approach also demands integration into traditional social and cultural interpretations, 'spotlighting both their disabling *and* abling aspects and intentionally disrupting the normative/non-normative binary' (Graham 2020, 34–5).

This focus on the medical and social models has led to a neglect of a third model, which could be described as a moral model involving the gods.[19] One 'deserves' good health by keeping on the right side of the gods, and, where the cause of a disease was unclear, divine or demonic agency could be blamed (Holmes 2010, 86; Oliver and Barnes 2012). In certain cases, a ritual confession was made when someone was stricken by illness or accident (Van Straten 1981, 101). Part of this practice involved the deposition of anatomical votives – this practice dates back to the Bronze Age (Morris and Peatfield 2014; Draycott and Graham 2017). Given to the gods as either bribes or thanks, one 'earned' one's healing. Some of these anatomical votives may serve as a memory aid for a lost part, such as an amputated leg (Van Straten 1981, 76). Anatomical votives could offer pilgrims a sense of regaining control over their bodies (Petsalis-Diomidis 2010, 260); they can therefore be viewed as psychological prostheses, or aids to feeling whole and normal (Adams 2019). Our increasingly secular society, where medics may be hoped to be omniscient and omnipotent (at least in times of stress), cannot offer a straightforward comparison to the ritual or moral model detectable in the ancient world, aside from praying for the sick.

Although the medical and social models offer intriguing ways to think about the relationship between the individual and the collective, we need to go beyond this dichotomy when applying disability studies to the Greco-Roman world.

First, all societies seem to have some combination of both at play, if weighed differently, which leaves the simple 'either … or' nature of the debate unhelpful. Second, the focus on this polarity has meant other forms of dealing with disabilities have been overlooked, notably appeals to divine support. Third, this focus on sociological models has resulted in another area, which has wrestled with what to do with disabled people for decades, being overlooked entirely: that of equality and human rights legislation. Arguably, Britain's 2010 Equality Act navigates a path between the medical and social models. It validates the medical model, involving the provision of technology and aids to 'fix' people and bring them in line with 'normal' modes of ability, but it also stipulates that society should help to provide these and adapt environments, rather than leaving individuals to fend for themselves.

Equality and anti-discrimination laws

Equality law offers a further opportunity to draw comparisons between different areas of identity studies (as explored above), and to expand further the nature and implications of impairments and disabilities. Whereas classicists have embraced philosophical, anthropological and theoretical literature on identity issues, there is less engagement with the law. We may consider it anachronistic to consider modern equality law, but it offers a deep and explicit philosophical and practical framework for such issues (just as an understanding of medical conditions may be useful for framing experiences, without having the simple end goal of retrospective diagnosis). Equality law is closely linked to human rights, which should clearly be of interest in Humanities disciplines. The nature of 'equality' itself is debatable. Various European and British theories of 'equality' have yielded seven meanings (Hepple 2014, 18): '1) respect for equal worth, dignity and identity as a fundamental human right; 2) eliminating status discrimination and disadvantage; 3) consistent treatment/formal equality; 4) substantive equality of opportunity; 5) equality of capabilities; 6) equality of outcomes; 7) fairness'. In Britain, the first formal equality legislation arrived with the 1965 Race Relations Act (followed by a further Act in 1968). The Equal Pay Act 1970 and the Sex Discrimination Act 1975 began the formal battle for equality on sex grounds (Hepple 2014, 11–3). The year 1970 also witnessed the passing of Alf Morris's Chronically Sick and Disabled Persons Bill into law, which committed the state to providing better support for those eligible. Its underlying aim was charitable in nature, so that they should be cared for; it did not grant full civil rights and protection against discrimination. The delay before disability discrimination law came in reflects society's general lack of awareness, and partly explains the unwillingness in some academic quarters to engage with disability studies alongside other disadvantaged groups.

The use of the modern term 'disability' is often linked to levelling structures aimed to provide some kind of equality in terms of opportunities and life experiences. This was first enshrined in British law in 1995,[20] under the Disability

Discrimination Act, which instructed certain spheres of life, such as employment, to provide reasonable adjustments for disabled people. The nature and extent of such adjustments were necessarily vague, so that sufficient support is made where possible, without bankrupting the supplier of that support. This Act made a fundamental change in how disabled people were to be treated and what they might expect. Instead of being left to deal with their short straw as best they may, responsibility for levelling up was cast out to wider society. Globally, this shift to human rights is marked by the 2006 United Nations Convention on the Rights of Persons with Disabilities.

Although certain aspects of disability law have been extended and developed, the main change in Britain's 2010 Equality Act was to bring all forms of discrimination under the same umbrella.[21] Disability discrimination was to be considered as unlawful as the other eight protected characteristics (PCs: race, age, sex, pregnancy and maternity, religion and belief, gender transitioning, marriage and civil partnership, and sexual orientation), and all fell under the banner of human rights. There was to be no hierarchy of discrimination: all are equally unacceptable. This measured approach should bring all on board – 'the single Commission and the single Act are less likely to be seen as representing only sectional interests, particularly since issues affecting White men – such as age, religion or belief and sexual orientation – are included' (Hepple 2014, 229). Being placed under the same law invites comparison with various identities and situations, which is a strong weapon against unconscious bias (e.g. consistently calling out racism, but failing to 'see' homophobia or indeed disability discrimination). The single law also faces head-on the potential clashes between interests and preferences, such as between religion and gay rights, or women's and trans rights. Only these nine PCs are protected in law, which may cause concern for disadvantages that fall outside them, particularly in terms of harassment (Hepple 2014, 21), or the notable absence of class.

In the 2010 Equality Act, the four main types of discrimination fall across all nine PCs in the same way. They are direct discrimination (e.g. refusing to allow a person into a restaurant because they are Jewish or have an assistance dog); indirect discrimination (e.g. maintaining working practices that fail to reasonably accommodate an employee on the grounds of religion or disability); harassment (e.g. name-calling or bullying on the grounds of one of the PCs); and victimization (punitive treatment of an individual who has claimed a form of discrimination). This Act offers a blueprint for civic life, as its main philosophy is that no individual, including those with PCs, may discriminate against another. This serves to discourage the weaponizing of PCs to an unreasonable extent: the law offers protection against another's unlawful behaviour, rather than empowering an individual to get whatever they want.

These obligations fall across areas of public and private life, such as education, transport and housing, and the duties vary. For example, educators have an anticipatory duty to expect and prepare for disabled students in advance, whereas employers have a responsive one, to act only when an employee requests reasonable adjustments. The scope of the 2010 Act is huge, and it is not just that it encourages comparisons between various PCs: in order to demonstrate a claim of discrimination, the claimant needs to present comparators. For example, a woman must demonstrate a pay gap by comparing herself with a man doing the same kind of job with the same experience.[22] This approach to equality therefore relies on data and evidence. For disability, the Equality Act prohibits direct discrimination, discrimination arising from disability (which abolishes the need for a comparator), indirect discrimination, and a failure to make reasonable adjustment (Connolly 2011, 388).

Of the nine PCs, only disability has this duty of reasonable adjustment, because this is the only characteristic based on impairments and special needs. The three situations in which reasonable steps must be taken to avoid any disadvantage are: (1) changes in practice, such as providing a BSL interpreter if needed; (2) changes in the built environment, such as ramps; and (3) provision of auxiliary aids, such as voice-activated software for blind people (Hepple 2014, 94–7). To not comply with these requirements amounts to discrimination against the disabled person. However, employers could argue that such an accommodation was not possible (Hepple 2014, 56, on *Mba v London Borough of Merton* 2014): 'the discriminator must show that "the treatment is a proportionate means of achieving a legitimate aim"' (Equality Act 2010, s15(1)(b)).

Even this brief survey of Britain's 2010 Equality Act indicates how identities can be set side by side, even while recognizing crucial differences between their natures. All of the PCs have been defined with a close, modern scrutiny – but there is no reason to feel that disability is the only characteristic that cannot be explored in the Greco-Roman world. In other words, the various legal, socio-political and even economic protections and provisions are clearly very different to the situation in antiquity (e.g. Adams 2020 on deafness). However, this is true of all PCs, and, as this Act instructs all PCs to be taken equally seriously, we should not single out disability as a no-go area for study in the past. I would also suggest that the law offers fruitful food for thought beyond the medical versus social models that are regularly referenced in the literature. Finally, there is a moral as well as intellectual argument for opening up classical scholarship to considerations of disability. A consideration of how equality and human rights law actually works in practice (specifically Britain as a case study here) offers a solid platform for such an approach.

This volume argues that an awareness of disability studies is essential in Classics and the Humanities more widely. The study of historical disabled people needs to engage with this and cognate fields, as we would expect with other identities, such as gender, sexuality and ethnicity. This dialogue between past and present will help combat the ableism of our scholarly work, and similar tensions encountered elsewhere lead the way, such as that between modern feminist views and the sexism of the Greco-Roman world. It should become unthinkable to explore the senses without bearing in mind sensory impairments, or 'the body' without remembering that it can, and often does, 'break'. Disabilities and ill health feature highly in identity and life, and, although being able-bodied may be taken for granted, it is not guaranteed to last. The final section explains how this volume seeks to persuade and convince the field of Classics of the benefits of this approach.

The layout of this book

There is a tension throughout this volume between the realities of the experiences of being disabled and how people with impairments are viewed, categorized, represented and treated. Disability studies offers insights into the former with obvious caveats, and modern accounts have more to offer than the assumptions arising from a scholar's imagination. In turn, Classics has played a major role in shaping Western bodily concepts, such as 'normal', 'ideal', 'beautiful' and even 'able', so this should be a two-way dialogue. This is an exploratory volume, which investigates the ways in which this conversation may be productive. The reader will note that a variety of approaches and methods are adopted.

This volume is divided into four parts, each of which has a more detailed introduction by the editor. Part 1, 'Communicating and controlling impairment, illness and pain', explores patient agency and voice. In Chapter 2, Michael J. Flexer and Brian Hurwitz actively engage with ancient authorities and Greek tragedy through the lens of modern medical case reports (MCRs). Georgia Petridou explores the challenges to articulating pain, ancient and modern, in Chapter 3. Clinical encounters demand precise communication, but is it always possible to represent such experiences in words?

As with all parts of this volume, these chapters are juxtaposed deliberately in order to explore the methodological and interpretive benefits of scholars from very different backgrounds engaging with both modern Western and ancient Greco-Roman treatments of disability. Flexer and Hurwitz are both from social science or medical humanities backgrounds, rather than Classics, and their resulting perspective of ancient authorities is fresh and insightful (see also King, Chapter 10, this volume for modern appropriations of such texts for medical or activist reasons). Petridou is an authority on ancient medicine and religion and has also sought inspiration from modern literature and case studies to consider perspectives not usually made explicit in classical evidence. This double reception (people from outside the field reinterpreting classical sources, and classicists investigating cross-cultural, especially modern, sources, in the creation of reception) was encouraged in the original conference and this volume. The pairing of these chapters increases their individual value even more.

These opening chapters address the medical side of disability head-on, which counters a growing trend to adopt a full social model to ancient disability (from Rose 2003 onwards). This is not a reactionary return to the dark days when disability was viewed solely in terms of what was wrong, missing and abnormal, nor does the focus on the relationship between patient and medic imply that an impairment must always be fixed. It is, however, a formal recognition of the practical side to illness and impairment; if the negative impact of a condition does not demand some kind of formal response and attention, then it is probably an inconvenience rather than a disability (according to the legal definition outlined above, set out within the parameters of the modern West). The chapters in this volume consider this medical–social tension on a case-by-case basis, with a greater consideration of the perspective of the disabled person (rather than just how they are represented and treated by others).

Part 2, 'Using, creating and showcasing disability supports and services', continues along similar lines to consider treatments in the form of props, prostheses and modes of communication that can substitute a missing body part or sense. In Chapter 4, Jane Draycott analyses the evidence for ancient prostheses, drawing out nuances in use and range in meaning, from functional to cosmetic. Sophie Goggins explores the modern context for these objects in Chapter 5, as staged in museums, particularly National Museums Scotland. Here, the issue of who gets to narrate the story carries particular resonance. In Chapter 6, Ellen Adams considers how blind and partially sighted people interact with visual culture in museums, drawing from a course based on the Parthenon galleries in the British Museum. This engages with the access practices of audio description and touch tours.

This part also juxtaposes three different kinds of expertise: ancient prostheses, museum curation and access programmes in museums. How can material culture and museum displays and events alleviate impairment and increase awareness about disability issues? Again, the dialogue between ancient and modern disability is tackled from different perspectives in all three chapters, so that the sum becomes more than their parts. The tension between medical and social is also navigated differently in each chapter for comparative purposes. Draycott explores one of the more obvious types of medical support, but also considers how they could be a social investment. Goggins discusses a medical exhibition, but in addition relates how personal responses also form part of the curatorial engagement. Adams investigates how museums have developed compensatory strategies for people with visual impairments, in response to disability law. She also explores how wider society might benefit from making these provisions more mainstream, which could in turn influence visual studies.

Part 3, 'Real bodies and retrieving senses: disability in the ritual record', is archaeological at heart. Continuing the engagement between sensory studies and disability studies (from Chapter 6), Emma-Jayne Graham anchors Chapter 7 not in a modern museum, but in the Roman sanctuary of Fortuna Primigenia at Praeneste. This convincing emic reconstruction of past experience invites us to reconsider our understanding of ancient religion beyond the issue of disability alone. From sanctuary to burial, Patricia Baker and Sarah Francis explore the mortuary treatment of people with evidence for significant impairments in Chapter 8. They argue that they were considered to be like children, supported by ancient authorities (using both literary and archaeological evidence, as most chapters in this volume do). Both chapters again explore the tension between the medical and social models (or Graham's use of interactional theory), while the explicit setting in the ritual sphere highlights the contrast between the everyday experience of disability and time spent engaging with other worlds (deities or the dead). As argued above, the ritual sphere offers a third avenue for dealing with disability beyond medical treatments and social accommodation, albeit in rather different ways, as illustrated here.

Graham's consideration of experiences of people with visual or mobility impairments highlights one issue that is often overlooked: it can be very time-consuming being disabled. One can still visit and participate, but movement is often slowed down, and the arrangements need to be better planned. This aspect adds to the phenomenological experience of including disabled people in collective events, past and present. In contrast, Baker and Francis highlight the *spatial* segregation that can occur, in this case in the mortuary sphere. This is becoming less common in societies such as Britain with the mainstreaming movement, but remains a sensitive subject: how and when should having special needs mean separate provision, rather than adjusting the mainstream environment?

Part 4, 'Classical reception as the gateway between Classics and disability studies', returns to elements of Part 1 that we never completely left. This volume began by exploring the voice of the forgotten othered, be it patient or person with impairment, and the challenges of articulating subjective experiences. Turning full circle, it returns to these themes, but with the added dimension of imagined stories and distorted dialogues between Greco-Roman antiquity and Western modernity. These illusions, filters and tensions generate a cognitive dissonance, whereby accounts of myriad and occasionally contradictory experiences present themselves simultaneously. Reality and representation do not sit as opposing ends of a spectrum, but rather fold into each other to produce the messiness of perception – including, and perhaps especially, that of the human body.

Who owns the narrative, who gets to set the scene? And how should we strike a balance between exploring cultural representations and human experience? In Chapter 9, Edith Hall explores modern engagements with disabled people from ancient myth, arguing that cultural representations can promote progressive values. Her central focus is Nicolas Poussin's landscape, *Blind Orion Searching for the Rising Sun* (1658), which acts as a springboard for considering the ripples of reinterpretation. Helen King completes the volume in Chapter 10, considering first how Classics has influenced modern medical and disability treatises, before turning to a modern invention of an ancient disabled woman in the form of Nydia, the blind flower-girl of Bulwer-Lytton's (1834) *Last Days of Pompeii*, rendered in 3D sculpture by Randolph Rogers (1853–4, 1859). As with all chapters in this volume, the wide range of approaches and methodologies reflect the broad church of Classics, and they demonstrate the myriad ways in which the voices of disabled people may contribute to the field.

As Classics seeks to decolonize its curriculum and research agendas in terms of marginalized voices, moving towards a more enriched, multivocal and sustainable future, this volume begins to consider how this may be achieved in terms of disability. In various ways, the chapters in this volume navigate a path between the three landmarks of: the Greco-Roman world, classical reception, and relevant modern fields such as disability studies and medical humanities. This necessitates a dynamic dialogue between past and present, as well as engagement with a wide range of sources (notably textual and visual) and scholars with diverse expertise. While the individual chapters achieve this independently, even more is gained when they are read side by side, as suggested in the introduction to each of the four parts.

Notes

1 Trentin (2013) also points out that disabled people have not formed part of the traditional teaching material of Classics.

2 Following Bolt (2014, 3), we may draw a distinction between ableism, which makes assumptions about normalcy and the default able-bodied person (equivalent to 'patriarchy'), and disablism, which refers to the exclusion of and hostile attitudes towards disabled people (equivalent to 'misogyny').

3 Note the use of 'Deaf' for people who use a sign language as their first or preferred language and have consequently built a strong community based on it, while 'deaf' refers to those with a significant medical hearing impairment.

4 Jütte (2005, 54) points out that this number of senses is shared by early Indian and Chinese cultures, which raises the question of whether this is a specifically Western phenomenon as is often stated (for example, Hamilakis 2011, 210).

5 See, for example, Kudlick (2003) on the impact of there being mainly White male leaders in the Deaf community and movement. This makes seeking the 'representative voice' problematic.

6 Aristotle defined the male as 'the one who is able', while the female was 'the one who is unable', and so the ability to do certain things was important: Aristotle, *Generation of animals* 765b 36. Aristotle has contributed so much to disability studies that he warrants an entry in the monumental *Encyclopedia of Disability Vol. 1* (Albrecht 2006), where this observation is described as 'quaint at best' (p. 124).

7 Anand (2013, 37) provides a very useful table of disability historiography, whereby the Greco-Roman contribution is summarised as: 'to find explanations for contemporary trends in discrimination against physical difference. To understand contemporary veneration of beauty and perfection'.

8 www.who.int/publications-detail/world-report-on-disability (accessed 7 May 2020).

9 Bourdieu warned against over-intellectualising the language of representation, especially concerning the body, but a self-conscious precision is essential given the complex relationship between impairment and identity (Bourdieu 1977, 120; see also Boivin 2008, 90).

10 www.gov.uk/definition-of-disability-under-equality-act-2010 (accessed 12 December 2019).

11 Medically, the impaired body formed a focus of Enlightenment interest in taxonomy: if one could classify the world, one could understand and control it (but see Bowker and Star 1999 for the contradictions and fuzziness in today's terminology).

12 These 'identity categories' have been explored in American literature and cultural assumptions regarding the physically impaired (Garland-Thomson 1997). The so-called Chinese encyclopedia is often referred to in order to demonstrate how cultural/natural taxonomies can vary. Here, animals are classified according to: those

belonging to the emperor; embalmed animals; fabulous animals; wild dogs; animals painted with a very fine brush of camel hairs; and those that seem to be flies when observed from a distance (Foucault 1970, xvi; Sonesson 1989, 67). See Bowker and Star (1999, 131), who compare this with the International Classification of Diseases.

13 'Why don't the WG questions use the word "disability"?': see the FAQ page here: www.washingtongroup-disability.com/resources/frequently-asked-questions (accessed 6 January 2021).

14 This kind of focus on aesthetics is directed towards the artist rather than the bodily experience of those at the time (for example, Porter 2010; see also Squire 2011).

15 It is notable, however, that Greek artists disliked showing impaired and mutilated bodies (Dasen 1993, 165–6). She argues that people with impaired growth in the ancient world were not 'seen as an irreducible monstrosity', as their bodies were at least complete.

16 www.britishmuseum.org/collection/object/G_1814-0704-277 (accessed 7 August 2020). Note that the earlier description has more in common with the freak show fascination with the so-called monstrosities and curiosities in the ancient world, particularly the Roman one.

17 Art reports from when the sculpture was sold suggest that a yoga guru was used for the pose, e.g. www.businessinsider.com/kate-moss-in-gold-fetches-900000–siren-by-marc-quinn-2011-10?IR=T (accessed 4 May 2020).

18 Perhaps the most successful protest against this interventionist approach to the body relates not to disability, but childbirth. For example, the British National Childbirth Trust actively discouraged professional assistance, including pain relief and doctors (particularly during the 1990s, but it is more relaxed today). Such movements arose from the oppressive medicalization of childbirth, with the mother often sedated and placed in stirrups (Conrad 2007, 157–8).

19 One exception is Horn (2013), but this relies in particular on early Christian Greek sources, where the concept of the individual's fault for his predicament becomes clear (p. 138): 'disability was the failure to receive healing: the ability in question was the ability of the person to muster sufficient faith in the power of the healer'. Similarly, the role of God and/or a divine plan in disabilities has been explored in biblical studies (Avalos, Melcher and Schipper 2007).

20 The year 1995 also witnessed the milestone publication of Garland's *Eye of the Beholder: Deformity and Disability in the Graeco-Roman World*, although Garland works in the American system, where the groundbreaking disability discrimination law was passed in 1990.

21 Because disability requires distinct consideration and treatment, it has a separate committee in the Equalities and Human Rights Commission (EHRC). The EHRC was established in the 2006 Equality Act as the authority required to implement the later legislation. This has since been starved of funds and is no longer able to perform its full remit. The 2010 Equality Act also followed the United Nations Convention on the Rights of Persons with Disabilities, which became effective in 2008 (Scully 2012, 118).

22 It also makes is virtually impossible for a claimant to work with two PCs at the same time – for example, a Black woman complaining about unequal pay would need to select one PC for a direct comparator in turn (Hepple 2014, 77–8; Sargeant 2018, 10–2).

References

ACAS [Advisory, Conciliation and Arbitration Service] (2020) 'Example of Equality and Diversity Monitoring Form.' www.acas.org.uk/job-application-form-templates (accessed 4 May 2020).

Adams, Ellen (2017) 'Fragmentation and the body's boundaries: reassessing the body in parts.' In Jane Draycott and Emma-Jayne Graham (eds) *Bodies of Evidence: Ancient Anatomical Votives Past, Present and Future*. London: Routledge, 193–213.

Adams, Ellen (2019) 'The psychology of prostheses: substitution strategies and notions of normality.' In Jane Draycott (ed.) *Prostheses in Antiquity*. London: Routledge, 180–208.

Adams, Ellen (2020) 'Deafness: sensory impairment as communication disability, past and present.' In Christian Laes (ed.) *The Cultural History of Disability in Antiquity*. London: Bloomsbury, 85–100.

Adams, Rachel, Benjamin Reiss and David Serlin (2015) 'Disability.' In Rachel Adams, Benjamin Reiss and David Serlin (eds) *Keywords for Disability Studies*. New York and London: NYU Press, 5–11.

Albrecht, Gary (ed.) (2006) *Encyclopedia of Disability*. Vol 1. Thousand Oaks and London: Sage.

Allan, Kathryn (ed.) (2013) *Disability in Science Fiction: Representations of Technology as Cure*. New York: Palgrave Macmillan.

Altman, Barbara (2001) 'Disability definitions, models, classification schemes, and applications.' In Gary Albrecht, Katherine Delores Seelman and Michael Bury (eds) *Handbook of Disability Studies*. Thousand Oaks: Sage, 97–122.

Anand, Shilpaa (2013) 'Historicising disability in India: questions of subject and method.' In Renu Addlakha (ed.) *Disability Studies in India: Global Discourses, Local Realities*. New Delhi: Routledge, 35–60.

Anderson, Julic and Ana Carden-Coyne (2007) 'Enabling the past: new perspectives in the history of disability.' *European Review of History* 14, 447–57.

Atack, Carol (2020) 'Plato's queer time: dialogic moments in the life and death of Socrates.' *Classical Receptions Journal* 12, 10–31.

Avalos, Hector, Sarah J. Melcher and Jeremy Schipper (2007) 'Introduction.' In Hector Avalos, Sarah J. Melcher and Jeremy Schipper (eds) *This Abled Body: Rethinking Disabilities in Biblical Studies*. Atlanta: Society of Biblical Literature, 1–9.

Bauman, H-Dirksen L. (2008) 'Introduction: listening to Deaf Studies.' In H-Dirksen L. Bauman (ed.) *Open Your Eyes: Deaf Studies Talking*. Minneapolis, MN: University of Minnesota Press, 1–32.

Baynton, Douglas C. (1996) *Forbidden Signs: American Culture and the Campaign against Sign Language*. Chicago and London: The University of Chicago Press.

Baynton, Douglas C. (2008) 'Beyond culture: Deaf Studies and the Deaf body.' In H-Dirksen L. Bauman (ed.) *Open Your Eyes: Deaf Studies Talking*. Minneapolis, MN: University of Minnesota Press, 293–313.

Bien, Christian G. (1997) *Erklärungen zur Entstehung von Mißbildungen im physiologischen und medizinischen Schrifttum der Antike*. Stuttgart: Franz Steiner Verlag.

Blackman, Lisa (2012) *Immaterial Bodies: Affect, Embodiment, Mediation*. London: Sage.

Boivin, Nicole (2008) *Material Cultures, Material Minds: The Impact of Things on Human Thought, Society and Evolution*. Cambridge: Cambridge University Press.

Boivin, Nicole, Adam Brumm, Helen Lewis, Dave Robinson and Ravi Korisettar (2007) 'Sensual, material, and technological understanding: exploring prehistoric soundscapes in south India.' *Journal of the Royal Anthropological Institute* 13, 267–94.

Bolt, David (2014) 'Introduction: perspectives from historical, cultural, and educational studies.' In David Bolt (ed.) *Changing Social Attitudes Toward Disability: Perspectives from Historical, Cultural, and Educational Studies*. London and New York: Routledge, 1–11.

Borić, Dušan and John Robb (2008) 'Body theory in archaeology.' In Dušan Borić and John Robb (eds) *Past Bodies: Body-Centered Research in Archaeology*. Oxford: Oxbow Books, 1–7.

Bourdieu, Pierre (1977) *Outline for a Theory of Practice*. Translated by Richard Nice. Cambridge: Cambridge University Press.

Bowker, Geoffrey C. and Susan Leigh Star (1999) *Sorting Things Out: Classifications and its Consequences*. Cambridge, MA: MIT Press.

Brady, Anita and Tony Schirato (2011) *Understanding Judith Butler*. London: Sage.

Breckenridge, Carol A. and Candace Vogler (2001) 'The critical limits of embodiment: disability's criticism.' *Public Culture* 13, 349–57.

British Museum (n.d.) British Museum Hunchback Catalogue: Townley Collection, 1814, 0704.277: https://www.britishmuseum.org/collection/object/G_1814-0704-277 (accessed 12 December 2019). The previous online entry at www.britishmuseum.org/explore/highlights/highlight_objects/gr/i/ivory_figure_of_a_hunchback.aspx (accessed 1 November 2015) is no longer live.

Brueggemann, Brenda (2009) *Deaf Subjects: Between Identities and Places*. New York and London: New York University Press.

Bull, Michael and Les Back (eds) (2003) *The Auditory Culture Reader*. Oxford: Berg.

Butler, Judith (1990) *Gender Trouble: Feminism and the Subversion of Identity*. London and New York: Routledge.

Butler, Judith (1993) *Bodies that Matter: On the Discursive Limits of "Sex"*. New York and London: Routledge.

Butler, Shane and Alex Purves (eds) (2013) *Synaesthesia and the Ancient Senses*. Durham: Acumen.

Cohen, Beth (ed.) (2000) *Not the Classical Ideal: Athens and the Construction of the Other in Greek Art*. Leiden and Boston: Brill.

Connolly, Michael (2011) *Discrimination Law* (2nd ed.). London: Sweet & Maxwell.

Conrad, Peter (2007) *The Medicalization of Society: On the Transformation of Human Conditions into Treatable Disorders*. Baltimore: Johns Hopkins University Press.

Coo, Lyndsay (2016) 'Sight and blindness: the mask of Thamyris.' In Michael Squire (ed.) *Sight and the Ancient Senses*. London and New York: Routledge, 237–48.

Crawford, Cassandra (2014) *Phantom Limb: Amputation, Embodiment, and Prosthetic Technology*. New York and London: New York University Press.

Crawford, Cassandra (2015) 'Body image, prostheses, phantom limbs.' *Body and Society* 21, 221–44.

Criado Perez, Caroline (2019) *Invisible Women: Exposing Data Bias in a World Designed for Men*. London: Chatto & Windus.

Cuny-Le Callet, Blandine (2005) *Rome et ses monstres: Naissance d'un concept philosophique et rhétorique*. Grenoble: Jérôme Millon.

Dasen, Véronique (1993) *Dwarfs in Ancient Egypt and Greece*. Oxford: Clarendon Press.

Davis, Lennard (1995) *Enforcing Normalcy: Disability, Deafness and the Body*. London: Verso.

Davis, Lennard (2005) 'Visualizing the disabled body: the classical nude and the fragmented torso.' In Mariam Fraser and Monica Greco (eds) *The Body: A Reader*. London and New York: Routledge, 167–81.

Davis, Lennard (2008) 'Postdeafness.' In H-Dirksen L. Bauman (ed.) *Open Your Eyes: Deaf Studies Talking*. Minneapolis and London: University of Minnesota Press, 314–25.

Davis, Lennard (2017) 'The ghettoization of disability: paradoxes of visibility and invisibility in cinema.' In Anne Waldschmidt, Hanjo Berressem and Moritz Ingwersen (eds) *Culture – Theory – Disability: Encounters between Disability Studies and Cultural Studies*. Bielefeld: Transcript Verlag, 39–49.

Day, Jo (2013) 'Introduction: making senses of the past.' In Jo Day (ed.) *Making Senses of the Past: Toward a Sensory Archaeology*. Carbondale and Edwardsville: Southern Illinois University Press, 1–31.

Dean-Jones, Lesley (2005) 'Review of: Martha L. Rose, *The Staff of Oedipus: Transforming Disability in Ancient Greece*. (2003: Ann Arbor: University of Michigan Press).' *American Historical Review* 110, 531–2.

Dillon, Matthew P.J. (1995) 'Payments to the disabled at Athens: social justice or fear of aristocratic patronage?' *Ancient Society* 26, 27–57.

Dolmage, Jay (2006) '"Breathe upon us an even flame": Hephaestus, history, and the body of rhetoric.' *Rhetoric Review* 25, 119–40.

Draycott, Jane (2011) 'Approaches to Healing in Roman Egypt.' PhD thesis, University of Nottingham.

Draycott, Jane and Emma-Jane Graham (eds) (2017) *Bodies of Evidence: Ancient Anatomical Votives Past, Present and Future*. London: Routledge.

Dunn, Lindsay (2008) 'The burden of racism and audism.' In H-Dirksen L. Bauman (ed.) *Open Your Eyes: Deaf Studies Talking*. Minneapolis, MN: University of Minnesota Press, 235–50.

DWP [Department for Work & Pensions] (2015) *Equality Analysis for the Future of Access to Work: May 2015*. DWP.

Ebenstein, William (2006) 'Toward an archetypal psychology of disability based on the Hephaestus myth.' *Disability Studies Quarterly* 26.4, https://dsq-sds.org/article/view/805/980

Edwards, Martha L. (1997) 'Constructions of physical disability in the ancient Greek world: the community concept.' In David T. Mitchell and Sharon L. Snyder (eds) *The Body and Physical Difference: Discourses of Disability*. Ann Arbor: University of Michigan Press, 35–50.

Foucault, Michel (1970) *The Order of Things: An Archaeology of the Human Sciences*. London: Tavistock.

Foucault, Michel (1973) *The Birth of the Clinic: An Archaeology of Medical Perception*. Translated by A.M. Sheridan Smith. London: Tavistock.

Foxhall, Lin (2013) *Studying Gender in Classical Antiquity*. Cambridge: Cambridge University Press.

Friedner, Michele and Stefan Helmreich (2012) 'Sound studies meets deaf studies.' *The Senses and Society* 7, 72–86.

Garland, Robert (2010) *The Eye of the Beholder: Deformity and Disability in the Graeco-Roman World* (2nd ed.). Bristol: Bristol Classical Press.

Garland-Thomson, Rosemarie (1996) 'Introduction: From wonder to error – a genealogy of freak discourse in modernity.' In Rosemarie Garland-Thomson (ed.) *Freakery: Cultural Spectacles of the Extraordinary Body*. New York and London: New York University Press, 1–19.

Garland-Thomson, Rosemarie (1997) *Extraordinary Bodies: Figuring Physical Disability in American Culture and Literature*. New York: Columbia University Press.

Garland-Thomson, Rosemarie (2002) 'The politics of staring: visual rhetorics of disability in popular photography.' In Sharon L. Snyder, Brenda J. Bruggemann and Rosemarie

Garland-Thomson (eds) *Disability Studies: Enabling the Humanities*. New York: Modern Language Association of America, 56–75.

Garland-Thomson, Rosemarie (2009) *Staring: How We Look*. Oxford: Oxford University Press.

Gertz, Genie (2008) 'Dysconscious audism: a theoretical proposition.' In H-Dirksen L. Bauman (ed.) *Open Your Eyes: Deaf Studies Talking*. Minneapolis, MN: University of Minnesota Press, 219–34.

Gilman, Sander L. (1999) *Making the Body Beautiful: A Cultural History of Aesthetic Surgery*. Princeton, NJ: Princeton University Press.

Goodey, Chris F. and M. Lynn Rose (2013) 'Mental states, bodily dispositions and table manners: a guide to reading "intellectual" disability from Homer to Late Antiquity.' In Christian Laes, Chris F. Goodey and M. Lynn Rose (eds) *Disabilities in Roman Antiquity: Disparate Bodies* A Capite ad Calcem. Leiden and Boston: Brill, 17–44.

Graham, Emma-Jayne (2013) 'Disparate lives or disparate deaths? Post-mortem treatment of the body and the articulation of difference.' In Christian Laes, Chris F. Goodey and M. Lynn Rose (eds) *Disabilities in Roman Antiquity: Disparate Bodies* A Capite ad Calcem. Leiden and Boston: Brill, 249–74.

Graham, Emma-Jayne (2020) 'Mobility impairment: identifying lived experiences in Roman Italy.' In Christian Laes (ed.) *A Cultural History of Disability in Antiquity*. London: Bloomsbury, 31–45.

Grosz, Elizabeth (1994) *Volatile Bodies: Toward a Corporeal Feminism*. Bloomington and Indianapolis: Indiana University Press.

Hall, Edith and Henry Stead (2020) *A People's History of Classics: Class and Greco-Roman Antiquity in Britain and Ireland 1689 to 1939*. London and New York: Routledge.

Hamilakis, Yannis (2011) 'Archaeologies of the senses.' In Timothy Insoll (ed.) *The Oxford Handbook on the Archaeology of Ritual and Religion*. Oxford: Oxford University Press, 208–25.

Hamilakis, Yannis (2013) *Archaeology and the Senses: Human Experience, Memory and Affect*. Cambridge: Cambridge University Press.

Hepple, Bob (2014) *Equality: The Legal Framework* (2nd ed.). Oxford and Portland, OR: Hart.

Holmes, Brooke (2010) 'Medical knowledge and technology.' In Daniel H. Garrison (ed.) *A Cultural History of the Human Body in Antiquity*. Oxford and New York: Berg, 83–105.

Holmes, Brooke (2012) *Gender: Antiquity and Its Legacy*. London: I.B. Tauris.

Horn, Cornelia B. (2013) 'A nexus of disability in ancient Greek miracle stories: a comparison of accounts of blindness from the Asklepieion in Epidauros and the shrine of Thecla in Seleucia.' In Christian Laes, Chris F. Goodey and M. Lynn Rose (eds) *Disabilities in Roman Antiquity: Disparate Bodies* A Capite ad Calcem. Leiden and Boston: Brill, 115–43.

Horstmanshoff, Manfred (2012) 'Disability and rehabilitation in the Graeco-Roman world.' In Rupert Breitwieser (ed.) *Behinderungen und Beeinträchtigungen/Disability and Impairment in Antiquity*. BAR Int. Series 2359. Oxford: Archaeopress, 1–9.

Hughes, Jessica (2008) 'Fragmentation as metaphor in the classical healing sanctuary.' *Social History of Medicine* 21, 217–36.

Hughes, Jessica (2017) *Votive Body Parts in Greek and Roman Religion*. Cambridge: Cambridge University Press.

Jackson, Ralph (2005) 'Circumcision, de-circumcision and self-image: Celsus's "operations on the penis".' In Andrew Hopkins and Maria Wyke (eds) *Roman Bodies: Antiquity to the Eighteenth Century*. London: The British School at Rome, 23–41.

Jütte, Robert (2005) *A History of the Senses: From Antiquity to Cyberspace*. Cambridge: Polity.

Kelly, Nicole (2007) 'Deformity and disability in Greece and Rome.' In Hector Avalos, Sarah J. Melcher and Jeremy Schipper (eds) *This Abled Body: Rethinking Disabilities in Biblical Studies*. Leiden: Brill, 31–46.

King, Helen (2019) *Hippocrates Now: The 'Father of Medicine' in the Internet Age*. London: Bloomsbury.

Kosut, Mary and Lisa J.Moore (2010) 'Introduction: not just the reflexive reflex: flesh and bone in the social sciences.' In Lisa J.Moore and Mary Kosut (eds) *The Body Reader: Essential Social and Cultural Readings*. New York and London: New York University Press, 1–26.

Kudlick, Catherine (2003) 'Disability history: why we need another "other".' *The American Historical Review* 108, 763–93.

Laes, Christian (2008) 'Learning from silence: disabled children in Roman antiquity.' *Arctos* 42, 85–122.

Laes, Christian (2018) *Disabilities and the Disabled in the Roman World*. Cambridge: Cambridge University Press.

Laes, Christian (ed.) (2020a) *A Cultural History of Disability in Antiquity*. London: Bloomsbury.

Laes, Christian (2020b) 'How and whether to say "disability" in Latin and Ancient Greek.' In Christian Laes (ed.) *A Cultural History of Disability in Antiquity*. London: Bloomsbury, 1–14.

Laes, Christian, Chris F. Goodey and M. Lynn Rose (2013) 'Approaching disabilities *a capite ad calcem*: hidden themes in Roman antiquity.' In Christian Laes, Chris F. Goodey and M. Lynn Rose (eds) *Disabilities in Roman Antiquity: Disparate Bodies* A Capite ad Calcem. London and Boston: Brill, 1–15.

Lane, Harlan (1992) *The Mask of Benevolence: Disabling the Deaf Community*. New York: Knopf.

Lardinois, Andre and Laura McClure (eds), (2001). *Making Silence Speak: Women's Voices in Greek Literature and Society*. Princeton and Oxford: Princeton University Press.

Leigh, Irene (2009) *A Lens on Deaf Identities*. Oxford: Oxford University Press.

Leshinskaya, Anna and Alfonso Caramazza (2014) 'Organization and structure of conceptual representations.' In Matthew Goldrick, Victor Ferreira and Michele Miozzo (eds) *The Oxford Handbook of Language Production*. Oxford: Oxford University Press: 118–33.

Letts, Melinda (2016) 'Questioning the patient, questioning Hippocrates: Rufus of Ephesus and the pursuit of knowledge.' In Georgia Petridou and Chiara Thumiger (eds) *Homo Patiens – Approaches to the Patient in the Ancient World*. Leiden and Boston: Brill, 81–103.

Linton, Simi (1998) *Claiming Disability: Knowledge and Identity*. New York and London: New York University Press.

MacFarlane, Patrick (2010) 'Health and disease.' In Daniel H. Garrison (ed.) *A Cultural History of the Human Body in Antiquity*. Oxford and New York: Berg, 45–66.

Masséglia, Jane (2015) *Body Language in Hellenistic Art and Society*. Oxford: Oxford University Press.
McCoskey, Denise E. (2012) *Race: Antiquity and Its Legacy*. London: I.B. Tauris.
Meskell, Lynn and Rosemarie Joyce (2003) *Embodied Lives: Figuring Ancient Maya and Egyptian Experience*. London and New York: Routledge.
Messinger, Seth (2008) 'Anthropology and its individual, social and cultural contributions to psychoprosthetics.' In Pamela Gallagher, Deirdre Desmond and Malcolm MacLachlan (eds) *Psychoprosthetics*. London: Springer, 107–17.
Mills, Steve (2014) *Auditory Archaeology: Understanding Sound and Hearing in the Past*. Walnut Creek, CA: Left Coast Press.
Mitchell, David T. and Sharon L.Snyder (2000) *Narrative Prosthesis: Disability and the Dependencies of Discourse*. Ann Arbor: The University of Michigan Press.
Mitchell, William J.T. (1994) *Picture Theory*. Chicago: Chicago University Press.
Mladenov, Teodor (2015) *Critical Theory and Disability: A Phenomenological Approach*. New York, London, New Delhi and Sydney: Bloomsbury.
Morris, Christine and Alan Peatfield (2014) 'Health and healing on Bronze Age peak sanctuaries.' In Demetrios Michaelides (ed.), *Medicine and Healing in the Ancient Mediterranean World*. Oxford: Oxbow Books, 54–63.
Mullins, Aimee (2009). www.ted.com/talks/aimee_mullins_prosthetic_aesthetics?language=en#t-333477 (accessed 24 February 2016).
Nagle, Stephen J., Margaret A. Fain and Sara L. Sanders (2000) 'The influence of political correctness on lexical and grammatical change in late-twentieth-century English.' In Dieter Kastovsky and Arthur Mettinger (eds) *The History of English in a Social Context*. Berlin and New York: De Gruyter, 257–78.
Nead, Lynda (1992) *The Female Nude*. London and New York: Routledge.
Nutton, Vivian (2012) *Ancient Medicine* (2nd ed.). London and New York: Routledge.
Ogden, Daniel (1997) *The Crooked Kings of Ancient Greece*. London: Duckworth.
Oliver, Michael and Colin Barnes (2012) *The New Politics of Disablement*. Basingstoke: Palgrave Macmillan.
Orrells, Daniel (2011) *Classical Culture and Modern Masculinity*. Oxford: Oxford University Press.
Orrells, Daniel (2015) *Sex: Antiquity and its Legacy*. London: I.B. Tauris.
Perry, Elizabeth and Rosemary Joyce (2005) 'Past performance: the archaeology of gender as influenced by the work of Judith Butler.' In Margaret Sönser Breen and Warren J. Blumenfeld (eds) *Butler Matters: Judith Butler's Impact on Feminist and Queer Studies*. Aldershot: Ashgate, 113–26.
Pestilli, Livio 2017. *Picturing the Lame in Italian Art from Antiquity to the Modern Era*. London and New York: Routledge.
Petridou, Georgia and Chiara Thumiger (2016) 'Introduction: towards a history of the ancient patient's view.' In Georgia Petridou and Chiara Thumiger (eds) *Homo Patiens – Approaches to the Patient in the Ancient World*. Leiden and Boston: Brill, 1–20.
Petsalis-Diomidis, Alexia (2010) *'Truly Beyond Wonders': Aelius Aristides and the Cult of Asklepios*. Oxford: Oxford University Press.
Porter, James (2010) *The Origins of Aesthetic Thought in Ancient Greece: Matter, Sensation, and Experience*. Cambridge: Cambridge University Press.
Quayson, Ato (2007) *Aesthetic Nervousness: Disability and the Crisis of Representation*. New York: Columbia University Press.

Riddle, Christopher (2013a) 'The ontology of impairment: rethinking how we define disability.' In Matthew Wappett and Katrina Arndt (eds) *Emerging Perspectives on Disability Studies*. New York: Palgrave Macmillan, 23–39.

Riddle, Christopher (2013b) 'Defining disability: metaphysical not political.' *Medical Health Care and Philosophy* 16, 377–84.

Rodaway, Paul (1994) *Sensuous Geographies: Body, Sense and Place*. London and New York: Routledge.

Rojas, Felipe (2015) 'Book review of *Archaeology and the Senses: Human Experience, Memory, and Affect*, by Yannis Hamilakis.' *American Journal of Archaeology* 119, https://www.ajaonline.org/book-review/2503.

Rood, Tim, Carol Atack and Tom Phillips (2020) *Anachronism and Antiquity*. London: Bloomsbury.

Rose, Martha L. (2003) *The Staff of Oedipus: Transforming Disability in Ancient Greece*. Ann Arbor: University of Michigan Press.

Sandell, Richard, Jocelyn Dodd and Rosemarie Garland-Thomson (eds) (2010) *Re-presenting Disability: Activism and Agency in the Museum*. London and New York: Routledge.

Sargeant, Malcolm (2018) *Discrimination and the Law* (2nd ed.). London and New York: Routledge.

Scarre, Christopher and Graeme Lawson (eds) (2006) *Archaeoacoustics*. Cambridge: McDonald Institute for Archaeological Research.

Schillmeier, Michael (2010) *Rethinking Disability: Bodies, Senses and Things*. New York and London: Routledge.

Scully, Jackie L. (2012) 'Deaf identities in disability studies: with us or without us?' In Nick Watson, Alan Roulstone and Carol Thomas (eds) *Routledge Handbook of Disability Studies*. London and New York: Routledge, 109–21.

Shakespeare, Tom (2006) *Disability Rights and Wrongs*. London and New York: Routledge.

Shakespeare, Tom (2014) *Disability Rights and Wrongs Revisited*. London and New York: Routledge.

Shakespeare, Tom, Sue Thompson and Michael Wright (2010) 'No laughing matter: medical and social experiences of restricted growth.' *Scandinavian Journal of Disability Research* 12, 19–31.

Silberman, Steve (2015) *Neurotribes: The Legacy of Autism and How to Think Smarter about People Who Think Differently*. London: Allen & Unwin.

Silverblank, Hannah and Marchella Ward (2020) 'Why does classical reception need disability studies?' *Classical Receptions Journal*, https://doi.org/10.1093/crj/claa009

Skeates, Robin (2010) *An Archaeology of the Senses: Prehistoric Malta*. Oxford: Oxford University Press.

Skinner, Marilyn B. (2013) 'Feminist theory.' In Thomas K. Hubbard (ed.) *A Companion to Greek and Roman Sexualities*. Oxford: Wiley-Blackwell, 1–16.

Snyder, Sharon L., Brenda J. Brueggemann and Rosemarie Garland-Thomson (eds) (2002) *Disability Studies: Enabling the Humanities*. New York: The Modern Language Association of America.

Sobchack, Vivian (2006) 'A leg to stand on: prosthetics, metaphor, and materiality.' In Marquard Smith and Joanne Morra (eds) *The Prosthetic Impulse: From a Posthuman Present to a Biocultural Future*. Cambridge, MA and London: Massachusetts Institute of Technology, 17–41.

Sonesson, Göran (1989) *Pictorial Concepts: Inquiries into the Semiotic Heritage and its Relevance to the Interpretation of the Visual World*. Aris Nova Series 4. Lund: Lund University Press.

Sørensen, Tim F. (2015) 'The continuity of the senses: *Archaeology and the Senses: Human Experience, Memory and Affect*. By Yannis Hamilakis.' *Current Anthropology* 56, 928–31.

Southwell-Wright, William (2013) 'Past perspectives: what can archaeology offer disability studies?' In Matthew Wappett and Katrina Arndt (eds) *Emerging Perspectives on Disability Studies*. New York: Palgrave Macmillan, 67–95.

Squire, Michael (2011) *The Art of the Body: Antiquity and Its Legacy*. London: I.B. Tauris.

Stahl, Johannes (2011) 'Physically deformed and disabled people.' In Michael Peachin (ed.) *The Oxford Handbook of Social Relations in the Roman World*. Oxford: Oxford University Press, 715–35.

Steiner, Wendy (1982) *The Colors of Rhetoric: Problems in the Relation between Modern Language and Painting*. Chicago and London: Chicago University Press.

Stiker, Henri-Jacques (1997) *A History of Disability*. Translated by William Sayers. Ann Arbor: University of Michigan Press.

Van Straten, Folkert T. (1981) *Gifts for the Gods*. Leiden: Brill.

Swain, John, Sally French and Colin Cameron (2003) 'Introduction: Enabling questions.' In John Swain, Sally French and Colin Cameron (eds) *Controversial Issues in a Disabling Society*. Oxford: Oxford University Press, 1–7.

Thomas, Carol (2007) *Sociologies of Disability and Illness: Contested Ideas in Disability Studies and Medical Sociology*. Basingstoke and New York: Palgrave Macmillan.

Trentin, Lisa (2013) 'Disability in class and Classics: towards a more nuanced understanding of Ancient History.' *Prandium: The Journal of Historical Studies* 2, 55–8.

Trentin, Lisa (2015) *The Hunchback in Hellenistic and Roman Art*. London: Bloomsbury.

Tringham, Ruth (2015) 'Review of *Archaeology of the Senses: Human Experience, Memory, and Affect*.' *European Journal of Archaeology* 18, 705–8.

Umachandran, Mathura and Tim Rood (eds) (2020) 'Introduction.' *Classical Receptions Journal* 12, 1–9.

UPIAS (1976) Union of the Physically Impaired Against Segregation: Foundation Statement. https://disability-studies.leeds.ac.uk/wp-content/uploads/sites/40/library/UPIAS-fundamental-principles.pdf (accessed 3rd February 2020).

Victoria and Albert (1999) www.vam.ac.uk/museumofsavagebeauty/mcq/prosthetic-legs/ (accessed 24 May 2016).

Vlahogiannis, Nicholas (1998) 'Disabling bodies.' In Dominic Montserrat (ed.) *Changing Bodies, Changing Meanings: Studies on the Human Body in Antiquity*. Routledge: London and New York, 13–36.

Vlahogiannis, Nicholas (2005) '"Curing" disability.' In Helen King (ed.) *Health in Antiquity*. London and New York: Routledge, 180–91.

Waldschmidt, Anne (2017) 'Disability goes cultural: the cultural model of disability as an analytical tool.' In Anne Waldschmidt, Hanjo Berressem and Moritz Ingwersen (eds) *Culture – Theory – Disability: Encounters between Disability Studies and Cultural Studies*. Bielefeld: Transcript Verlag, 19–27.

The Warnock Report (1978) Special Educational Needs. Report of the Committee of Enquiry into the Education of Handicapped Children and Young People. London.

Yeames, A.H.S. (1907) 'An ivory statuette.' *Papers of the British School at Rome* 4, 279–82.

Zurhake, Laurien (2020) 'Chronic pain and illness: pain and meaning: interpreting chronic pain and illness in Greco-Roman antiquity.' In Christian Laes (ed.) *A Cultural History of Disability in Antiquity*. London: Bloomsbury, 47–65.

Part 1

Communicating and controlling impairment, illness and pain

Ellen Adams

Part 1 considers the patient's role in the context of clinical consultations. It also demonstrates the benefits of a three-way dialogue between antiquity, modernity and classical reception – a theme that runs throughout this volume. Another running theme, explicitly picked up again in the final section, Part 4, is that of the tension between representation and reality – for example, how the narratives constructed in clinical exchanges shape the experience of ill health and disability. The contributors (from medical humanities in Chapter 2, Classics in Chapter 3) have engaged with their more unfamiliar discipline very constructively, mainly centred around narrative-based medicine.

This is one area where medical humanities overlap with disability studies. Although the clinical encounter is a fundamental theme of the former, the importance of the patient or disabled person in decision-making processes is one of the key concerns of disability activism. For this reason, it seemed apt to ease classical readers into disability studies through the more familiar door of medical humanities. It was also a deliberate choice to take a wide definition of 'disability', to include chronic ill health and pain, as the debilitating impact of these can be as significant as any sensory, mobility or mental impairment. Pain in particular is a condition for which no magic wand can be conjured up, although medical intervention may be able to alleviate the problem. Pain and ill health are also conditions that all of us have experienced to a degree (excepting the rare few who have congenital insensitivity to pain) and so offer a more familiar platform to start with. This may produce a more medicalised approach to disability than sometimes advocated, but this volume seeks to explore a balance between medical and social models (Adams, Chapter 1, Introduction).

Flexer and Hurwitz (Chapter 2) have set the performance of a clinical encounter against the tragic stage with all its palliative catharsis, where a medical case report (MCR) is described as a play script, and 'simulated patients' are deployed in medical training. The process of *pathos* (suffering), *anagnorisis* (diagnosis) and *peripeteia* (reversal or cure) is compared in both arenas to striking effect. Ancient authorities, notably Aristotle and Sophocles, become 'good to think with', comparable with how disabled people are so often used as a prop by theorising Humanities scholars (see Chapter 6 regarding the blind man with his cane). We therefore witness the creation of classical reception by those placed in the medical world, as explored by King (Chapter 10, this volume). In contrast, Petridou (Chapter 3) explores Aristides's use of narrative therapy, with rhetoric, literature and music – human cultural processes that support and shape individual perceptions of their predicaments. It seems, as Petridou further demonstrates, that exploring minorities and non-traditional groups outside that of male, able-bodied elites is best conducted through triangulation of antiquity, classical reception and the present day.

Flexer and Hurwitz emphasise the performative nature of this engagement. Creating a representation, or mimesis, of conditions is one matter; communicating symptoms and experiences is another. And Petridou asks the pertinent question: how can we articulate a pain for which there are no words? She explores the ineffability of pain, and pain as a socially negotiated subjectivity. Petridou draws from Emily Dickinson's poem in her title, where the double meaning of 'utter' ('overwhelming' or 'to articulate') is so apt. Both chapters explore the tension between the singularity of the individual experience and the clinical, statistical generalisations needed for reliable diagnoses. The focus on 'narrative' humanises the topic of illness, pain and disability, as it is grounded in the experience of those involved and reinforces how responses to impairment are subjective and wide-ranging. Approaching the subject through the lens of storytelling indicates how, despite the vast differences in diagnostic categorisation and healing know-how between the Greco-Roman and modern Western worlds, disability remains an appropriate or even necessary topic.

Petridou mentions PIP (Personal Independence Payment), which is issued by the British government. State support offered by rich nations is a modern phenomenon, and perhaps therefore irrelevant for antiquity. But exploring the process of applying for such support helps to pin down this evasive term 'disability'. Applying for PIP requires three key components: (1) diagnosis of condition/impairment; (2) measure of severity of condition/impairment; and (3) assessment of the impact of the condition on day-to-day life and mobility. First, a medical diagnosis is required, which immediately places people with some conditions at a disadvantage (for example, people with chronic fatigue syndrome or fibromyalgia have had to fight for recognition that these conditions are 'real'). Biases in medical research have led to certain conditions being dismissed as spurious, imagined or a consequence of life-style choices rather than a disability, such as endometriosis (King, Chapter 10, this volume). Second, an assessment of the severity of the condition is required – mild or even moderate levels of most conditions are unlikely to entitle the bearer to state support. For example, people who wear glasses will not be recognised as 'disabled' unless they are on a register for being blind or visually impaired (under British law, they are then automatically identified as disabled).

The third stage concerns the impact of this disability on one's daily life and/or mobility, as set out in a 'how your disability affects you' form. This is not an easy form to work through, especially if you have a congenital disability and so have no personal comparator to set one's case against. It requires raking over the hurdles and challenges faced in all aspects of life and can be a very negative process to navigate. Those who need it (for example, those having learning or mental health difficulties) are allowed help with the form, but most people will tackle this form independently, unlike the conversational exchanges described in the chapters in this Part. The only human exchange is with an assessor from one of the private companies to which the government outsources such responsibilities. Their brief appears to be to keep the numbers of awards down; successful applications are steadily falling over time, while appeal tribunal success rates are increasing, with 75% upheld in 2019. The antagonism and suspicion inherent in this process reveal a rather more hostile dialogue than those discussed in the following two chapters.

Some feel that disability cannot be explored in the ancient world, because of anachronism and the problems with applying modern experiences, but I suggest that understanding this assessment procedure offers useful unpacking. 'Disabled' is a term that demands further qualification, even in the modern context, and is generally very fluid. It does not mean 'unable', and most conditions, impairments and illnesses have an impact in certain situations, while falling into the background in others. To understand this, the observer can only listen, while the disabled person attempts to explain. However, as Flexer and Hurwitz note regarding MCRs, when the patient is the object, they can be othered to the point that he, she or 'it' is ironically forgotten.

Chapter 2

Two troubles

The dramatic tragedy of Western medicine

Michael J. Flexer and Brian Hurwitz

Abstract

This chapter employs the familiar temporal constraints of the clinical encounter, and the asymmetries in power in relation to medical authority between patients and clinicians. From there, it deploys the literary critical writings of Aristotle, Nietzsche's idiosyncratic Romantic reinterpretation of Greek drama and Socratic knowledge, and the possible dialectical interplay of influence between Attic dramatic tragedy and the healing cult of Asclepius, as heuristics for understanding and interrogating the contradictions and shortcomings in Western medical practice, specifically the clinical encounter and its textual analogue, the published medical case report (MCR). In so doing, this chapter argues that the spatiotemporal and narrative imperatives of the clinical encounter (and MCR) share strong genre similarities with dramatic tragedy and progress through the devices of *pathos, anagnorisis* and *peripeteia.* As such, the dominance of this genre has created a lineage of 'forgotten others': the antecedent influence of dramatic tragedy, and its antagonistic narrative structure, on the clinical encounter; the possibility of disease experienced across the life course according to the temporal expansiveness and heterogeneity of action common to the epic genre; the silenced narrative of the patient, as mutual agonist rather than vanquished antagonist. This chapter concludes with a look towards ways in which new forms of clinical encounter and collaboration can develop between clinicians and patients as cooperative agents operating outside the genre dictates of the medical case qua dramatic tragedy.

While Ajax was distraught,
He at least found happiness in his obsession:
We, sane, were pained to see him. Now he is well,
And free of the sickness, bitter grief torments him,
And ours is none the less. Are there not here
Two troubles in place of one?

Soph. *Aj.* (270–5)

Duality and unity within the tragic drama and the medical case

Anyone who has ever waited to see a British general practitioner (GP) has been subject to a distinctly Aristotelean exhortation to stick to a unity of plot: 'one problem per consultation'.[1] This imperative is handed down by receptionists, on websites and shouted out from posters, such as Fig. 2.1.

Despite aspirations for a 'person-centred care approach' to consulting that 'gives people more choice and control in their lives by [...] a shift from asking "what's the matter with you" to "what matters to you"', the Royal College of General Practitioners holds the ability to negotiate priorities addressed during consultations to be a core clinical competence of the GP (Royal College of General Practitioners 2016, 31–3; Royal College of General Practitioners n.d.). For them, a GP ought to be in control of the dramatic narrative. There are good and obvious reasons for the one plot request (if not, necessarily, for the aggressive, exasperated tone in which it is often couched): economic, and even-handed, management of the GP's scant time;[2] clarity and focus of the clinical encounter to ensure the correct diagnosis; and an unavoidable prioritising of the most pressing, and potentially most time-dependent, illnesses. Inconveniently, however, comes stacked against this an incontrovertible truth about medicine

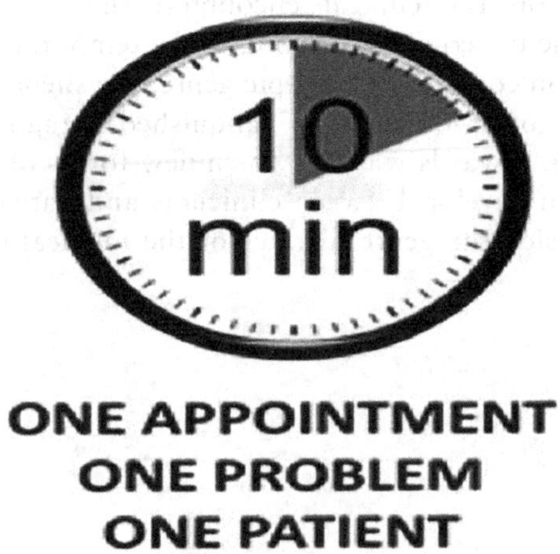

Figure 2.1 Image from the newsletter of the Alvaston Medical Centre, *The Boulton Bugle* (9), October 2019. Reproduced with permission from Alvaston Medical Centre (2019)

generally and general practice more specifically: who ever had just one problem? Whatever counts as a problem, there needs to be consensus on the matter across patients and doctors.[3] Co-morbidity is the very essence of ill health, and complexity, ambiguity and even singularity are the wild, unruly characteristics of medicine, as lived on the frontline of medical practice, in contrast to its modern underpinnings: medical science, as a reified, aloof and abstracted system of categorisation and algorithmic therapeutics. It is only necessary to look at the debates, current at the time of writing, over the possibly meaningful differences between dying 'with' or 'from' the COVID-19 virus to realise that not even a pandemic reduces health to just 'one problem'.

This contradiction raises two core areas of interest for this chapter: the construction of the clinical encounter and the construction of the medical case, with its analogue, the published medical case report (MCR). From the outset, we will work from the principle that the case and the clinical encounter mutually co-establish each other and the norms of thinking they are informed by, embody and propagate. In terms of the steps of reasoning, of interaction, of engagement, of interpretation, whatever can be identified in the encounter can be – perhaps transformed or translated to some extent – found within the case and MCR. Of course, this dialogic relationship makes sense given the pedagogic role – within formal medical training and during ongoing learning in the workplace – of the MCR. What we have here is the genre of the case in two different media: the written form of the MCR and the performance of the clinical encounter. Just as the comic tale and the comic sketch have a mixture of different and shared conventions, tropes and rhetorical devices, so it is with the case. And the case itself has, as we have identified, a difficult relationship with health, illness and disease: 'one problem per case'.[4]

Why, though, begin with Aristotle and with Sophocles's *Ajax*? We are presenting here an imagined intellectual lineage. We do not make any strong claims for its veracity. Rather, we have found Aristotle's *Poetics*, Attic dramatic tragedy and the contemporaneous healing cult of Asclepius, and possible intertextual, cross-cultural exchanges between them, to be a useful set of heuristics for opening up MCRs and the clinical encounter in twentieth and twenty-first century Western medicine. As such, we know that we are taking considerable liberties with the classical material, and we hope that readers will appreciate the spirit of the engagement: we are positing a playful rhizome of influence – occasionally tendentious – to support a rather more hardnosed critique of current cultural forms of medical knowledge and authority. As scholars from outside the classics, we ask your indulgence while we weave this argument. We hope that there might be something in our readings and associations that also, by naïve accident, sparks the interest of the professional classicist and offers, obliquely, some novel outlook on very familiar texts. If there can be a simple justification for using Aristotle, and specifically, his *Poetica*, it might be that, contra Aristotle, there are valuable similarities – structurally, aesthetically, thematically – between MCRs, the lived experience of medicine and poetic forms such as tragedy and epic. Aristotle disparaged the tendency to designate medical writers as 'poets', disagreeing that what characterised poets was merely the technical approach of composing in verse:

> not from the fact that they are making imitations, but indiscriminately from the fact that they are writing in metre. For it is customary to describe as poets even those who produce medical and scientific works in verse.
>
> Arist. *Poet.* (1.1447b)

Implicit in our argument is that there is indeed *mimesis* occurring, in the MCR, and, similarly, a *mimetic* relationship of influence between Greek dramatic tragedy and the clinical encounter as it exists today. Of course, though, this is our repurposing of Aristotle's terms and theories and hardly an analysis he would have recognised. Yet, in some ways, the gap we are bridging in our argument was narrower for Aristotle already. In his *Rhetorica* (1.2.1355b–1357a), he placed medicine firmly within the *technê* – a category spanning our contemporary dichotomised categories of 'arts' and 'sciences' – and medicine appears as an illustrative model for virtuous (or non-virtuous) character in the *Ethica Nicomachea* (5.10.25):

> But to play the coward or to act unjustly consists not in doing these things, except incidentally, but in doing them as the result of a certain state of character, just as to practise medicine and healing consists not in applying or not applying the knife, in using or not using medicines, but in doing so in a certain way.

These words of Aristotle's prompt us to hypothesise a connection between 'a certain state of character' and what constitutes the essence of practising medicine and healing, and this will form an important point later in the argument. Suffice it now to state that we will be reasoning about medicine through analogy with poetry and through the prism of Aristotle's writing, albeit in a way that might appear rather non-Aristotelean in approach.

Ajax, 'a man diseased' (Soph. *Aj.*, 662), is a well-worn example of the influence of medical problems and modes of thinking on Athenian dramatic tragedy, and specifically the representation and artistic elucidation of madness – understood varyingly as a medico-clinical illustration of madness, revealing a philosophical truth about the diseased state of the world, or a psychoanalytical case study of suicidal ideation – and Sophocles has been characterised for at least 50 years as a dramatist of pathology (Biggs 1966; Holt 1980; Lansky 1997).[5] In recent years, there has been extensive scholarship on the relationship between *Ajax* and the diagnostic category of post-traumatic stress disorder (Kamieński 2012; Doerries 2015; Cole 2019).[6] The objective here is not to contribute to the considerable diagnostic literature on *Ajax*, Ajax or Sophocles, but rather to invert the familiar narrative and ask not how medicine informed tragedy in fifth-century BCE Athens, but rather how tragedy's dialogue with medicine then established a lineage of influence on clinical practice and case formation that endures to the present. Applying to the play Aristotle's critical frameworks, as laid out in the *Poetica*, for diction and plot – in terms of complexity, duration and subject focus – immediately brings out some important structural, thematic and dramatic similarities between Attic tragedy and MCRs. These similarities might be considered as genre characteristics, and so what are the formal genre relations across the two media?

Ajax seems remarkably in step with our GP surgery poster. In the clinical encounter, the patient is called upon to tell 'a story which is solid, like the hero himself; short and intense' (Zoja 2017, 2). Part of the problem, then, with the clinical encounter is this genre dissonance. Health and illness are complex, changeable, and speak with the many different voices of epic poetry, but the clinic is the scene of dramatic action. That Ajax is perfectly suited for the short, sharp (instructive) shock of tragedy and so poorly suited for the endurance, compromises and vicissitudes of the epic narrative captures the essence of this problem. Both the play and the eponymous protagonist continually cycle back to the 'one problem' of his madness, and the fallout from this, with dogged single-minded pursuit of a diagnosis and therapy for resolution: 'Dirges and canticles are no prescription / For ills that need the knife' (Soph. *Aj.*, 579–80). There is a dramatic imperative at work for Ajax, within the 'reality' of the play, which itself is the psychological manifestation of the formal imperatives of the drama: there must be a unified course of action towards resolution of the underlying malady. When the remedy must be instantaneous – both in space and time, as the unities of the Attic stage demand – then pause, palliation, reflection, all longitudinal approaches, are out of reach. Like Ajax, who as a figure on the stage exists only at that time and place, the remedy becomes a pointed moment – the sword of Hector jutting from the ground. It is necessary here to draw a distinction between Ajax and *Ajax*: the drama continues beyond Ajax's violent resolution, as the survivors – both friends and family of Ajax and his political opponents – have to manoeuvre towards some position of resolution and cure. First, we have the strictly time- and space-bound drive to conclusion experienced by Ajax the character: a rush to suicide. Second, something structurally similar – although with a distinctly restorative and curative resolution – occurs for the play as a whole: the healing of the social wounds between the Greek kings and Ajax's entourage.

The point we are trying to make is that this is a quality of *genre* rather than of psychological, physiological or pathological need, or of the representation of any such need. Other genres allow for other representations of what may be called pathology and other modes of playing out trauma that do not rush to conclusion, be it destructive as for Ajax, or restorative as for *Ajax*. Consider, for example, how Aeneas's chronic condition of finding *lacrimae rerum* (Virg. *Aen.*, 1.462). contrasts with the acute *peripeteia* seen in *Ajax*. The tragic drama, like the clinical encounter, is necessarily acute – regardless of the nature of the illness – because of the temporal constraints and the need to create a resolution.

Structurally, the resolution of the clinical encounter does not have to be a 'cure' per se, but some kind of closing off of the encounter itself. Even a suggestion to a patient to 'watch and wait' and the promise of a form of enduring care, extending beyond the temporal and physical bounds of the clinical encounter, still function as a dramatic end to that particular consultation and urge the departure of the patient from the scene.[7]

At this juncture, it is important to raise the concept of 'disability' and how 'being disabled' – either according to a medical, mechanistic conception of an intrinsic impairment or a social model of a person being disabled by a society unwilling to accommodate their access needs or sensory requirements, or any mixture of these two positions – fits into this argument about the interrelated, genre-defined temporality and narrative shape of the clinical encounter, the clinical case and Greek dramatic tragedy. Certainly, on the Athenian stage, what we might term disability is displaced either into the past, as given circumstances, or into the future, as consequence. Textual and archaeological evidence suggests that people with mobility and visual impairments were involved in all aspects of classical life, such as sanctuaries (for example, see Graham, Chapter 7, this volume). The supposedly shameful burden – 'that dreadful mark' or 'stigma' (Soph. *OT*, 1035) – of some kind of lameness is woven through Sophocles's *Oedipus Rex*.[8] The resonances of mobility impairment in both the tragic protagonist's name and the riddle of the Sphinx – from which his glory, wealth and power derive – belong to the myth and are obviously not Sophocles's invention, and they find no place or moment in the drama on the stage, belonging to the 'cradle' (Soph. *OT*, 1035). Similarly, the 'brand of shame' (Soph. *OT*, 246) to come, the chronic condition of blindness and impaired wandering to which Oedipus is dooming himself, is only glimpsed in a final tragic tableau. Sophocles might have Oedipus hubristically declare '[L]et that man drag out / His life in agony, step by painful step' (Soph. *OT*, 246–7), but there is no space, no possible narrative accommodation within the drama, for seeing him live with his impairments.[9] Oedipus's enduring 'marks' – his literal and figurative visual and mobility impairments – cannot constitute the 'one problem' proper of the tragic plot; this has to be the space- and time-bound presenting problem of the identity of the culprit responsible for the curse afflicting Thebes. The genre tendency of tragic drama, and the clinical encounter, towards the acute and away from the chronic, forecloses the possibility – within these narratives – of telling a rich story of a life lived with impairments. We shall see this in more detail when we turn to contemporary published MCRs.

Is it reasonable to read across these forms? Yet what is the MCR if not an exercise in mimesis? Allow us another liberty with Aristotle, whereby we reinterpret his words as describing the aesthetic and instructive value of medical case-based reasoning when he writes:

> They enjoy seeing likenesses because in doing so they acquire information (they reason out what each represents, and discover for instance, that 'this is a picture of so and so'); for if by any chance the thing depicted has not

> been seen before, it will not be the fact that it is an imitation of something that gives the pleasure, but the execution or the colouring or some other such cause.
>
> Arist. *Poet.* (1.1448b)

In all *technê*, mimesis is subordinated to 'some other such cause', and, in Aristotle's account, aesthetic pleasure, intellectual development and the creation of new knowledge are all folded into each other. To place the case within an Aristotelean typology of poetic forms is to reveal its adjacency to the tragic drama. In its performance medium of the clinical encounter, the case involves a temporally and spatially bound investigation of 'one problem', where 'one problem' stands for something(s) isolable, discrete and unitary. Only by being such does it qualify as a case, so to speak. A clinical encounter without a clinical problem is not a case; there is no thing for the encounter to resolve, other than the patient's physical presence and, perhaps, their misprision that there is a case to solve. It is the very essence of the case that the 'one problem', as symptom(s) brought into the encounter by the patient, has been recognised as 'one problem' in medical terms by the clinician. If this does not happen, then the encounter fails to be a case. In the semiotic terms of Roland Barthes, the cluster of phenomenological, subjective symptoms brought into the time–space by the patient has proven impossible to translate into medical signs that can be incorporated into a functioning single signifying narrative unit: the case (Barthes 1994).

This adjacency of tragic drama and medical case is not just topological, but also topographical. Permit us something fanciful: we are now casting our eyes out across from our seat in the theatre and up at a new structure above us where other germs of the modern clinical encounter and MCR are gently sprouting, and – so we suggest – will enter into a creative dialectic with the dramatic tragedies taking place only a short distance away. Within four or five years of the arrival of the cult of Asclepius in Athens in 420 BCE, the healing sanctuary – the Asclepieion – 'was inaugurated on the southern slope of the Acropolis in Athens, above the Theatre of Dionysus' (Steger 2018, 47). This spatial arrangement was then exported across Greece in the Hellenistic period, with examples seen at Pergamon, Dion, Corinth and, most famously, at Epidaurus, where the theatre and shrine are separated by barely 500 metres (Mitchell-Boyask 2008, 117). Unity of place is a part of the healing offered by Asclepius:

> [T]o think of the healing encounter solely in terms of medical techniques is to miss the context in which it takes place – the physical setting, the sacred spring, the sacred grove (even if, as at the Asclepieion at Athens, it could hardly have amounted to more than three or four trees), the sacrifices and the reassurance offered by the memorials, whether inscriptions or cultic recitations, that this was a place where healing was available.
>
> Nutton (2004, 110)

The visual, spatial, sensorial rhetoric of the Asclepieion and the healing it performs resonate with those conventions of the abutting theatres: a unity of place, with conventionalised, symbolic spaces, ritualised music and set sequences of moving between these states, to ensure a particular outcome of catharsis. This spatial proximity was complemented by proximities in time and action. The *Asclepieia* formed part of the Athenian festival, the Great Dionysia, in Elaphebolion (Petridou 2014). Mitchell-Boyask provides a persuasive account of the significance this relationship has for theatre, growing from the pre-Attic interlinked associations of music, ritual and healing into a multilayered, formalised theatricalising of (ill) health, as a pre-eminent dramatic (and social) concern (Mitchell-Boyask 2008, 117):

> the situation of an Asklepieion near a theatre, following the model of Athens, is so common, surprisingly so, that the relationship between healing, music and theatre becomes all the more apparent, and Asclepius himself begins to resemble something like a theatre god.

This association stands. Sophocles endures as the tragedian of pathology, providing the mythological framework for twentieth-century psychopathology, and similarly it is Sophocles who is often credited with having introduced Asclepius into Athens (Mitchell-Boyask 2008, 110).[10]

Asclepian healing offered a complementary counterpart to the concurrent Hippocratic practice of medicine. Though the Hippocratic corpus is heterogeneous and diverse, across the different texts there is a commonality of purpose: the understanding of disease, underpinned by a humoral, mechanistic conception of the body as a holistic 'system of fluids and conduits' and the application of this understanding back to individual instances of illness (Nutton 2004, 77). Health is defined as the achievement, reacquisition and maintenance of *eukrasia*, an act of balance aggregated over various complex elements in combination (Nutton 2004, 80). As such, this sounds much more akin to the narrative shape of epic poetry, and both *The Iliad* and *The Odyssey* are polyphonic, complex tales of the restoration of a troubled equilibrium (whether that be the tensions between Greek kings on the beaches outside Troy or the honour, peace and property rights of the house of Odysseus).

By way of contrast, attending the Asclepieion was a process of tragic-dramatic healing, reliant on ritual performance, physical co-presence, dialogue and an emphatic assertion of resolution. By tragic-dramatic, we refer to the structural components of the genre, rather than the content. A successful instance of Asclepian healing is still of the tragic drama genre, regardless of whether it ends in successful or unsuccessful cure. A surviving testimonial epigram to the god Asclepius from Marcus Iulius Apellas, who attended the sanctuary at Epidaurus in the second century CE, shows the dialogic call-and-response of the process, where instructions or insights from the god prefigure the actions and events to come (M. Iulius Apellas IG IV^2 1.126, translations from Steger 2018, 123):

> When I arrived at the temple, he told me for two days to keep my head covered,
> And for these two days it rained.

The structure of the encounter is one of assessment, instruction and cure, driven by verbal diktats, most often indicating an opaque deviation from Marcus Iulius Apellas's own habits and, on one occasion, constituting a clear instance of antagonism:

> The god told me [...]
> [...] to take milk with honey.
> When one day I drink milk alone he said, 'Put honey in the milk so that it can get through.'

The narrative entails itemised, real-time responses to the demands of a god and is topped and tailed by an explicit *parados* and *exodos*, the summoning to and the dismissal from the scene of healing by the god:

> In the priesthood of Publius Aelius Antiochus
> I, Marcus Iulius Apellas, an Idrian from Mylasa, was sent for by the god,
> For I was often ill and suffering from dyspepsia.
> [...]
> He bad me also inscribe this. Full of gratitude I departed well.

The genre difference between the Hippocratic/epic and Asclepian/tragic is evident, remembering that Apellas being healed does not make this case any less a tragic drama, in terms of structure. Whereas the opening retrospective invocations to the Muses in *The Iliad* and *The Odyssey* immediately proclaim their respective subjects – 'the rage of Peleus' son' (Hom. *Il.*, 1.1) or the journey of 'a complicated man' (Hom. *Od.*, 1.1) – and point to the eventual reconciliation of Agamemnon and Achilles and the return home as *things already done*, the dramatic tragedy – like the clinical encounter – is lived in the present tense. For audience, Chorus and characters alike in *Ajax*, '[t]here is no escaping / From the awful thing you are telling' (Soph. *Aj.*, 221–2). Ajax himself writes no epigram of 'gratitude' to the gods – who have destroyed him, as tragic *peripeteia* are 'engines of the gods / Designed against mankind' (Soph. *Aj.*, 1035–6) – and so the closing departure is funereal, as Ajax's brother Teucer elides grave-digging with departure from the literal stage, and the close of performance and narrative with the close of life: 'Let us make an end' (Soph. *Aj.*, 1408). There is no other time or space or life outside the bounds of the performance.

The obvious, and non-trivial, exceptions to this dichotomy between Hippocratic medicine as epic poetry and Asclepian cultic healing as dramatic tragedy are the *Epidemics*. However, even within these seven books, there are two distinct genres: prototypical MCRs and broader accounts of specific epidemics.

The case accounts certainly share more genre characteristics with dramatic tragedy and have as single subject the singular expression of illness (within a particular, individual body), whereas the epidemics are broader in their scope, with a more numerous cast of characters, and are unified around the subject of the depersonalised, roaming and developing disease itself. Significantly, the *Epidemics* do not address impairments, as the Hippocratic practitioner was to exclude incurable ailments; the chronic and the enduring could not constitute a medical case (Kelley 2007, 33). Temporally, too, these correspond, respectively, to the truncated, urgent timescale of the drama and the wider canvas of the epic: the cases rapidly count off the passing of each day; the accounts of epidemics progress at the pace of seasons with lengthy descriptions of the changing weather, times of year and geographies. So, we need to refine our distinction, or, rather, to allow that the MCRs within the *Epidemics* belong properly to the Asclepian dramatic tragedy category, and not the Hippocratic epic (Lloyd 1978).

Ideally, perhaps, the clinical encounter should play out like an inverted Attic tragedy, proceeding from *pathos* (the patient bringing their suffering, their 'undeserved misfortune', to be witnessed by the clinician; Arist. *Poet.*, 3.1453a) to *anagnorisis* (the discovery by diagnosis)[11] through to curative *peripeteia* (where the disease is reversed). Considering how the theatres of Greece faced off against and reflected the neighbouring *Asclepieia*, this might make good sense.[12] The complex cultural network, in which developed Athenian tragic drama and Asclepian cultic healing, offers an example of rhizomatic rather than causal relation across strands that are dialectic and cross-pollinating. As we will see, as we move rapidly forward in time, the intrinsic dramatic antagonism, the time- and space-bound imperatives and the aesthetic of cruel voyeurism of Athenian tragedy continue to act themselves out in the clinical encounters and MCRs of Western medicine nearly two and a half millennia later.

Diagnosis or *anagnosis*: a tension in the case between discovery and knowledge

> The whole of our modern world is caught in the net of Alexandrian culture and takes as its ideal the *theoretical man* who is equipped with the highest powers of knowledge, works in the service of science, and whose archetype and progenitor is Socrates.
>
> Nietzsche (2008 [1872], 97; original italics)

Nietzsche's thesis in *The Birth of Tragedy* – composed in 1871 in response to the *Gesamtkuntswerk* of Wagner and the recent Prussian military victory over France – is idiosyncratic to say the least, and better read as a manifesto for German Romanticism than as a scholarly work on Attic drama or society. One of its central insistences is that the exact period we have taken as our point of departure – the arrival of Asclepius on the slopes of the Athenian Acropolis in the final decades of the fifth century BCE – is the moment of rupture, when the powerful dynamic tension between Apollonian representation through bounded forms and the Dionysian formless spirit of inspiration, constitutive of Greek tragedy, broke apart, to be supplanted by a Socratic rationalism. Nietzsche's text is an appeal to reintegrate the Apollonian and the Dionysian and to recover a balance lost under the ever-greater intellectual hegemony of so-called (by Nietzsche) Socratic Enlightenment rationalism sweeping late nineteenth-century Europe. Within this intellectual hegemony sit core empirical achievements (or 'discoveries') of medical science of his day: ether anaesthesia (1840s); Louis Pasteur's germ theory (1850s–60s); and Joseph Lister's work on antisepsis (from 1867). No doubt, consciously or not, Nietzsche had his sights set on the burgeoning German tradition of scientific medicine in particular and the university system that produced novel – but, to use our terms, biologically reductionist – modes of medical science, such as Jakob Henle and histology or Rudolf Virchow and cellular pathology (Risse 1993, 17).

Certainly, Nietzsche's distinction between the Socratic scientific *knowledge* and Dionysian revelatory *discovery* reinforces our prior inclusion of Hippocratic cases within our Asclepian dramatic tradition of medical healing. There is considerable performance in this *mock* therapy proposed for earache:

> If the ear aches, wrap wool around your fingers, pour on warm oil, then put the wool in the palm of the hand and put it over the ear so that something will seem to him to come out. Then throw it in the fire. A deception.
>
> Hippoc. *Epidemics* (6, 5.7)

Recommended here is what today we may think of as *mock* therapy for earache. It specifies how to enact what we might call a *pretend* therapy – acknowledged as a deceit – one, moreover, that is closely aligned to the real treatment regimen usually recommended for the condition. In the Hippocratic text *Places in Man*, the following therapy and rationale are given for treating earache:

> When there is a flux to the ears, first it produces pain, for the flow is violent; this distress continues until the flux gains a pipe through which to escape; when flow is once established, there is no longer distress.
>
> For the patient afflicted with this pain warm a naturally warming medication, dissolve it in oil of bitter almonds, and infuse it into the ear. Also apply a cupping-instrument behind it, if the pain is in the left ear, on the right side, and if in the right ear, then on the left. Do not make incisions, but let the cup alone draw. If with this treatment the pain does not stop, cool some naturally cool substance and infuse it into the ear ... (Always change from a course of management that is not leading to recovery; if some measure is making things worse, move to its opposite ...) If a pipe

> has already formed, and purulent fluid is flowing out, copious and ill-smelling, do the following. Moisten a sponge, and, drying it with a dry medication, apply it as tightly as possible to the ear, then apply a cleaning medication to the nostrils, in order that what is flowing into the ears will be carried forward into the nose and not move back into the head, for it is peccant.
>
> Hippoc. *Places in Man* (G.12.298–300)

As this treatment is recounted, it is related in detail to the circumstances of the pain: which sides different treatments are offered; the stage of associated clinical phenomena; its effects on fluxes and directions of flows in vessels – 'pipes' – and how resolution takes place by encouraging discharges that later require to be dried up.[13]

The overall impression is of a treatment aimed at *aiding and abetting* the bodily processes, by nudging them in certain directions – for example, by infusing oil into the ear to help the humour to discharge, first through the ear and then the nose. Either way, not only do we hear plausible advice about how to monitor the effects of treatment and modify it depending on progress, we also *see* – visually *sense* – an elaborate bodily interior comprised of anatomical inside and outside connections, pipes, fluid build-ups, flows and discharges.

Why, then, in *Epidemics* Book 6 does the author set out both a pretend treatment *and* a pretend cure for earache: 'so that something will seem' – presumably to the patient – 'to come out'? The deception seems to correspond to elements of the real performance of such therapy set out in *Places*, the implication being that an elaborate pose in *Epidemics* Book 6 accomplishes what a true treatment achieves. It would appear that the *mock* treatment is modelled on and as effective as the real treatment. But in which circumstances is it offered? Tantalisingly, we are not told. But we have here an instance of the insistence to action that characterises the clinical encounter as dramatic tragedy. There is the triumvirate of time, space and problem, and these demand a narrative of action. Therapy is the staging of this action, and it is more than just a quirk of language that the agonist forces the action in both therapeutics and dramatics.

Pain and therapy as a performance, rather than (solely) a ministering to biochemical, mechanical somatic 'realities', may seem to problematise the supposed certainties of the Socratic knowledge approach. However, in his fourth-century BCE *Philebus* dialogue between Socrates, Philebus and Petarchus, Plato argues that, just as there can be unfelt pains stemming from disruptions below the threshold of perception and as a consequence of certain mental states, so too there can be false pleasures and false pains not merely grounded in false testimony, but in a pain that is not the result of the bodily disruption believed to cause pain, and yet it is felt *as if it is* – in today's terms, when there is a fault in the representation of the body, as in phantom pain.[14]

Epidemics Book 6 and Plato's dialogue suggest the Greeks knew of cases in which there is a dissociation between the bodily disruption and painful disease;

that there are circumstances in which the symptomatic realm has an existence *free* from its otherwise underlying physical substratum, for which the treatment was to mimic standard treatment for the condition, including some of the bodily visualisations that go with it. Both the performance and theory of the standard treatment for ear pain from physical disruption are embodied and *imprinted* on the mock treatment for pain in the ear that does not seem to be caused by physical disruption. What is this, if not the catharsis of the Greek tragedy re-performed as placebo effect in a clinical encounter? Arguably, this is a positive borrowing from theatre by healing, but it raises worrying questions about a practice of care that remains built upon the quasi-mystified powers of performance residing in the clinician. As Hippocrates notes, the therapy is absolutely and integrally a 'deception', and one that can only be achieved through systematic exclusion of the patient *qua* antagonist from the position of agency and knowledge occupied by the clinician. Here we see that 'certain state of character' we discussed earlier, although we are taking the meaning further than Aristotle intended; the clinician is – whether applying real or mock therapies – simultaneously the performance of the role of clinician. It is the *character* of the clinician, or the *character* assumed by the thespian in embodying the dramatic text, that wields power. Even an understanding of the underlying craft – be it stagecraft or healthcare – or a recognition that it is a practice, rather than a power, does not dispel the clouds of illusion or necessarily weaken the affective impact. We lament, with the Chorus, Ajax's fate, even though we know it was only magicked up for the moment of performance. The complicit mysticisms of our cultural representations are the self-same suspensions of disbelief that imbue the clinician (and – more perniciously – more esoteric quack healers) with their power.[15]

Nietzsche might insist upon an essential antagonism between Socratic abstracted science and the Dionysian formless spirit, and we might be tempted to follow his distinctions and place modern, Western medicine firmly within the former, as a Rationalist exercise, driven by theory, in contrast to inspirational, ritualised, individualised healing as a Romantic practice. But then the waters are considerably muddied, given that Asclepius is both the son of Apollo – and so intimately associated with Dionysus to be almost a god of theatre – and yet simultaneously functions as an occasional point of reference for Socratic and Neoplatonic thought (Slaveva-Griffin 2016). Similar conflict and uncertainty reside in the troubled, dynamic epistemological status of the MCR. Nietzsche may wish to consign medical science to the sterile 'modern world' of the Alexandrian theoretical man, but Richard Cabot, who ushered case-based reasoning into medical education at Harvard Medical School in the early years of the twentieth century and inaugurated the publishing of the Case Records of the Massachusetts General Hospital, was demonstrably a man of Aristotelean *phronesis* according to medical historian John Forrester (1996; see also Cabot 1906).

This contradiction is the tension between the case as a text or performance or genre of discovery (*anagnorisis*) and one of knowledge (*anagnosis*). *Anagnorisis* is a dramatic discovery and central to the Aristotelean model we have been building, whereas *anagnosis* is a (re)reading. Both are forms of identificatory recognition, but the former is revelatory, whereas the latter is routine. Is the act of diagnosis – the preliminary act in the clinical encounter and that which typifies the case, both in terms of form (it is a process of diagnosis) and in content (it is a case of that diagnostic type) – an active, novel and individual event led by the singular subject or rather a passive, patterned and repetitive sequence enacted on a universal object? In the following section, we will turn to a close examination of MCRs published by the *New England Journal of Medicine* as part of Cabot's Case Records of the Massachusetts General Hospital, reading them through the prism of this established genre-genetic sharing between Asclepian healing and dramatic tragedy. Indeed, the problem of the specificity and singularity of the individual MCR versus its capacity for generalisability and clinical utility is well expressed by Aristotle: 'the art of medicine does not specify what is healthful for Socrates or Callias but for persons of a certain sort (this is a matter of art, while particulars are limitless and not knowable)' (Arist. *Rh.*, 1.2.11.1356b).

We see the problem posed here also by Nietzsche, if we allow his reference to 'music' to extend to tragic drama (as he himself intends it) and from there to the clinical encounter and medical case (as he most certainly did not; Nietzsche 2008 [1872], 88–9):

> This reality, then, the world of individual things, supplies the visible, the particular and individual, the individual case, both to the universality of concepts and to the universality of melodies, these two universalities being united but also in a certain respect opposed; while the concepts contain only the forms which are abstracted in the first place from the visible world, the outer shell of things as it were once it has been removed, and so are completely genuine *abstracta*, music on the other hand gives the innermost core which preceded all assumption of form, or the heart of things.

What a remarkable vindication of the dramatic tension that comprises the particular case or clinical encounter. Its very shortcomings are its manifestation as the heart of things. It is to the heart of things we now turn.

The forgotten other of the medical case

> It is a less serious fault not to know that a female deer has no horns than to make an unrecognisable picture of one.
>
> Arist. *Poet.* (4.1460b)

This quotation from the *Poetica* expresses a curious truth of mimesis: we can have recognisable representations that will pass a test of *anagnosis* and have no actual correlative object outside the realm of representation. Simply: we all know what a unicorn looks like and could recognise it, regardless of the fact that no unicorns exist. (Indeed, our familiarity with the representation might mean we often fail, at least at the level of reflex thinking, to remember that unicorns are not real objects out in the world, *except* as representations, for representations still circulate in the world as objects.) To the unicorn, we could easily add the names of past 'diseases' that have vanished out of objective reality on greater empirical investigation and now lurk in the gloom of representation only: railway spine, wandering womb, the 'English sweate'. More uneasily, we might wonder what current 'disease' signs will prove to be signifiers without signified objects.[16] As mentioned earlier, the clinical act of diagnosis is a rendering of reported symptoms into a recognisable sign that is validated by a body of medical knowledge, itself mutually constituted by medical education practices, medical science research programmes and institutions, professional bodies and working clinical services. But, at the heart of this complex, rhizomatic network is the diagnostic entity and its moment of recognition in the clinical encounter – a foundational act, we are arguing, that is structurally, aesthetically and attitudinally indebted to (or, rather, co-developed with) Athenian dramatic tragedy. At this point we can ask, what traces of this conjoined development can we see in current medical cases?

We recently constructed a corpus of nearly 500 MCRs published between 1945 and 2019 in the *New England Journal of Medicine* (*NEJM*), the *British Medical Journal* (*BMJ*) and *The Lancet*, and we have drawn some examples of MCRs taken specifically from Cabot's Case Records of the Massachusetts General Hospital for analysis here. One of the immediately striking features of these – beyond the remarkably unchanging conventions of narrative structure and appearance, in contrast to MCRs published in the *BMJ* or *The Lancet* – is that these all contain at least one section laid out like a play script, capturing (or constructing) a discussion of possible diagnoses between various clinicians. These very evidently demonstrate a fundamentally discursive and, not infrequently, oppositional and dialectic progression towards (or, sometimes, away from) a moment of *anagnorisis*, the reveal – through diagnosis – of the identity of the 'complaint' that has brought the patient to the clinic. This is an interpretive – and creative – act: the clinicians are asking themselves of the patient: 'if there is any meaning in his words / His bitter cries?' (Soph. *Aj*., 324–5) Inscribing this meaning is the semiotic process of diagnosis, but dramatic tragedy gives the form and narrative to this process.

The dramatic and aesthetic imperatives are to create the most recognisable picture of what is – at the moment of arrival in the clinic – unseen and waiting to be uncovered, and to strive for an economy of narrative. In the discussion of a case from 1947, discussant Dr Aub emphasises that the discussion – and the process of discovery – is also a process of creating a narrative representation composed of clean lines: 'In these discussions I do not like to put in every possible diagnosis so as to be sure to include everything that was wrong with the patient' (Mallory, Castleman and Parris 1947a, 39). It is the clinician's representation – as constituted medical sign – rather than the patient's representation – as heterogeneous and complex phenomenological symptoms – that must prevail at the end of the clinical drama. What is curious about this case is that Dr Aub's diagnosis of bronchiogenic neoplasm – provided as a dramatic commentary staged after the actual clinical encounter – is in conflict with the clinical diagnosis of metastatic hypernephroma, which was subsequently confirmed by specimen analysis. Although it was initially the diagnosis he considered most likely, Dr Aub, in response to an ill-defined instinct, and from considering the combination of the patient's history and chest X-ray signs, discounted hypernephroma as less likely than a primary bronchial tumour. However, Dr Mallory opens the pathological discussion by asserting 'that although Dr Aub's logic is excellent, the specimen does not bear it out in any way'. The discursive logic of the clinician is 'excellent', and rather it is the failure of the tissue specimen to 'bear [...] out' this excellence; the specimen falls flat dramatically, delivering what Dr Aub (grudgingly, perhaps) calls 'the obvious diagnosis' (Mallory, Castleman, and Parris 1947a, 40). There is no negative clinical outcome here, as this is a retrospective discussion, but what is interesting is that the heroic, dramatic character of the clinician here drove him from the correct diagnosis, pursuing the novel, dramatic *anagnorisis* rather than the more pedestrian *anagnosis*.

These case records, as written documents, recreate the temporality and the quotidian dramas and frustrations of the diagnostic discussions they represent, while at the same time – given their brevity and their formal and very *written* language (indicated by the absence of agrammatisms, abbreviations, lapsus) – they are very apparently not verbatim transcripts. However, if Aristotle were to be judging some of this diction, he would criticise the clinical jargon of riddles and barbarism (Arist. *Poet.*, 3.1458a). The degree of editorial liberty taken is unclear, and exchanges such as the following from another case in 1947 are not uncommon:

DR ROPES: [...] I do not know the result.
DR AUB: I have seen amyloid disease with involvement of the whole small intestine.
DR ROPES: With symptoms?
DR AUB: I cannot remember.

Mallory, Castleman and Parris (1947b, 77)

This staging, with its representation of clinicians being uncertain and unable to access their own accumulated *phronesis*, is initially puzzling. We would argue it serves three purposes, which themselves fold into an overarching objective. First, there is the casting of clinical reasoning as fallible and its knowledge as provisional. Second, there is the creation of suspense, a self-conscious and dramatic experiencing of the temporality of diagnostic reasoning. Third, there is the creation of character. Within this temporally bounded drama, the clinicians have unexplored and only hazily represented personal and professional pasts. All these primarily aesthetic purposes are subordinate to the construction of clinical diagnostics as a narrative of labour and adversity, comprising clashes between agonists. Pointedly, in these cases, the patient has no voice, no agency and no presence within the discussion – except as atomised in various images, test results, statistics and so on. The *real* and meaningful drama of medicine, even of the clinical encounter, is displaced from the engagement between patient and healer to the domain only of the clinicians. The patient as other is not just forgotten, but vanquished, ushered from the stage and dissected (at least, figuratively; sometimes literally) for the mutual edification and celebration of medical authority, as embodied in these clinicians offering up a representation of their practice.

For the person living with an impairment, there is a double displacement. The patient is not only atomised, made invisible and silenced, but the dramatic narrative conventions – as with *Oedipus* – push their impairment and, by extension, their lived experience of (ill)health, outside the story proper. Even when pertinent, perhaps even of pre-eminent importance, to the MCR, the form struggles to give discursive space to disability. Disability as a term rarely features in the MCRs in our corpus, and most commonly refers to acquired mobility impairments or other irreversible limb damage. A case series of agricultural accidents from 1969 is typical in this regard, where 'disability' recurs throughout as a consequence, but is excluded from the dramatic action of the individual case studies embedded within the larger paper (Cooper, 1969). Consider this example taken from the series (Cooper 1969, 195):

> Case 58. Possibly the most serious accident in this group was experienced by a 47-year-old woman who worked on a turkey farm. While operating a tendon-pulling machine – a device which amputates the feet and avulses the long tendons of the legs of turkeys – her right hand became caught in the machine, resulting in the avulsion of the index finger and second metacarpal, partial avulsion of the thumb, and extensive damage to the middle finger … A grossly comminuted fracture of the first metacarpal was associated with avulsion of the thenar and interosseus muscles arising from that bone.
>
> Several other tendons, nerves, and muscles were injured in the metacarpal region. On the day of admission an extensive operation was performed to try to salvage as much of the hand as possible, and in particular the thumb. Thrombosis occurred, however, in the surviving vessels in the thumb, necessitating amputation of the thumb some three days later. Some eight and a half months after her accident she returned to work part-time. She was able to make a fairly good grip using her three remaining fingers. A thumb prosthesis was being considered when she was last seen.

The MCR narrative is the twin dramatic narrative of the acute problem and its remedial, diagnostic clinical correlate. The unity of plot depends on the presenting moment conjoining a very recent past – that of the accident in this case – to its puzzle-solving clinical instance. The bulk of the MCR text concerns the dramatic details of that one problem in that one instant. The vastly expanding future time in the final sentences that exponentially moves from 'three days' to 'eight and a half months' and then to a possible, open-ended future with a thumb prosthesis, constitutes a temporal exit from the stage into an outstretched future of 'disability' that, like Oedipus's wanderings, falls mostly outside the real tragic drama. It is deeply telling that more space is given over in the case series to 'a most exciting history' of a farmer's wild tussle with an escaped bullock, which proves full of thrilling incident but is completely free of any clinical or medical detail, than is afforded to a consideration of what it might mean for the 'cases' to live beyond the confines of these short narratives with their newly acquired impairments (Cooper 1969, 196).

The genre demands of the clinical encounter and the MCR, as inherited from dramatic tragedy, contribute to a situating of 'disability' outside the sphere of healthcare. In a 1995 clinical problem-solving report in the *NEJM*, the clinician's commentary only turns to 'disability' when musing on the tendency of patients to seek solace in alternative remedies and treatments (Kreisberg 1995, 843):

> Maybe part of the problem is that patients have unrealistic expectations about health and the relief of symptoms because of the dramatic medical advances that are featured in the media. Some patients are unable or unwilling to live with pain or disability and are continually seeking physicians or healers, whereas other patients wish only to be reassured that they do not have a serious or life-threatening illness and, once reassured, are willing to live with discomfort or disability.

The implicit position here is that 'disability', like the chronic 'pain' or 'discomfort', is something that patients take away to live with, and that 'continually seeking physicians or healers' for such things is quixotic and a product of overexuberant media or a culture that imagines healthcare has answers and tools it does not. Although writing with compassion and even-handedness about complementary medicine, Kreisberg does not seem to see that the distinction between the clinical problem-solving of the acute dramatic narrative of the clinic or MCR and the epic narrative of a life lived with chronic pain and 'disability' is not a distinction experienced in the life of the patient, but one produced by the genre characteristics that clinical medicine has developed. For the patient, this is one life and one ongoing, epic story.

Even in a contemporary online case report where the authors explicitly identify the value of early diagnosis of a specific virus – human T-cell lymphotropic virus type-1 (HTLV-1) – in order to prevent or at least limit future 'disability', the MCR does not position the 'significant physical disability' as anything other than a destiny to be avoided and one that resides outside the temporal, dramatic framework of the MCR itself (Andrade, Diaz and Buestan 2016). The 'disabled' or chronic patient is forgotten and othered and temporally thrown into a future that is beyond the immediate concerns of the clinician, or back into an aetiological past that is of interest only insofar as it elucidates the present (and presenting) clinical puzzle, such as the supposed clinical and narrative relevance of 'intellectual disability' in a case of peduncular psychosis: 'The presence of documented intellectual disability from a young age is relevant because mental illness, including psychotic disorders, has been reported to have a higher prevalence in intellectually disabled populations' (Andrews et al. 2016, 2). An integral part of the patient's character, of their lived experience, of their reality of being in the world is considered 'relevant' purely as it serves as an identifiable risk factor for successfully navigating the differential diagnosis process. The patient's character is subordinated to the narrative demands of the central drama – in which the clinician, not the patient, and certainly not the 'disabled' patient, enjoys the status of protagonist.

These MCRs display a split temporal perspective that echoes that of the Athenian tragic drama. In a case taken from 2016, shifts in tense emphasise the deliberate composition of the narrative. The text moves abruptly from a clinician announcing 'Management decisions were made' to a section entitled 'Discussion of Management', which combines a present-tense representation of being *in media res* with an analytical, reflective perspective of hindsight in the past tense (Choy et al. 2016, 781–2):

> For this patient we recommend en bloc excision [...] We performed a two-stage operative procedure to remove the L6 giant-cell tumour. During the first stage [...] After the spinal decompression, a partial diskectomy was performed.

The case is something that is both unfurling before us as audience, and something that is, at the same time, already done.[17] As with the tragedy of Ajax, the moment being represented in and as the present, and reliant on co-presence, is also definitively located in the past. In contrast to the earlier MCRs, this 2016 example withholds the outcome for the patient until the final moments of the text. It balances enough narrative uncertainty and suspense to propel us through the drama, but, tastefully, not so much that our sense of aesthetic pleasure is readily apparent to us. At least, to some small extent, the subjective experience of the patient, as a figure moving through time and through the clinical encounter(s) without firm knowledge of how the illness will resolve, is sketchily represented in this narrative structure. So too, in these 2016 MCRs, do the titles include both the phenomenological symptoms of the patient and the validated medical signs of the clinicians, as well as an embodiment, or silhouette, of the patient: 'A 28-year-old woman with back pain and a lesion in the lumbar spine'; 'A 71-year-old woman with Müllerian Carcinoma, fever, fatigue and myalgias' (Manian et al. 2016). The forgotten other is enjoying something of a (partial) resurrection.

These MCRs are not the only trace, in the material of contemporary medicine, of the cross-pollination with performance and tragedy. The objective structured clinical exams (OSCEs) have become, over the past 30 years, an integral part of the testing and validating of medical knowledge of students in the US and UK. First used in clinical neurology exams in 1964 in the US, OSCEs are roleplayed clinical encounters with trained actors assuming the patient roles, to be treated by trainee medics (Wallace, Rao and Haslam 2002). That standardised patients (SPs) are simultaneously known as 'simulated patients' demonstrates the ongoing, systemic dance between universal consistency on the one hand and unique, time- and space-bound performance on the other (Hodges et al. 1996). What could better exemplify the formal dramatic *antagonism* Attic drama incepted within Western medicine than SPs marking down trainee medics (Mazor et al. 2005)?

As suggested by Fig. 2.2 this re-staging of the clinical encounter hinges on two antagonistic forces: the patient's telling of their story and the clinicians re-writing of this passive tale of suffering with their active one of discovery, remedy and resolution (FourteenFish 2018). Elucidating this duality within the heart of the clinical encounter and tracing its origins in Western orthodox medicine's dialectical early relationship with tragic drama have not been an exercise in intellectual *jouissance*. We believe there are some valuable and practical implications for clinical practice and medical education. There exists a chain of forgotten others that we hope to bring to light. First, Attic drama has been a forgotten other embedded within the early structuring of the clinical encounter, through the cross-pollination between the rituals, narrative structures and social functions of the twin cults of

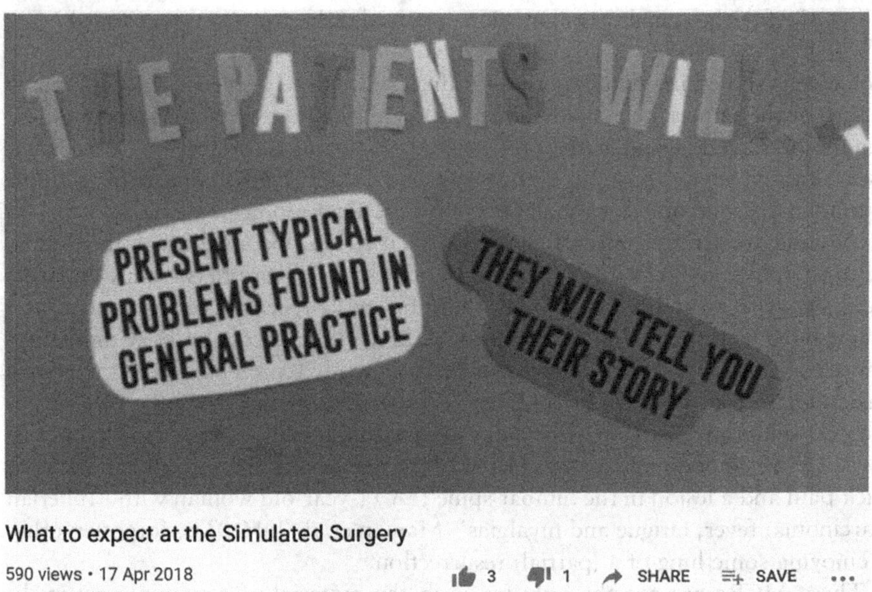

Fig. 2.2 Still from YouTube video explaining the procedures for the NHS England's GP Induction and Refresher Scheme's simulated surgery test. Reproduced with permission from FourteenFish (2018)

Dionysus and Asclepius in the fifth century BCE. Second, the clinical encounter as drama has a forgotten other in the form of the disease life course as an epic. This has led to the third forgotten other of the *epic* life narrative of the patient, which finds no suitable means of expression and realisation within the tight genre restrictions of the tragic dramatic clinical encounter. This structural exclusion is exacerbated by the (concealed) antagonisms imported from the dramatic form, to the extent that – until recent 'patient-centred' reforms – the patient themselves, as agonist, has been forgotten, as they were overwritten, silenced and objectified within the encounter and within the written form of the MCR. At the same time as establishing these forgotten others, we have also observed two important dichotomies. The first is structural and is between the genre forms of the tragic drama (the case and clinical encounter) and the epic (the life of the patient and the course of a disease), and the second is aesthetic and is between two modes of diagnosis and narrative: *anagnorisis* (as a discovery or reveal) and *anagnosis* (as reading back knowledge already had).

In examining how these dichotomies and forgotten others remain (and have hardened) as conventions within medical education, medical practice and the communication and discovery of new medical knowledge in the form of MCRs, we find important questions and lacunae rather than answers and solutions, and embracing these uncertainties and this lack of resolution might serve as an effective attitudinal counterpoint to the dramatic imperatives of the case and clinical encounter. What might a clinical encounter built on the collaboration of mutual agonists, rather than conflicting antagonists, look like? How might the different temporal and spatial scopes of the clinical encounter and the broader human life of the patient be better reconciled and constructively integrated? What disadvantages are there to a medical epistemology that, through the use of OSCEs and MCRs, is built upon inherent conflict and dramatically heightened constraints of time, space and resources? What can be done to unriddle and demystify the central figure of the healer and address the enduring asymmetries of power and agency that define the clinical encounter? This analysis has only been an exercise in learning to see the questions. The answers lie beyond. As the Chorus concludes in the exodos of Sophocles's *Ajax* (1416–20):

> Many are the things that man
> Seeing must understand.
> Not seeing, how shall he know
> What lies in the hand
> Of time to come?

Notes

1 '[T]he plot of a play, being the representation of an action, must present it as a unified whole.' (Arist. *Poet.* 2.1451a).

2 Numerous studies worldwide show that in the West, length of consultation varies by patient age, gender, class, and diagnosis, and also by GP gender (Deveugele et al. 2002; Irving et al. 2017; Hobbs et al. 2016). We acknowledge the perennial struggle to lengthen UK consultation time over the past 50 years, and to decrease the number of patients a GP sees daily.

3 If a symptom counts as a problem, the reasonableness of the policy needs to be judged against how polysymptomatic populations at large have been found to be. Many community-based surveys have characterised the profile of symptoms experienced in non-consulting populations as an 'iceberg'. One study of several thousand people found the mean number of symptoms in a 2-week period to equal 3.7, of which 'many ... were complex or potentially complex such as "feeling tired/run down and headaches"' (McAteer, Elliott and Hannaford 2011). Similarly, the higher the number of symptoms experienced, the more likely people were to consult in primary care (Elliott, McAteer and Hannaford 2011). A New Zealand survey found 90% of the population had one or more sumptoms in the previous 7 days (Petrie et al. 2014).

4 Just how problematic this relationship can be – especially in general practice – is brought out by the GP journalist Michael O'Donnell: 'The blinding flash of revelation came not on the road to Damascus but in a BBC studio. "When you left hospital medicine and became a GP", said my interrogator, "what was the most difficult lesson you had to learn?" Even as my brain processed the question, I heard my voice deliver the answer, as if in reflex response. "I had to learn the difference between disease and illness." ... I discovered illness, the "customised" disease suffered by individuals whose physical and emotional states determine the way disease affects their lives, can even determine the nature and severity of their symptoms. I'd encountered illness in hospital but hadn't the time to recognise it. In general practice I couldn't avoid it' (O'Donnell 2007).

5 Of course, Ajax's madness has an overtly divine agent – Athena – but the clinical encounter and case do not often speculate on origins and causes, except where they impact on diagnosis.

6 We are indebted to Professor Michael Trapp for drawing our attention to this literature.

7 Michael Flexer would like specifically to acknowledge the influence on our argument here of his colleagues on the *Waiting Times* research project, and particularly: Baraitser (2017) and Baraitser and Brook (2020).

8 Stigma, impairment, affliction and a fatalistic mark are all conflated in two popular twentieth-century English translations by Watling (1947) and Fagles (1982) respectively: '[T]hat old trouble ... / I have carried the stigma from my cradle' and '[T]hat old affliction ... / That dreadful mark – I've had it from the cradle' (Soph. *OT*, 1033–35).

9 Again, the Watling and Fagles translations together provide the sense of these impairments as deserved external marks of internal moral failing: 'may wear the brand of shame / For their shameful act, unfriended to their life's end / Nor do I exempt myself' and 'let that man drag out / His life in agony, step by painful step – I curse myself as well' (Soph. *OT*, 246–8). The old, despicable canard that physical 'flaws' indicate spiritual flaws is shown here to be ancient. Though if Sophocles is not exactly refuting the supposed connection, he is certainly ironising it. See Kelley (2007, 40) for an account of the pernicious 'influence of physiognomy in the ancient'.

10 Many thanks again to Michael Trapp for directing us to the primary sources for this association between Sophocles and Asclepius: the *Etymologicum Magnum* (256.10 ff.) and Plutarch (*Numa* 4.6; *Moralia* 1103a) – T67–69 in *Tragicorum Graecorum Fragmenta* (*TrGF*).

11 No worry that this form of anagnorisis is the 'least artistic [...] by means of visible signs or tokens' (Arist. *Poet.* 3.1454b).
12 The opposition implied here by saying they 'face off' is the nature of the creative dialectic exchange between the two.
13 When Brooke Holmes (2010, 3) writes that the Greek attitude to symptoms transformed 'stories ... about human suffering and also about *human nature*' (our italics), her focus is on a transformation that revolves around making bodily interiors conceptually visible. But here no disrupted structure or process seems to be required in order to accept that an indistinguishable pain can occur in the absence of it.
14 A person can be pained 'even if [the person's pain] is not about something ... that is the case' (Pl. *Philebus* 40d4–10; see Evans 2020, 80). 'Socrates introduces a "second type of pleasure and pain," belonging to "the soul alone" (Pl. *Philebus* 32b6-c5)'; see Tuozzo 1996, 500.
15 Mattern (2020) traces a line of influence from the Galenic case stories to the Case Records of the Massachusetts General Hospital. Though she does not comment on the performed character of the clinician, she identifies the survival of the 'diagnostic-puzzle theme' (p. 12) as a main component of the 'drama of the Case Records' (p. 14). Although Mattern is clearly employing a wider lay definition of the term 'drama' than we are here, we certainly subscribe to her conclusion: 'every medical drama is also a moral drama, with winners and losers, heroes and villains, and the most complex characters of all, the patients, who may or may not deserve their fate' (Mattern 2020, 25).
16 Such claims are made about diagnostic entities such as loneliness, chronic fatigue syndrome, or irritable bowel syndrome.
17 For the role of retrospective narrative construction and hindsight in formulating contemporary published cases, see Hurwitz 2017.

References

Primary sources

Aristotle, 'On the Art of Poetry.' Translated by T.S. Dorsch (1965), *Classical Literary Criticism*. Harmondsworth: Penguin, 29–75.

Aristotle, *On Rhetoric: A Theory of Civic Discourse*. Translated by George A.Kennedy (2007, 2nd ed.). Oxford: Oxford University Press.

Aristotle, *Nicomachean ethics*. Translated by David Ross (2009). Oxford World's Classics. Oxford: Oxford University Press.

Hippocrates, *Epidemics 2, 4–7*. Translated by Wesley D. Smith (1994). Loeb Classical Library. Cambridge, MA: Harvard University Press.

Hippocrates, *Places in Man*. Translated by Paul Potter (1995). *Places in Man. Glands. Fleshes. Prorrhetic 1–2. Physician. Use of Liquids. Ulcers. Haemorrhoids and Fistulas*. Loeb Classical Library. Cambridge, MA: Harvard University Press, 13–100.

Homer, *The Iliad*. Translated by Robert Fagles (1991). London: Penguin.

Homer, *The Odyssey*. Translated by Emily Wilson (2018). New York: W.W. Norton.

Plato, *Philebus*. Translated by Benjamin Jowett (2008). Project Gutenberg. Available at: www.gutenberg.org/files/1744/1744-h/1744-h.htm

Sophocles, *King Oedipus*. Translated by Edward F. Watling (1947), *The Theban Plays*. Harmondsworth: Penguin.

Sophocles, *Ajax*. Translated by Edward F. Watling (1953), *Electra and Other Plays*. Harmondsworth: Penguin.

Sophocles, *Oedipus the King*. Translated by Robert Fagles (1982), *The Three Theban Plays*. Harmondsworth: Penguin.

Virgil, *The Aeneid*. Translated by Cecil Day Lewis (1986). Oxford: Oxford University Press.

Secondary sources

Alvaston Medical Centre (2019) https://alvastonmedicalcentre.nhs.uk/website/CO1047/files/newsletter.pdf (accessed 2 October 2020).

Andrade, Maria J.M., Edgar P.C. Diaz and Maria E. Buestan (2016) 'HTLV-1-associated myelopathy in a solid organ transplant recipient.' *BMJ Case Reports*, 1–5. http://dx.doi.org/10.1136/bcr-2016-215243

Andrews, John P., Joseph Taylor, David Saunders and Zheala Qayyum (2016) 'Peduncular psychosis.' *BMJ Case Reports*, 37–40. http://dx.doi.org/10.1136/bcr-2016-216165

Baraitser, Lisa (2017) *Enduring Time*. London and New York: Bloomsbury.

Baraitser, Lisa and William Brook (2020) 'Watchful waiting: temporalities of crisis and care in the UK National Health Service.' In Victoria Browne, Jason Danely and Doerthe Rosenow (eds), *Vulnerability and the Politics of Care*. Oxford: Oxford University Press, 230–47.

Barthes, Roland (1994) *The Semiotic Challenge*. Translated by Richard Howard. Berkeley and Los Angeles: University of California Press.

Biggs, Penelope (1966) 'The disease theme in Sophocles' *Ajax*, *Philoctetes* and *Trachiniae*.' *Classical Philology* 61(4), 223–35.

Cabot, Richard C. (1906) *Case Teaching in Medicine: A Series of Graduated Exercises in the Differential Diagnosis and Treatment of Actual Cases of Disease*. Boston, MA: Heath.

Choy, Edwin, Francis J. Hornicek, Yen Lin Chen, Daniel I. Rosenthal and Darcy Kerr (2016) 'Case 26–2016: a 28-year-old woman with back pain and a lesion in the lumbar spine.' *New England Journal of Medicine* 375(8), 779–88.

Cole, Emma (2019) 'Post-traumatic stress disorder and the performance reception of Sophocles' *Ajax*.' In David Stuttard (ed.), *Looking at Ajax*. London: Bloomsbury Academic, 151–160.

Cooper, David K.C. (1969) 'Agricultural accidents: a study of 132 patients seen at Addenbrooke's Hospital, Cambridge, in 12 Months.' *British Medical Journal* 4(5677), 193–8.

Deveugele, Myriam, Anselm Derese, Atie van den Brink-Muinen, Jozien M. Bensing and Jan De Maeseneer (2002) 'Consultation length in general practice: cross sectional study in six European countries.' *British Medical Journal* 325(7362), 1–6.

Doerries, Bryan (2015) *The Theatre of War: What Ancient Greek Tragedies Can Teach Us Today*. New York: Knopf.

Elliott, Alison M., Anne McAteer and Philip C. Hannaford (2011) 'Revisiting the symptom iceberg in today's primary care: results from a UK population survey.' *BMC Family Practice* 12, 16.

Evans, Matthew (2020) 'Plato and the meaning of pain.' *Apeiron* 40, 71–94.

Forrester, John (1996) 'If p, then what? Thinking in cases.' *History of the Human Sciences* 9 (3), 1–25.

FourteenFish (2018) What to expect at the Simulated Surgery. www.youtube.com/watch?v=Moyii-p7Pis (accessed 23 September 2020).

Hobbs, F.D. Richard, Clare Bankhead, Toqir Mukhtar, Sarah Stevens, Rafael Perera-Salazar, Tim Holt and Chris Salisbury (2016) 'Clinical workload in UK primary care: a retrospective analysis of 100 million consultations in England, 2007–14.' *The Lancet*, 2323–30.

Hodges, Brian, Jeffrey Turnbull, R. Cohen, A. Bienenstock and Geoffry Norman (1996) 'Evaluating communication skills in the objective structured clinical examination format: reliability and generalizability.' *Medical Education* 30, 38–43.

Holmes, Brooke (2010) *The Symptom and the Subject: The Emergence of the Physical Body in Ancient Greece*. Princeton, NJ: Princeton University Press.

Holt, Philip (1980) 'Ajax' ailment.' *Ramus* 9(1), 22–33.

Hurwitz, Brian (2017) 'Narrative constructs in modern clinical case reporting.' *Studies in History and Philosophy of Science Part A*, 62, 65–73.

Irving, Greg, Ana Luisa Neves, Hajira Dambha-Miller, Ai Oishi, Hiroko Tagashira, Anistasiya Verho and John Holden (2017) 'International variations in primary care physician consultation time: a systematic review of 67 countries.' *BMJ Open* 7 (10), 1–15.

Kamieński, Łukasz (2012) 'Helping the postmodern Ajax: is managing combat trauma through pharmacology a Faustian bargain?' *Armed Forces and Society* 39, 395–414.

Kelley, Nicole (2007) 'Deformity and disability in Greece and Rome.' In Hector Avalos, Sarah J. Melcher and Jeremy Schipper (eds), *This Abled Body: Rethinking Disabilities in Biblical Studies*. Atlanta: Society of Biblical Literature, 31–46.

Kreisberg, Robert (1995) 'Clinical problem-solving: we blew it.' *New England Journal of Medicine* 332(14), 945–9.

Lansky, Melvin R. (1997) 'Shame and suicide in Sophocles' *Ajax*.' *The Psychoanalytic Quarterly* 65(4), 761–86.

Lloyd, Geoffrey E.R. (ed.) (1978) *Hippocratic Writings*. Translated by J. Chadwick and W.N. Mann. Harmondsworth: Penguin.

Mallory, T.B., Benjamin Castleman and E.E. Parris (1947a) 'Case Records of the Massachusetts General Hospital: Case 33012.' *New England Journal of Medicine* 236 (1), 38–40.

Mallory, T.B., Benjamin Castleman and E.E. Parris (1947b) 'Case Records of the Massachusetts General Hospital: Case 33021.' *New England Journal of Medicine* 236 (2), 75–8.

Manian, Farrin A., Miriam Barshak, Kathryn Lowry, Kristen Basnet and Christopher P. Stowell (2016) 'Case 27–2016: a 71-year-old woman with Müllerian carcinoma, fever, fatigue, and myalgias.' *New England Journal of Medicine* 375(10), 981–91.

Mattern, Susan P. (2020) 'Structure and meaning in the case records of Massachusetts General Hospital.' In Markus Asper (ed.), *Thinking in Cases: Ancient Greece and Imperial Chinese Case Narratives*. Berlin: Walter de Gruyter, 9–30.

Mazor, Kathleen M., Judith K. Ockene, H. Jane Rogers, Michele M. Carlin and Mark E. Quirk (2005) 'The relationship between checklist scores on a communication OSCE and analogue patients' perceptions of communication.' *Advances in Health Sciences Education* 10(1), 37–51.

McAteer, Anne, Alison M. Elliott and Philip C. Hannaford (2011) 'Ascertaining the size of the symptom iceberg in a UK-wide community-based survey.' *British Journal of General Practice* 61(582), 1–11.

Mitchell-Boyask, Robin (2008) *Plague and the Athenian Imagination: Drama, History, and the Cult of Asclepius*. Cambridge: Cambridge University Press.

Nietzsche, Fredrich (2008 [1872]) *The Birth of Tragedy*. Translated by Douglas Smith. Oxford: Oxford University Press.

Nutton, Vivian (2004) *Ancient Medicine*. London: Routledge.

O'Donnell, Michael (2007) 'Ultimate achievement.' *British Medical Journal* 334 [online]: www.bmj.com/content/334/7601/s170

Petridou, Georgia (2014) 'Asclepius the divine healer, Asclepius the divine physician: epiphanies as diagnostic and therapeutic tools.' In Demetrios Michaelides (ed.), *Medicine and Healing in the Ancient Mediterranean World*. Oxford: Oxbow Books, 297–307.

Petrie, Keith J., Kate Faasse, Fiona Crichton and Andrew Grey (2014) 'How common are symptoms? Evidence from a New Zealand national telephone survey.' *BMJ Open* 4(6), 8–13.

Risse, Guenter B. (1993) 'Medicine and disease: an overview.' In Kenneth F. Kiple (ed.) *The Cambridge World History of Human Disease*. Cambridge: Cambridge University Press, 9–19.

Royal College of General Practitioners (2016) 'The RCGP Curriculum: Core Curriculum Statement.' https://www.gmc-uk.org/-/media/documents/RCGP_Curriculum_1_Being_a_GP_Jan2018.pdf_73517306.pdf

Royal College of General Practitioners (n.d.) 'About Person-Centred Care.' https://www.rcgp.org.uk/clinical-and-research/our-programmes/about-person-centred-care.aspx (accessed 23 September 2020).

Slaveva-Griffin, Svetla (2016) 'Socrates' debt to Asclepius: physicians and philosophers with Asclepian souls in Late Antiquity.' *Numen* 63(2–3), 167–95.

Steger, Florian (2018) *Asclepius: Medicine and Cult*. Translated by Margot M. Saar. Stuttgart: Franz Steiner.

Tuozzo, Thomas M. (1996) 'The general account of pleasure in Plato's Philebus.' *Journal of the History of Philosophy* 34(4), 495–513.

Wallace, Jeremy, Ranga Rao and Richard Haslam (2002) 'Simulated patients and objective structured clinical examinations: review of their use in medical education.' *Advances in Psychiatric Treatment* 8(5), 342–8.

Zoja, Luigi (2017) *Paranoia: The Madness that Makes History*. Translated by Jonathan Hunt. London and New York: Routledge.

Chapter 3

'There is a pain – so utter –'

Narrating chronic pain and disability in antiquity and modernity

Georgia Petridou

Abstract

Although chronic pain subjugates and fragments the body, it is rarely categorised as a form of disability, as it is thought of as a symptom rather than a medical condition. Yet, chronic pain demands far more complex communication and signification processes that often defy established biomedical taxonomies. Moreover, individualised pain-related terminology, cultural barriers, and defective pain communication often create a dissonant relationship between chronic pain sufferers and healthcare providers. This chapter is a comparative study of chronic pain as a hidden disability in antiquity and modernity. It divides its attention between two modern chronic pain sufferers, the nineteenth-century American poetess Emily Dickinson and the twentieth-century police lieutenant Howard Harris (whose case was examined and reported by Arthur Kleinman in his seminal book *Illness Narratives: Suffering, Healing and the Human Condition*), and one ancient sufferer, the second-century CE Mysian orator Aelius Publius Theodoros Aristides. Extra emphasis is placed on the paradoxical co-existence of chronic pain's ineffability and the effective verbalisation of pain as the ultimate litmus test of literary genius. The argument in a nutshell is that effective patient–physician resonance was and still is a *sine qua non* for the communication and curing of chronic pain, while narrative-based medicine (NBM) was and still is a powerful tool that enables the development of such a relationship between the patient and the physician (ancient and modern alike).

Introduction: chronic pain as disability and patient–physician resonance

I must admit, I feel a heavy weight on my shoulders: the weight of writing about disability, albeit in a historical context, while being able-bodied.[1] Nonetheless, I feel compelled to be part of this conversation because I fully subscribe to Tobin Siebers's famous statement that 'able-bodiedness is a temporary identity at best' (Siebers 2008, 5). Moreover, as a historian, I firmly believe that debating the very concept of 'normal' and 'normalcy' (Davis 2013) and employing disability studies as a basic analytical framework force us to be conscious of how we construe, use, and abuse our own 'othering' processes. Kim Nielsen (2008, n.p.) puts this issue more aptly:

> Using disability as an analytical framework simply means that the historian asks questions about past definitions of 'fit' and 'unfit' bodies and minds. How did social institutions attempt to create and enforce adherence to those definitions? What were the consequences of those definitions for social relationships, legal institutions, democracy, education, medicine, bodies, epistemological frameworks, foreign policy, social welfare, and on and on? Who is excluded and why?

In many ways, Nielsen's approach to disability highlights some of the key questions of this volume: who determines what is a 'fit' or 'unfit' body? How were these un/fit bodies framed and understood in the Classical world and how do they compare to modern un/fit bodies? In an attempt to provide tentative answers to the questions set above, this chapter offers a comparative study between ancient and modern un/fit bodies crippled by chronic pain. Extra emphasis is placed on: (a) the ineffability of pain; (b) the integral role empathy and careful listening play in unearthing the patient's lived experience of chronic pain; and (c) chronic pain's 'socially negotiated subjectivity' (Derbyshire 2016; cf. also Eisenberger 2012; Giummarra, Tracy, and Young 2016).

But why should ancient historians be interested in chronic pain? How does chronic pain relate to disability? This study looks at pain as a hidden disability and a universal – that is, an element that unites us and the Classical world (Wilson 2013). As decades of anthropological research have shown (e.g. Moore Free 2002; Wierzbicka 2012; Throop 2010; 2015), pain unites large, industrialised societies with small, pre-industrialised societies. Whether we grew up in Manchester in the UK or in the island of Yap in Micronesia, we are all bound to experience and express pain at some point of our lives. More to the point, as the clinical psychologist Ephrem Fernandez and the anaesthesiologist and psychiatrist Ajay Wasan (2010, 451), note: 'pain is a global problem, with one in five persons suffering moderate to severe levels of chronic pain (World Health Organization 2004)' (on the relationship of chronic pain and suffering, see Schleifer 2014). Yet, the communication of sensations of chronic discomfort and agony to laypeople and medical professionals alike is often impeded by pain's complex nature: pain is both personal and communal; it is both culture-specific and universal. In addition, pain communication is inhibited by pain's inherent ontological dualism: pain is both a biological and a cultural phenomenon (Melzack 1973; Scarry 1985; Duncan 2017; van Rysewyk 2016–19).

When we talk about pain as a cultural construction, we refer to pain's diverse cultural framings. Although, for biomedicine, pain is a more or less unvarying procedure (Osterweis, Kleinman, and Mechanic 1987; Derbyshire 2016; Meugnot and Jackson 2016), recent studies in socio-anthropology and the anthropology of pain (e.g. Moore Free 2002; Wierzbicka 2009; 2012; Meugnot and Jackson 2016) have proved that the ways we conceive, communicate, and control pain are always culture-specific. The ways we experience, communicate, and respond to pain depend very much on our personal experiences and our experiences of observing other pain sufferers in our immediate or wider social environment (DelVecchio Good, Brodwin, Good, and Kleinman 1992). The anthropologist Jason Throop (2010, 2) puts it more concisely:

> pain itself may be transformed through the particular meanings, values, ideals, and expectations that we bring to bear in dealing with the existential possibilities and limitations that it evokes. As much as pain is a foundational aspect of our existence as humans, it is variegated in its forms of manifestation and significance.

This premise holds true for both modernity and antiquity. In a recent study of pain, pain representation, and communication in the Antonine Era, Daniel King (2018) has shown how the cultural specificity of bodily knowledge, pain representation, and communication has had wider implications for the cognitive, emotional, and affective aspects of lived pain experience of sufferers in the same period.

In the Western world, chronic pain's inherent biocultural identity impacts severely on welfare provision. Chronic pain's complex, dual nature often evades the classificatory attempts of health organisations and committees (such as the Social Security Administration and the Institute of Medicine in the US, or the Department for Work and Pensions, the Disability Service Centre, and the Department of Health and Social Care in the UK), namely the main organisations that are responsible for setting the statuary standards defining disability resulting from chronic pain. The controversial replacement of the DLA with the PIP (Personal Independent Payment) in the UK and the subsequent reassessment of hundreds of thousands of claimants, which resulted in loss of some income or income altogether for some of them, is a good example of how vulnerable chronic pain patients really are to the so-called 'purging of disability rolls' that gets engineered every now and then in modern societies, often in response to financial crises. The failure of these controversial reforms to re-evaluate pain-related disability is partly down to the long and labyrinthine evaluation processes claimants must survive in order to persuade the committees that they are worthy of income support, and partly is down to chronic pain's complex biocultural nature and inherent ineffability (Schott 2004).

Pain in general, and chronic pain in particular, defy articulation (Melzack and Torgerson 1971; Moore Free 2002; Schott 2004). In fact, articulating pain fully and adequately has often been considered the litmus test of literary genius and/or rhetorical eloquence (see the famous case of Emily Dickinson discussed in the following section). More importantly, putting pain into words is a *sine qua non* for effective pain communication between sufferer and healthcare provider, which is in turn an integral constituent of the *patient–physician resonance*. Having borrowed the term resonance from the sociologist Hartmut Rosa (2019), I employ the terms patient and physician with the widest possible meaning to include sufferers of all ages and genders and healthcare providers of all possible backgrounds and levels of expertise. By patient–physician resonance, I refer to a special kind of successful rapport that develops between the chronic sufferer and her or his healthcare provider. Patient–physician resonance is of the essence for both the timely diagnosis and the effective treatment of chronic and life-limiting pain. Unsurprisingly enough, a great percentage of this rapport rests on narratives constructed by those partaking in the medical encounter. This is precisely why, in turn, narrative-based medicine (NBM) is a *desideratum* for the development of patient–physician resonance. NBM puts the patient at the centre of the medical encounter and values patient narratives, instead of treating them simply as a diagnostic tool (Greenhalgh and Hurwitz 1998; Charon 2005; Hurwitz and Charon 2013).

Nonetheless, individualised pain-related terminology, in particular, and defect pain communication, in general, often create a discordant rapport between chronic pain sufferers and healthcare providers (Kenny 2004). This discordance, the lack of fruitful communication and rapport between the main agents of the therapeutic encounter, could be conceptualised as patient–physician dissonance and is particularly prevalent among migrant and refugee communities in the large melting-pot populations in North America and Northern and Southern Europe. Patient–physician dissonance can be the result of what anthropologists of pain describe as 'culture clash' in the healthcare systems (Galanti 1992; Moore Free 2002; Kenny 2004), or it could occur *despite* the patient's and physician's shared social roles and expectations, shared, communicated, and mediated via common cultural symbols (e.g. language, literature). As recent studies in ancient patient history have shown (e.g. Roby 2016; van Schaik 2016; King 2018), the ancient patient's experience of chronic pain was not unlike that of modern patients. While examining pain representation in Galen of Pergamum and Aretaeus of Cappadocia, King (2018, 43–102) lays extra emphasis on pain-related terminology and patient–physician communication or lack thereof. Both physicians present themselves as listening to and learning from their patients. However, they differ in that, whereas Aretaeus presents himself as engaging closely with the patient's voice and views in diagnosing and treating pain, Galen insists on preserving the traditional image of the patient, one that is familiar to the reader of the Hippocratic texts, as an unreliable witness (cf. Webster 2016). King highlights the role of language as the semiotic system par excellence employed in negotiating pain and power dynamics between the sufferer and their attending physician in the Antonine period. The following section reiterates this idea of language playing a key role in pain communication and negotiation in the early modern era and delves further into the concept of patient–physician resonance.

Narrating chronic pain and patient–physician resonance

> There is a pain – so utter –
> It swallows substance up –
> Then covers the Abyss with Trance –
> So Memory can step
> Around – across – upon it –
> As One within a Swoon –
> Goes safely – where an open eye –
> Would drop Him – Bone by Bone –
> Emily Dickinson (1863)

'There is a pain – so utter –' was written by Emily Dickinson in 1863 (see Franklin 1999). This poem is only one of the poems in which the author, while being in pain herself, engages closely with self-observation and narration of pain in all its all-conquering nature (note the second line, 'It swallows substance up') and pervasiveness. Above all, Dickinson, in this poem, triumphs over pain by conquering its elusive materiality and ineffability (on the elusive materiality of pain, see Schleifer 2009). Dickinson was no stranger to severe and chronic pain (i.e. pain that lingers for longer than 6 months), with recurrent infections of the respiratory system and, according to some biographers (Hirschhorn 1999; Mamunes 2007), bouts of tuberculosis too. The reader may be familiar with Dickinson's most famous poem on pain, 'Pain has an element of blank', a minimalist masterpiece on the ubiquity and the enormity of chronic pain in the life of pain sufferers. She also suffered from serious ophthalmological illness during her thirties and indeed feared blindness. However, she is most famous for withdrawing gradually from the public eye and even from close friends and only agreeing to speak to visitors through closed doors. Despite these superimposed or self-inflicted limitations (biographers disagree especially as to what extent she withdrew from the public to focus on her work or had already, in her twenties developed a serious anxiety disorder that made human interaction difficult and problematic), she continued writing her poems, diaries, and letters and, through them, continued to make sense of a world whose fragmentariness was punctuated by severe, long-lasting pain (see, for example, her Lyman letter no. 290, Sewall 1965).

Emily Dickinson and her prolific literary production not only despite, but also because of, pain bring to mind another chronic pain patient, Aelius Aristides. Aristides, one of the most prolific and well-known representatives of the so-called Second Sophistic, produced a unique first-person narrative in six books, the *Hieroi Logoi* ('Sacred Discourses'), in which he chronicled his battles with putting chronic suffering into words (King 1999). In Aristides's case, chronic pain seems to be the result of an unidentified illness or various illnesses (depending on how one reads the text; cf. Downie 2016; Israelowich 2012) that spanned more than 20 years. Charles Behr (1968, xiii) described the *Hieroi Logoi* as the 'voluminous and faithful record of dream world and waking life', which if properly employed could reveal:

> for the first time unequalled possibilities ... to break the barriers of anonymity which surround the inner life of even the best known figures of antiquity, and without qualification or conjecture, to penetrate to the subconscious level of one of them.

The *Hieroi Logoi* is essentially an illness narrative with distinct aretalogical overtones; although extremely self-conscious and highly idiomatic, it conveys successfully the intensity of Aristides's lived experience of chronic suffering. Unlike Emily Dickinson's poetic renderings of chronic pain, however, Aristides has been suspected of insincerity and exaggeration of his pain experience (Petridou 2019a, with further bibliographical references). More importantly, his close engagement with narrating his bodily functions and changes has been repeatedly interpreted as a sign of hypochondria (e.g. Harris 2009; 2016).

Yet, as Rita Charon (2005, 261) maintains rather fittingly, 'sick persons and those who care for them become obligatory story-tellers and story-listeners'. Dickinson and, to an extent, Aristides (see later section) were two of these few 'privileged' chronic pain sufferers who, armed with literary charisma, were able to face the challenge of putting pain into words head-on. For the vast majority of us, to quote Byron Good (1992, 37), 'bodily experience assumes enormous proportions' that often defy words. Patients describe their pain as 'shattering' and 'world-destroying'. Chronic pain subjugates and fragments body and mind (Geniusas 2016). It demands complex signification and communication processes between the sufferers, their carers, and healthcare providers. This precisely why there is so much scholarly and clinical interest in NBM – or simply narrative medicine, as it is also called – the last 40 years or so.

Brian Hurwitz and Rita Charon provide a good definition of NBM in their 2013 contribution to the *The Lancet* as follows: 'Narrative medicine practices are bringing the power of story-based telling, appreciation, and analysis into the routines of scientific clinical work'. Narrative medicine strives to put the patient at the centre of the medical encounter and, as such, stands in opposition to 'Evidence-based medicine (EBM)', which in the case of diagnosis and treatment of chronic pain relies mostly on neuroscientific evaluations of pain. NBM places emphasis on the narrative structure of both medical knowledge and patient experience and employs narrative as a tool to gain access to the perspectives of both patient and caregiver. The epistemic value of the patient's voice, and of the narrative he or she can construct, has risen to prominence in modern clinical praxis especially in the area of palliative care, the area of healthcare focusing on preventing and relieving the patients' lingering, life-limiting suffering – an increasingly significant aspect of Western medicine, especially in connection with the management of age-related and chronic diseases, which affect a larger part of the population than before (van Schaik 2016).

Putting pain into words, though, is not an easy task, and this has wider repercussions for the patient–physician resonance. 'The merest schoolgirl, when she falls in love, has Shakespeare or Keats to speak her mind for her', Virginia

Woolf (2002, 6–7) asserts in her well-known 1930 essay *On Being Ill*, 'but let a sufferer try to describe a pain in his head to a doctor and language at once runs dry'. In fact, pain eludes not only the communication between patient and physician, but also often the historian of disability, the ancient historian, the archaeologist, and often even the palaeopathologist, who may perhaps be able to recognise ancient disease and its physical signs on human remains – let us say, the deformity and dysplasia in skeletal structures caused by infectious diseases such as tuberculosis and syphilis, arthropathies, such as osteoarthritis and gout – but miss altogether the pervasiveness of chronic suffering in one's lived experience and relationships. Even pain specialists, who rely exclusively on quantitative neuroscientific exploration of pain, such as functional magnetic resonance imaging, cannot quite fully comprehend or qualify its impact on the individual's everyday life, as argued by the majority of the contributors to the first of two collected volumes on the *Meanings of Pain*, edited by Simon van Rysewyk (2016).

The problem(s) with Howard Harris

Crucially, chronic pain in both its diagnosis and treatment defies established biomedical taxonomies. Back in 1988, in a volume that changed the face of medical humanities, Arthur Kleinman debated and argued against the medical construct of '*the* chronic pain patient' by focusing on multiple manifestations of chronic pain in several different sufferers. Despite the common denominator of chronic pain, each of the sufferers embodied their pain and disability in very different ways. One of them was the police lieutenant Howard Harris, or Howie, who although in his late fifties and severely disabled, refuses to retire and claim disability pension out of fear of how that would impact his family finances and power dynamics. While discussing Howie's case in a sensitive and respectful manner, Kleinman (1988, 56–74) highlights the ultimate paradox of lived or felt pain, as he called it: pain has been perceived and described as this subjective and private experience par excellence, which nonetheless demands clear and adequate communication of its intensity and its impact on the sufferer's functionality and quality of life to vouchsafe its timely and efficacious management and/or treatment. Kleinman has intentionally chosen a case of chronic lower back pain-induced disability induced by chronic pain so utter (to be reminded of Dickinson's words) that it has ended up dominating the patient's entire family life and wider social circle. Howie indicates his vulnerability by being overcautious and constantly anxious that his spine will 'break', as he puts it, not only throughout their consultations, but, as his family and friends report, throughout his entire day, and by being in a perpetual state of preparation for the next major pain attack.

The medical tests have failed to verify the extent and the intensity of the problem – as it is often the case – and, sadly, his attending physician ('Wilber Mason, Howie's former primary care physician') is reluctant to spend more time with a patient whom he regarded implicitly as a typical case of hypochondriasis. This is how Mason describes his patient (Kleinman 1988, 71):

> He is pathetic. He's half his own problem. He's basically given up. What can I do? He comes to me in pain, I've got to give him something. I don't feel there is much we can do, really. I can't bear to see his name on the list of patients in my clinic. I think in the year I have seen him regularly he has never once said he was feeling better or smiled or been optimistic. This pain problem is getting him down and has clearly gotten to his family and is getting to me, too. I feel up against the wall. I've sent him to all the specialists and used all the latest drugs. I don't think we are any longer dealing with a disease; this pain has become his way of life.

If we were ever trying to find a good example of a dissonant patient–physician relationship, then this is it. Although both physician and patient agree on the severity, ubiquity, and omnipotence of pain in Howie's life, neither of them seems to be able to completely connect with the other and communicate their frustration and helplessness in the face of chronic pain and resulting disability. For 20 years, Howie has tried every available orthodox and alternative treatment for lower back chronic pain, which has, as he put it in Kleinman's transcriptions of their taped interviews, 'screwed up my life' (Kleinman 1988, 61). The high intensity of this unending pain that Howie often describes as 'radiating', 'burning', 'pulsing', 'flashing', 'stabbing', 'sharp', 'hot', 'stinging', 'punishing', among other things, has often, by his own admission, forced him to think of death as a preferable solution, although his Christian faith forbids suicide (Kleinman 1988, 62–3). His primary care physician, on the other hand, in his respective interview with Kleinman, openly accuses him of failing to manage what ironically is the very definition of chronic suffering: 'this pain has become his way of life', he exclaims indignantly. As in Emily Dickinson's and Aelius Aristides's cases, pain leads Howie to social withdrawal and self-imposed seclusion, which in turn impacts heavily on the family dynamic. Howie's wife, Ellen, and their three children feel rather embittered about their respective absent husband and father and openly accuse him of hypochondria and lying:

> 'He stays by himself. I know he's in pain. But every day? Can it always be that bad? I think he is part of the problem. He's a bit of a hypochondriac. Once he starts worrying about pain, he can't get off it. We have no personal life.'
>
> Kleinman (1988, 67)

And: '"I can't stomach hearing about pain," complaints one of the twins. "How do we know it's as serious as he says? I mean, I believe him, but you can't see it. He isn't dying or anything like that"' (ibid., 68).

'Where is the illness?', Kleinman asks and concludes:

> In the back, all right. But what about its presence in Howie's sense of self, in his relationship with his wife and mother, in the reactions of his

> children, in his work setting, in his doctor? The pain is the central idiom of a network of communication and negotiation. In a sense, the network is in pain.
>
> Kleinman (1988, 72)

It takes a lot of time (the interviews with Howie were conducted over a period of 2 years), a reasonable amount of personal investment from the two principal parties involved in the process of deciphering and signifying pain (i.e. the patient and the physician), and, above all, a highly functional, open, bidirectional line of communication between the patient and the physician, what we called earlier patient–physician resonance, to offer such an in-depth analysis (Kleinman most notably calls it an 'interpretation' and not diagnosis) of the complex biocultural nature of chronic pain suffering that both respects the patient and simultaneously reveals, respectfully, fundamental aspects of their network pathology. Narrative medicine has been of cardinal importance in the process of recording this chronic patient's voice and employing it as a heuristic tool.

Rita Charon, who in 2000 founded the Program in Narrative Medicine at Columbia University, maintains that teaching narrative-based therapy to healthcare providers enhances their empathic receptors and helps them become aware of their cultural bias and effectively fight against it. In an informative and moving article (Charon 2005, 264), she explains how practising narrative medicine has changed her ways of taking a patient's history and enhanced her rapport with them:

> I find that I have changed my routines on meeting with new patients. I simply say, 'I'm going to be your doctor. I need to know a lot about your body and your health and your life. *Please tell me what you think I should know about your situation*' (emphasis mine). And patients do exactly that – in extensive monologues, during which I sit on my hands so as not to write or reflexively call up their medical record on the computer. I sit and pay attention to what they say and how they say it: the forms, the metaphors, the gaps and silences. Where will be the beginning? How will symptoms intercalate with life events? I listen, not with Freudian or Lacanian or gestalt frameworks of meaning-making, but with narratological ones. The first time I did this, the patient started to cry after a few minutes. 'Why are you weeping?' I asked him. He answered, 'No one ever let me do this before'.

The description of the patient's reaction to the procedure in the final two lines of the extract constitute, at least to my mind, the epitome of modern patient–physician resonance. But what about the ancient sufferer from chronic and life-limiting pain (the kind of pain the Greeks would describe as *epiponos, epiponotatos*, or *polychronios* or simply refer to as *chronion/aniaton algema*: King 1999, 279; Wilson 2013)? And what about patient–physician resonance in the Classical world?

The problem(s) with Publius Aelius Aristides Theodoros

Notwithstanding the well-known limitations of our sources and their fragmentariness, which I have discussed elsewhere (Petridou and Thumiger 2016), I am reluctant to agree with Robert Garland (2010, xi), who wrote in his influential *The Eye of the Beholder: Deformity and Disability in the Graeco-Roman World* that there are 'no memoires written by the disabled in classical antiquity – the classical world was anything but confessional and there would have been no market for such revelations'. If one was willing to cast one's net wider and look especially at authors dating to the Imperial Era, one might be surprised by the wealth of personal testimonies of patients who detail their bodily processes and chronicle their long-lasting illnesses.

> In general, in the Imperial Age and in Late Antiquity, the pattern of the 'suffering self' was widespread among both Christians and pagan writers: as has been recently pointed out, the references to their own diseases by authors like Aristides and Marcus Aurelius or, on the Christian side, Ignatius of Antioch, should be read as expressions of a culture which was using representations of bodily pain and suffering to construct a new subjectivity of the human person.
>
> Perkins (1995, 173; cf. also Perkins 1992; Miletti 2017, 11; Petridou 2018a)

Aristides's *Hieroi Logoi* ('Sacred Discourses'), in particular, offer us an inimitable opportunity to witness: (a) the chronic pain patient's active involvement in the diagnosis and treatment of chronic pain and life-limiting suffering; (b) the centrality of narrative construction in chronic pain management; and (c) the resonant and dissonant relationships between Aristides and his physicians (earthly and divine alike).

Of course, part of the problem in both Garland's discussion and, generally, in discussions of disability in the Classical and post-Classical world, is that chronic pain that induces disability is a very different kind of suffering; it is an invisible and silent one, certainly one that does not necessarily meet *The Eye of the Beholder*. Indeed, no chapter devoted to chronic pain as hidden disability is included in the book. If, on the other hand, we bundle all these authors together and put their individual expressions of sorrow and agony in the face of either chronic illness such as gout, chronicled in Marcus's correspondence with his teacher Fronto (1.2 [1 Hout; 1.80 Haines] and 5.13 [74 Hout; 1.200 Haines] in Bowersock 1969, 71–5; Perkins 1992, 267–72; Brabant 2006, 67; Várhelyi 2010, 88–9), or prolonged torture during martyrdom, as in Ignatius's case, in the same basket, we are again missing the point. To my mind, grouping together all these individual expressions of chronic anguish detracts attention from the real pain and urges the reader to view their suffering as part of an elaborate stance, part of the façade of the 'suffering scriptor' (Petridou 2019a). But how can we do justice to these authors without committing the primordial sin of adopting over-realistic interpretations (King 1999; 2014; Petsalis-Diomidis 2010) of these texts?

First, we ought to properly contextualise them and discuss them individually, judging each of these narratives against the modes and registers of their respective literary discourse. Just as, in Kleinman's discussion of Howie's case, there is no such thing as *the* chronic pain patient, and everyone embodies debilitating pain differently, so must we be equally suspicious of the concept of *the* suffering self or *the* suffering scriptor in the Second Sophistic. There may be parallels to be drawn between Aristides's *Hieroi Logoi* and Lucian's *Podagra*, for example – both narratives emphasise chronic suffering and portray life-limiting illness as initiation into mysteries of the highest order – but they are essentially very different texts, the first a narrative of illness and religious individualism with a distinct aretalogical flavour, and the latter a tragicomedy (the title in manuscripts is given as either *Tragodopodagra* or *Tragopodagra*; see Petridou 2018b; 2020). Second, special attention needs to be paid to each work by the same author, and even each individual passage within the same work.

Although it is true that modern readers may find it hard to unravel the genuine pain behind the rhetorical tropes and literary artifice (Petridou 2019b), it is also important to remember that embedding unutterable chronic pain in words would have constituted a literary achievement for these authors of the Antonine period. As mentioned above, Aristides, just like Howard Harris, has been repeatedly suspected of disingenuous and hyperbolic expressions of pain. In a recent study, Downie (2016) remarks on the idiosyncratic style of the *Hieroi Logoi*, which does not contain any of the linguistic tropes (especially metaphors) often found in pain sufferers' narratives. In his intricate chronicle of chronic suffering, Downie maintains, Aristides adopts the stance of both the patient and the physician, of both the sufferer and the observer. Moreover, according to Downie, Aristides often circumnavigates pain expression by declaring his inability to put such a multitude of pains into words. However, this is hardly surprising for an orator who often retorts to rhetorical schema of *aposiopesis* when it comes to putting his physical and mental anguish into words, to showcase precisely the enormity of that anguish. This is, after all, a patient who, like Howard Harris, withdrew from the world and took refuge in the complex of the Pergamene Asclepieion to convalesce under the supervision of physicians such as Satyrus, the teacher of the famous Pergamene physician Galen. It is quite possible that, during that period, Aristides internalised this sort of medical discourse used by the professional health carers of the temple. More significantly, Aristides is a member of the sociocultural elite whose members, as authentic advocates of the Greek *paideia*, would have familiarised themselves with popularised medical treatises and debates (van Nuffelen 2014). In fact, Aristides consciously cultivates the image of the informed patient who is not only in possession of the basics of the medical discourse, but also functions occasionally as a physician of sorts, taking both his own life and the lives of others into his hands (Petridou 2016).

The medical practitioners operating at the Asclepieion seem to have been energetically involved in the lives of the patients (Israelowich 2012, 90, cf. also 88–91):

> The world of the *Sacred Tales* has physicians offering medical care to the convalescents of the Asclepieion, providing them with authoritative advice with regard to the interpretation of dreams, performing medical procedures such as enemas and phlebotomies and even joining them in their journeys to undergo purges in certain divinely designated sites.

Aristides mentions some of his physicians (Asclepiacus in 48.35; Heracleon in 48.20; Porphyrion in 51.12; and Satyros in 49.8), but the majority of them remain anonymous (e.g. *Or*. 48.39 and 49.27). Among his attending physicians, Aristides seems to have developed a closer relationship with the physician Theodotos who features more than the others in the narrative (*Or*. 47.13 and 55–7; 48.34; 50.21; and 51.57). Let us observe more closely Theodotos's sympathetic approach to Aristides's narrative in *Or*. 47.56–7, one of the episodes that dates to 'Cathedra' (145–147 CE), the 2-year period in which Aristides resided at the Asclepieion complex:

> (Winter 146) and after this there was wormwood, made clear in some way. It [sc. the remedy] was revealed in the clearest way possible, just as countless other things also made the presence of the god manifest. For I seemed almost to touch him and to perceive that he himself had come, and to be halfway between sleep and walking and want to get the power of vision and to be anxious lest he depart beforehand, and to have turned my ears to listen, sometimes as in a dream, sometimes as in a waking vision, and my hair was standing on end and tears of joy, and the weight of knowledge was no burden – what man could even set these things into words? But if he is one of the initiates, then he knows and understands. After these things had been seen, when it was dawn, I summoned the doctor Theodotos. And when he came, I recounted my dreams to him. He marvelled at how divine they were and was at a loss as to what he should do, since he feared the excessive weakness of my body in Wintertime. For I lay indoors during many successive months (ὀφθέντων δὲ τούτων, ἐπειδὴ ἕως ἐγένετο, καλῶ τὸν ἰατρὸν Θεόδοτον· καὶ ὡς ἧκε, διηγοῦμαι τὰ ὀνείρατα. ὁ δ' ἐθαύμαζε μὲν ὡς εἶχε δαιμονίως, ἠπόρει δὲ ὅ τι χρήσοιτο, χειμῶνός τε ὥρᾳ καὶ ἅμα τὴν ἄγαν ἀσθένειαν τοῦ σώματος δεδιώς· μηνῶν γὰρ ἤδη συχνῶν ἐκείμην ἔνδον.). Therefore, we thought that it was no worse to send also for the temple warden Asclepiacus.

Aristides has just narrated the double vision he shared with the *neokoros* (one of the temple wardens) Philadelphos. The vision urged him to drink wormwood or Artemisia Absinthium, one of the medicinal substances that appear often in medical authors, from the Hippocratics (e.g. *Morb.* 3.11; *Mul.* 1.74) to Aretaeus (*CD* 1.13) and Alexander of Tralles (1.10). The orator equates his extremely vivid healing experience to a religious one. His ecstatic joy at the manifest presence of the divine healer Asclepius is unbridled. The god appears to be not only in clear sight, but also almost within reach. This healing epiphany comes at a pivotal time (Petridou 2015, 171–94), when the orator has been laying incapacitated for several months and his body is extremely weak. Aristides is extremely eager to share his experience with the doctor Theodotos, whose opinion Aristides respects and admires. In a picture-perfect paradigm of patient–physician resonance, Theodotos listens carefully and marvels at the divine origins of Aristides's visions (ὁ δ' ἐθαύμαζε μὲν ὡς εἶχε δαιμονίως), thus empathising with his patient and generously validating Aristides's interpretative skills. However, unlike Aristides, Theodotos is not filled with joy; he is filled with worry about the lack of strength of his patient and *aporia*. Theodotos is at a loss regarding the recommended course of action (ἠπόρει δὲ ὅ τι χρήσοιτο) and, given the weakness of his patient's body, requests the help of the temple warden Asclepiacus, who may also have been a physician (*Or.* 49.25).

Aporia is not a cognitive state exclusively related to Theodotos. Instead, in the *Hieroi Logoi, aporia* ('being at a loss', 'embarrassment', 'perplexity') or *amechanie* ('want of means or resources', 'helplessness') is the modus vivendi of Aristides's earthly doctors. On every single occasion where the human doctors cannot help, Aristides takes refuge with Asclepius or other healing deities. Apparently, he was not alone in doing so. Asclepius was known as the last refuge of those who were plagued by incurable illnesses and insufferable pain (Wickkiser 2009, 58–61; Renberg 2017, 22–4, 175–6).

Indeed, being *derelictus a medicis* (lit. 'being abandoned by earthly physicians') and taking refuge in the temple of Asclepius form a *topos* in narratives (epigraphic, papyrological, and literary) that account for patients' experiences with chronic pain and long-term illness (Horstmanshoff 2004). Compare here the well-known second-century inscription from Rome (Dittenberger, *Syll.*^{3} III, 1173.7, 11 = *IG* XIV, 966), where Lucius, who has pleurisy, refers to Asclepius having being despaired of by his human physicians (Λουκίῳ πλευρειτικῷ ἀφηλπισμένῳ ὑπὸ παντὸς ἀνθρώπου ἐχρημάτι|σεν ὁ θεὸς ἐλθεῖν κτλ.); or the second-century inscription from the Athenian Asclepieion (*IG* II^2 4514), in which Diophantos, a temple attendant, honours Asclepius for curing him of gout, which he calls 'a painful incurable ailment' (ἀνίατον κακὸν ἕλκος, l. 23; see Edelstein and Edelstein 1998, vol. 1, 242, n. 428; Aleshire 1991, 111; Girone 1998, 31–5, Prêtre and Charlier 2009, 199–202). In a passage from Galen's *De curandi ratione per venae sectionem* (4.23 = 11.314–315 K), which aims at self-promotion by glorifying Galen's expert knowledge in venesection, we learn about a *therapeutēs* of Asclepius in Pergamum (i.e. a member of the cultic group of *therapeutae* in Pergamum: Petridou 2017a), who had been relieved from chronic pain (*chronion algēma*) by means of arteriotomy by the thumb prescribed by Asclepius (ἀπηλλάγη δι' ἀρτηριοτομίας). Finally, Asclepius of

Epidauros is credited with saving a female patient from incompetent mortal healers who operated on her in his absence in Aelian *NA* 9.33 (καὶ ὑπὸ χειρὸς θνητῆς ἐς ἄκεσιν ἥκειν ἀδυνάτοις).

Aristides himself refers often, in the six books of the *Hieroi Logoi*, to the false views held by human doctors (e.g. in 47.13, 57, 62–8; 48.5, 38–9, 69; 49.8, 18–9; 50.38; 51.9, etc.) and contrasts them to Asclepius's right views and diagnoses. Earthly physicians often appear completely baffled by both the origins and the nature of chronic suffering. Theodotos, however, who features more prominently (e.g. *Or*. 47.13; 47.55–7; 48.34; 50.21; 51.57) than any other named physician in these books (Israelowich 2012, 88–91), is very different in that, although he often disagrees with Aristides's interpretations of his symptoms and the god-sanctioned courses of action, he appears to be taking note of what his patient says – very much like Arthur Kleinman in Howie's case, and Rita Charon in her practice of NBM. Theodotos is also set apart from the rest of Aristides's physicians in that he also seems willing to modify his prescriptions and recommendations to fit closely the needs of his patient. The following extract from the fifth book of the *Hieroi Logoi* (*Or*. 50.38–9) will flesh this premise out:

> Tale follows tale, and let us say again that along with other things, Asclepius, the Saviour, also commanded us to spend time on songs and lyric verse, and to relax and maintain a chorus of boys. There would be no end of saying in how many other ways we benefited from this advice in contentment and self-sufficiency. But the children sang my songs; and whenever I happened to choke, if my throat were suddenly constricted, or my stomach became disordered, or whenever I had some other troublesome attack, the doctor Theodotos, being in attendance and remembering my dreams, used to order the boys to sing some of my lyric verse. And while they were singing, there arose unnoticed a feeling of comfort, and sometimes everything that pained me went completely away.

As I have argued elsewhere (Petridou 2017b; 2019b), narrative therapy and literary therapy – that is, therapy centred on the creation and performance of narratives – lay at the heart of Aristides's resonant relationship with Asclepius. Aristides is, in fact, far more mainstream in using rhetoric, literature, and music to cure bodily ailments than we have previously thought. Narrative therapy in general and literary therapy in particular were not exceptional measures taken simply in the case of Aristides. They may sound peculiar to us but, nonetheless, they were common practice in the temples of Asclepius. It is true, of course, that, although Aristides works with previously well-attested healing practices (e.g. in Plutarch, Galen, Antyllus), he elevates them to a whole new level of efficacy by making them sound tailor-made and exclusive.

Alexia Petsalis-Diomidis, in her pioneering study on the *Hieroi Logoi* and the cult of Asclepius in Pergamum, has argued that, in his other orations (e.g. *Or*.

24.5; *Or.* 33. 9; and *Or.* 34.53), Aristides does not compare the earthly doctors with the divine one as unfavourably as he does in the *Hieroi Logoi*. Nonetheless, if we are to look carefully at these passages, we would realise that this is not quite so. In *Or.* 4.5, for example, Aristides does not necessarily extol doctors or their achievements; he simply makes a point about novelty, which is not always better than tried and trusted medical recipes. Likewise, in *Or.* 33.9 Aristides remarks that the doctors should always be ready to help, but it is up to the patients to ask for their help. The only positive remark made here is the fact that he compares the medical art (*technē iatrikē*) to his own (*technē rhetorikē*) and, effectively, himself to one of the doctors. However, being a doctor is a role that Aristides occasionally assumes even in the *Hieroi Logoi* (Petridou 2016). In the same vein, Aristides also compares himself to a good doctor in *Or.* 34.53, who, although having the means to gratify their patient, does not do so, instead choosing the more difficult course of action, which is fairer and more beneficial to that patient.

Most scholars believe that the earthly physicians Aristides consulted in Smyrna, Pergamum, and elsewhere naturally compare unfavourably with Asclepius, their patron deity, and that Aristides was particularly drawn to Asclepius because he provided a kind of holistic treatment that built on the elite patient's sociocultural standing and professional demands, thus preparing him for a victorious return to vigorous reading, writing, and uninhibited declaiming. Others, such as André Jean Festugière (1954) and Patricia Cox Miller (1998), have chosen to focus more on the signification process of pain and how Asclepius facilitated this process for Aristides – that is, provided meaning for an otherwise nonsensical suffering. I wonder, though, whether the comparison would always be in favour of Asclepius, not just because he specialised in the treatment of chronic pain and illnesses (as seen above), but because he sought to develop a resonant relationship with his patients. At least, this is what Galen would have us believe in his *De Sanitate Tuenta*, his treatise on hygiene, where he clearly demonstrates that literary therapy lay at the heart of a wide range of treatments administered to the more literary minded of the occupants of the Pergamene Asclepieion in order to regulate their bodily warmth and help them deal with both physical and psychological disorders:

> No mean witness of this opinion is our ancestral divinity Asclepius [ὁ πάτριος ἡμῶν θεὸς Ἀσκληπιός], who caused not a few odes to be written and humorous mimes and songs to be composed [οὐκ ὀλίγας μὲν ᾠδάς τε γράφεσθαι καὶ μίμους γελοίων καὶ μέλη τινὰ ποιεῖν ἐπιτάξας] by those in whom the excessive activity of passion made the constitution of the body.
>
> *De Sanitate Tuenta* (1.8.17–23 Koch 1923 = 6.40–2 Kühn 1821–33)

There are countless examples in Greek literary and documentary sources that make this connection, between incurable and/or long-lasting pain, Asclepian therapeutics, and patient–physician resonance. It comes as no surprise, then, that, when faced with the constant uncertainty and recurring agony of chronic pain, Aristides makes the obvious choice to trust the healer who offers a greater rapport with patients, employs narrative therapy, and specialises in treatment of chronic pain. Aristides's resonant relationship with Asclepius is the reason why he so proudly declares in *Or*. 28.132:

> Even when we were physically stricken, we did not come to ignoble supplication to the doctors. But although, to speak by the grace of the gods, we possessed the friendship of the finest doctors, we took refuge in the temple of Asclepius, in the belief that if it was fated for us to be saved, it was better to be saved by his agency, and that if it was not possible, it was time to die.

Conclusion

This study's attention has been divided between two modern sufferers and one ancient sufferer from chronic pain. Two of those sufferers, namely the nineteenth-century American poetess Emily Dickinson and the second-century Mysian orator Aelius Publius Theodoros Aristides, were renowned for their eloquence. For this reason, it is fascinating to see how they dealt with the problem of verbalising chronic suffering. The first was praised for her eloquence, whereas the second was suspected of insincerity. The third case is the twentieth-century police Lieutenant Howard Harris (aka Howie), whose case was examined by Arthur Kleinman and included in his seminal book *Narratives of Illness* as a cautionary tale against underrating and misappropriating the voice of the sufferer. As Michael Fletcher and Brian Hurwitz argue very aptly in this volume (Chapter 2), suppressing the voice of the patient is, by necessity, the prevalent trait in clinical practice in the UK (see especially their informative discussion of the pressure put on NHS patients to focus on one symptom per medical consultation with their GP). The same holds true for the medical case reports (MCRs) published in several prestigious medical journals. Published MCRs, Fletcher and Hurwitz maintain, often report on the patients' narratives by focusing selectively on one medical plot that drives the 'clinical drama', complete with the obligatory Aristotelian *peripeteia* and *anagnorisis*, as it is directed and staged by the reporting physicians. The patient's voice is thus reframed so radically that the published report refracts rather than reflects the original medical encounter.

Unlike Dickinson and Aristides, Howie was plagued by what seems to be a complete inability to convey the extreme nature of his suffering to both his internal social circle and his attending physician. The lack of rapport between patient and physician in Howie's case – what we referred to before as patient–physician dissonance – comes into sharp contrast with the empathetic stance Aristides's divine physician Asclepius and human physician Theodotos choose to adopt in their treatment of the orator's chronic ailments – the latter being an exemplary case of patient–physician resonance.

Perhaps we could finish this comparative study of chronic pain as a hidden disability with a modern chronic pain sufferer, the American investigative journalist Cathryn Jacobson Ramin, whose recent book, *Crooked: Outwitting the Back Pain Industry and Getting on the Road to Recovery* (2017), not only chronicles her personal struggles with chronic lower back pain, but also examines the impact of extreme medicalisation and commercialisation of chronic back pain in modern Western societies. The chronic pain narrative of Cathryn Jacobson Ramin, who, like Emily Dickinson and Aelius Aristides, is a writer by trade and thus endowed with eloquence and persuasiveness, could be thought as the ultimate foil to Howie's fragmented and untrustworthy narrative about his problems with chronic lower back pain. However, even Jacobson Ramin's narrative focused on encounters with healthcare givers that clearly demonstrate the power of patient–physician resonance in treating effectively and alleviating chronic pain. Patient–physician resonance was, and still very much is, a *sine qua non* in communicating and curing chronic pain.

Note

1 I would like to thank wholeheartedly Ellen Adams and Emma-Jayne Graham for inviting me to the conference, where a first draft of the paper was presented. I am indebted to Ellen Adams and the anonymous referee for their careful editing and insightful comments on an earlier draft of this chapter. I am indebted to Jörg Rüpke and the Max-Weber Kolleg, University of Erfurt, for the generous Mercator fellowship I received in 2020 under the auspices of the DFG and FWF-funded International Research Training Group (IGS) 'Resonant World Relations in Ancient and Modern Socio-Religious Practices' project (shared between the University of Erfurt, Germany, and the University of Graz, Austria), which allowed me to work on the revisions of this chapter.

References

Aleshire, Sara B. (1991) *Asklepios at Athens: Epigraphic and Prosopographic Essays on the Athenian Healing Cult*. Amsterdam: J.C. Gieben.

Behr, Charles A. (1968) *Aristides and the Sacred Tales*. Amsterdam: Adolf M. Hakkert.

Birn, Anne-Emanuelle (2018) 'WHOse health agenda? 70 years of struggle over WHO's mandate.' *The Lancet* 391(10128), 1350–1.

Bowersock, Glen (1969) *Greek Sophists in the Roman Empire*. Oxford: Clarendon Press.

Brabant, Dominique (2006) 'Persönliche Gotteserfahrung und religiöse Gruppe – die Therapeutai des Asklepios in Pergamon.' In Andreas Gutsfeld and Dietrich-Alex Koch (eds), *Vereine, Synagogen und Gemeinden im kaiserzeitlichen Kleinasien*. Tübingen: Mohr Siebeck, 61–75.

Charon, Rita (2005) 'Narrative medicine: attention, representation, affiliation.' *Narrative* 13(3), 261–70.

Cox Miller, Patricia (1994) *Dreams in Late Antiquity: Studies in the Imagination of a Culture*. Princeton, NJ: Princeton University Press.

Davis, Lennard J. (2013) *The End of Normal: Identity in a Biocultural Era*. Ann Arbor: University of Michigan.

DelVecchio Good, Mary-Jo, Paul E. Brodwin, Byron J. Good and Arthur Kleinman (eds) (1992) *Pain as Human Experience: An Anthropological Perspective*. Berkeley: University of California Press.

Derbyshire, Stuart W.G. (2016) 'Pain and the dangers of objectivity.' In Simon van Rysewyk (ed.), *Meanings of Pain*. Cham: Springer, 23–36.

Downie, Janet (2013) *At the Limits of Art: A Literary Study of Aelius Aristides' Hieroi Logoi*. Oxford: Oxford University Press.

Downie, Janet (2016) 'The experience and description of pain in Aelius Aristides' Hieroi Logoi.' In John Wee (ed.), *The Comparable Body: Analogy and Metaphor in Ancient Mesopotamian, Egyptian, and Greco-Roman Medicine*. Leiden: Brill, 247–74.

Duncan, Grant (2017) 'The meanings of "pain" in historical, social, and political context.' *The Monist* 100, 514–31.

Edelstein, Emma J. and Ludwig Edelstein (1998) *Asclepius: Collection and Interpretation of the Testimonies* (2nd ed.). Baltimore: Johns Hopkins Universities Press.

Eisenberger, Naomi I. (2012) 'The neural bases of social pain: evidence for shared representations with physical pain.' *Psychosomatic Medicine* 74(2), 126–35.

Fernandez, Ephrem and Ajay Wasan (2010) 'The anger of pain sufferers: attributions to agents and appraisals of wrongdoings.' In Michael Potegal, Gerhard Stemmler and Charles Spielberger (eds), *International Handbook of Anger*. New York: Springer, 449–64.

Festugière, André J. (1954) *Personal Religion Among the Greeks*. Berkeley and Los Angeles: California University Press.

Franklin, Ralph W. (ed.) (1999) *The Poems of Emily Dickinson: Reading Edition*. Cambridge, MA: Belknap Press.

Girone, Maria (1998) *Ἰάματα. Guarigioni Miracolose di Asclepio in Testi Epigrafici*. Bari: Levente editori.

Galanti, Geri-Ann (1992) *Caring for Patients from Different Cultures: Case Studies from American Hospitals*. Philadelphia: University of Philadelphia Press.

Garland, Robert (2010) *The Eye of the Beholder: Deformity and Disability in the Graeco-Roman World* (2nd ed.). London: Bristol Classical Press.

Geniusas, Saulius (2016) 'Phenomenology of chronic pain: de-personalization and re-personalization.' In Simon van Rysewyk (ed.), *Meanings of Pain*, Vol. 1. Cham: Springer, 87–106.

Giummarra, Melita J., Lincoln M. Tracy and Kurtis A. Young (2016) 'The social side of pain: what does it mean to feel another's pain?' In Simon van Rysewyk (ed.), *Meanings of Pain*, Vol. 1. Cham: Springer, 355–76.

Good, Byron J. (1992) 'A body in pain – the making of a world of chronic pain.' In Mary-Jo DelVecchio Good, Paul E. Brodwin, Byron J. Good and Arthur Kleinman (eds), *Pain as Human Experience: An Anthropological Perspective*. Berkeley: University of California Press, 29–48.

Greenhalgh, Trisha and Brian Hurwitz (eds) (1998) *Narrative-Based Medicine: Dialogue and Discourse in Clinical Practice*. London: BMJ Books.

Harris, William V. (2009) *Dreams and Experience in Classical Antiquity*. Cambridge, MA: Harvard University Press.

Harris, William V. (2016) 'Popular medicine in the classical world.' In William V. Harris (ed.), *Popular Medicine in the Graeco-Roman Antiquity: Explorations*. Leiden: Brill, 1–66.

Hirschhorn, Norbert (1999) 'Was it tuberculosis? Another glimpse of Emily Dickinson's health.' *The New England Quarterly* 72, 102–18.

Horstmanshoff, Manfred (2004) 'Aelius Aristides: a suitable case for treatment.' In Barbara Borg (ed.), *Paideia: The World of the Second Sophistic*. Berlin: DeGruyter, 277–90.

Hurwitz, Brian and Rita Charon (2013) 'A narrative future for health care.' *The Lancet* 381, 1886–7.

Israelowich, Ido (2012) *Society, Medicine and Religion in the Sacred Tales of Aelius Aristides*. Leiden: Brill.

Jacobson Ramin, Cathryn (2017) *Crooked: Outwitting the Back Pain Industry and Getting on the Road to Recovery*. London: Harper Collins.

Kenny, Dianna T. (2004) 'Constructions of chronic pain in doctor–patient relationships: bridging the communication chasm.' *Patient Education and Counselling* 52, 297–305.

King, Daniel (2018) *Experiencing Pain in Imperial Greek Culture*. Oxford: Oxford University Press.

King, Helen (1999) 'Chronic pain and the creation of narrative.' In James I. Porter (ed.), *Constructions of the Classical Body*. Michigan: University of Michigan Press, 269–86.

King, Helen (2014) 'The art of medicine. Narratives of healing: a new approach to the past?' *The Lancet* 383, 946–7.

Kleinmann, Arthur (1988) *Illness Narratives: Suffering, Healing and the Human Condition*. New York: Basic Books.

Koch, Konrad (1923) *Galeni De sanitate tuenta* in CMG V.4.2. Leipzig and Berlin: Teubner.

Kühn, Carolus Gottlob (1821–33) *Claudii Galeni opera omnia*. 20 vols. Hildesheim: Georg Olms.

Mamunes, George (2007) *"So has a Daisy vanished": Emily Dickinson and Tuberculosis*. Jefferson, NC: McFarland.

Melzack, Ronald (1973) *The Puzzle of Pain*. New York: Basic Books.

Melzack, Ronald and Warren S. Torgerson (1971) 'On the language of pain.' *Anaesthesiology* 34, 50–9.

Meugnot, Aurore and Philip L. Jackson (2016) 'The contribution of new technological breakthroughs to the neuroscientific research of pain communication.' In Simon van Rysewyk (ed.), *Meanings of Pain*, Vol. 1. Cham: Springer, 87–106.

Miletti, Lorenzo (2017) '"I also have to dialogue with the posterity." Aelius Aristides' legacy to the Late Antiquity.' In Alberto J. Quiroga Puertas (ed.), *Rhetorical Strategies in Late Antique Literature. Images, Metatexts and Interpretation*. Leiden: Brill, 7–25.

Moore Free, Mary (2002) 'Cross-cultural conceptions of pain and pain control.' *Baylor University Medical Centre Proceedings* 15(2), 143–5.

Nielsen, Kim E. (2008) 'Historical thinking and disability history.' *Disability Studies Quarterly* 28(3), https://dsq-sds.org/article/view/107/107

Osterweis, Marian, Arthur Kleinman and David Mechanic (eds) (1987) *Pain and Disability: Clinical, Behavioral, and Public Policy Perspectives*. Institute of Medicine (US) Committee on Pain, Disability, and Chronic Illness Behavior. Washington, DC: National Academies Press.

Perkins, Judith (1992) 'The "self" as sufferer.' *Harvard Theological Review* 85, 245–72.

Perkins, Judith (1995) *The Suffering Self: Pain and Narrative Representation in the Early Christian Era*. London: Routledge.

Petridou, Georgia (2015) *Divine Epiphany in Greek Literature and Culture*. Oxford: Oxford University Press.

Petridou, Georgia (2016) 'Aelius Aristides as informed patient.' In Georgia Petridou and Chiara Thumiger (eds), *Homo Patiens: Approaches to Patient in the Ancient World*. Leiden: Brill, 451–70.

Petridou, Georgia (2017a) 'Contesting religious and medical expertise in the Hieroi Logoi: the therapeutai of Pergamum as religious and medical entrepreneurs.' In Richard L. Gordon, Georgia Petridou and Jörg Rüpke (eds), *Beyond Priesthood: Religious Entrepreneurs and Innovators in the Roman Empire*. Berlin and New York: De Gruyter, 183–208.

Petridou, Georgia (2017b) 'Poésie pour l'esprit, rhétorique pour le corps: Remèdes littéraires et cautions épistolaires dans les Hieroi Logoi d'Aelius Aristide.' *Mètis* 15, 69–94.

Petridou, Georgia (2018a) '"One has to be so terribly religious to be an artist": divine inspiration and theophilia in Aelius Aristides' Hieroi Logoi.' *Archiv für Religionsgeschichte* 20(1), 253–68.

Petridou, Georgia (2018b) 'Laughing matters: chronic pain and bodily fragmentation in Lucian's Podagra.' *Illinois Classical Studies* 43, 488–506.

Petridou, Georgia (2019a) 'The curious case of Aelius Aristides. The author as sufferer and illness as "individualizing motif".' In Eve-Marie Becker and Jörg Rüpke (eds), *Autoren in religiösen literarischen Texten der späthellenistischen und der frühkaiserzeitlichen Welt. Zwölf Fallstudien*. Tübingen: Mohr Siebeck, 199–219.

Petridou, Georgia (2019b) 'Literary therapies and rhetorical prescriptions in Aelius Aristides: medical paradoxography or common practice?' In George Kazantzidis (ed.), *Medicine and Paradoxography in the Ancient World*. Berlin and New York: De Gruyter, 183–97.

Petridou, Georgia (2020) 'The "lived" body in pain: illness and initiation in Lucian's Podagra and Aelius Aristides' Hieroi Logoi.' In Valentino Gasparini, Maik Patzelt, Rubina Raja, Anna-Katharina Rieger, Jörg Rüpke and Emiliano Urciuoli (eds), *Lived Religion in the Ancient Mediterranean World*. Berlin and New York: De Gruyter, 237–59.

Petridou, Georgia and Chiara Thumiger (2016) 'Introduction: towards a history of the ancient patient's view.' In Georgia Petridou and Chiara Thumiger (eds), *Homo Patiens: Approaches to the Patient in the Ancient World*. Leiden: Brill, 1–20.

Petsalis-Diomidis, Alexia (2006) 'Sacred writing, sacred reading: the function of Aelius Aristides' self-presentation as author in the Sacred Tales.' In Brian McGing and Judith Mossman (eds), *The Limits of Ancient Biography*. Swansea: University of Wales Press, 193–211.

Petsalis-Diomidis, Alexia (2010) *Truly Beyond Wonders: Aelius Aristides and the Cult of Asklepios*. Oxford: Oxford University Press.

Prêtre, Clarisse and Philippe Charlier (2009) *Maladies humaines, thérapies divines: analyse épigraphique et paléopathologique de textes de guérison grecs*. Archaiologia. Villeneuve-d'Ascq: Presses universitaires du Septentrion.

Renberg, Gil (2017) *Where Dreams May Come: Religions in the Graeco-Roman World*, Vol. 2. Leiden: Brill.

Roby, Courtney (2016) 'Galen on the patient's role in pain diagnosis: sensation, consensus, and metaphor.' In Georgia Petridou and Chiara Thumiger (eds), *Homo Patiens: Approaches to the Patient in the Ancient World*. Leiden: Brill, 304–22.

Rosa, Hartmut (2019) *Resonance. A Sociology of Our Relationship to the World*. Translated by James Wagner. Cambridge and Medford, MA: Polity. [Originally published in 2016 as *Resonanz. Eine Soziologie der Weltbeziehung*. Berlin: Suhrkamp.]

Scarry, Elaine (1985) *The Body in Pain: The Making and Unmaking of the World*. New York: Oxford University Press.
Schleifer, Ronald (2009) *Intangible Materialism: The Body, Scientific Knowledge, and the Power of Language*. Minneapolis: University of Minnesota Press.
Schleifer, Ronald (2014) *Pain and Suffering*. London and New York: Routledge.
Schott, Geoffrey D. (2004) 'Communicating the experience of pain: the role of analogy.' *Pain* 108(3), 209–12.
Sewall, Richard B. (1965) *The Lyman Letters: New Light on Emily Dickinson and Her Family*. Amherst: University of Massachusetts Press.
Siebers, Tobin (2008) *Disability Theory*. Ann Arbor: University of Michigan Press.
Throop, Jason C. (2010) *Suffering and Sentiment: Exploring the Vicissitudes of Experience and Pain in Yap*. California: University of California Press.
Throop, Jason C. (2015) 'Sacred suffering: a phenomenological anthropological perspective.' In Kalpana Ram, Christopher Houston and Michael Jackson (eds), *Phenomenology in Anthropology: A Sense of Perspective*. Bloomington, IN: Indiana University Press, 68–89.
van Nuffelen, Peter (2014) 'Galen, divination, and the status of medicine.' *Classical Quarterly* 63, 337–52.
van Rysewyk, Simon (ed.) (2016–2019) *Meanings of Pain*, Vol. 2. Cham: Springer.
van Schaik, Katherine D. (2016) '"It may not cure you, it may not save your life, but it will help you".' In Georgia Petridou and Chiara Thumiger (eds), *Homo Patiens: Approaches to the Patient in the Ancient World*. Leiden: Brill, 471–96.
Várhelyi, Zsuzsanna (2010) *The Religion of Senators in the Roman Empire. Power and the Beyond*. Cambridge: Cambridge University Press.
Webster, Colin (2016) 'Voice pathologies and the "Hippocratic triangle".' In Georgia Petridou and Chiara Thumiger (eds), *Homo Patiens: Approaches to the Patient in the Ancient World*. Leiden: Brill, 166–99.
Wierzbicka, Anna (2009) 'Language and metalanguage: key issues in emotion research.' *Emotion Review* 1, 3–14.
Wierzbicka, Anna (2012) 'Is pain a human universal? A cross-linguistic and cross-cultural perspective on pain.' *Emotion Review* 4(3), 307–17.
Wickkiser, Bronwen L. (2009) *Asklepios, Medicine, and the Politics of Healing in Fifth-Century Greece: Between Craft and Cult*. Baltimore: Johns Hopkins University Press.
Wilson, Nicole (2013) 'The semantics of pain in Greco-Roman antiquity.' *Journal of the History of the Neurosciences* 22, 129–43.
Woolf, Virginia (2002) *On Being Ill*. Introduction by Hermione Lee. Ashfield, MA: Paris Press.

Part 2

Using, creating and showcasing disability supports and services

Ellen Adams

Part 2 brings together three chapters that explore support mechanisms devised for disabled people, such as physical prostheses or compensatory strategies (e.g. audio description for blind people). This is sociopolitical, as prostheses may enhance status if made of elite materials, economic, if time and resources have to be invested, and ethical, from the decision-making process of what supports should be put in place, to how they might be displayed to the world in a museum context. This topic follows naturally from the previous Part on narrative medical histories and how these are owned, (mis)represented, diagnosed, and treated. Issues of individual versus state responsibility for investing in such supports are also relevant in this Part. Disability aids and services can be received in a wide range of ways by their users, from enthusiastic assimilation to full rejection.

Draycott (Chapter 4) opens this Part with an account of ancient prostheses. Classicists will be used to the issues encountered in assessing reliable sources and adequate contextual information. By focusing on a neglected body of evidence and presenting it with as much contextual information as possible, she is able not only to extract a much more nuanced understanding of the evidence (e.g. concerning trends based on gender), but also to explore this kind of replacement support in a variety of ways – is the benefit cosmetic or functional? Does the prosthetic device aim to achieve 'normality' or to enhance the person's status in some way? Goggins (a museum Senior Curator; Chapter 5) also explores these questions concerning the display of modern prostheses, and we are reminded that the use of tools, supports, and enhancements is a key aspect of Being Human. The contrast between these two chapters highlights the importance of considering what impact the museum context has on how we view particular objects.

Drawing from a range of archaeological and literary evidence, Draycott is able to present an etic account of prostheses and their users – personal experience is not represented, and she notes that references to prostheses are often made in the rather objective terms of material – 'shoulder of ivory'. But archival documentation and contextual background are a challenge for modern prostheses as well, as Goggins explains. The users' experience can also be difficult to fathom here, or even the identity of the user. Credit and acknowledgements are given primarily to the inventors and donors, but there is, at times, room for an emic account, as generated from the users. Perhaps a museum context automatically presents a more face-to-face engagement with individual users than written accounts ever would. And the modern context demands ethical considerations, as Goggins relates – encountering an image of oneself as a museum-worthy specimen could clearly be taken in a variety of ways. I felt more than slight unease at observing Frida Kahlo's prostheses in the stunning 2018 V&A exhibition, when it is known that she did not want such private possessions to be displayed.

Perhaps the main difference between Draycott's and Goggins's consideration of prostheses is that of context. Draycott notes that all classical examples come from tombs and burials – with the additional intriguing detail that all extremity prostheses come from male ones, and all facial prostheses from female. They were encased with their owners, a very personal piece of property, possibly to serve in an afterlife. They were not meant to be seen, but instead taken out of circulation. In contrast, Goggins showcases prostheses in glass tombs, actively encouraging engagement in a variety of ways. They are juxtaposed with the 'cool' motorbikes and technology (under the theme of *Technology by Design*), interactive computer programmes have been set up, and videos show insights from users. Goggins describes how the decision was taken to incorporate biomedical objects throughout the museums, a form of inclusion meant to entice visitors put off by the term 'biomedical'.

The museum context is extraordinary, a modern space designed to explore, challenge, and enrich visitors' worlds. Goggins (Chapter 5) and Adams (Chapter 6) explore this setting explicitly, in terms of a permanent exhibition on prosthetic replacements and a series of activities including audio description and handling, respectively. Both chapters invite the reader to compare the original context/use and the current exhibit, demonstrating how museums do not so much decontextualize artefacts, but reframe them in a completely innovative way. For example, the National Museums Scotland case with Kelly Knox's Vine Arm has a photograph of Knox set in the background, with the arm itself presented in the foreground (Chapter 5, Fig. 5.1), whereas the British Museum has taken the architectural Parthenon sculptures and presented them as works of art in a purpose-built space.

Museums do not present artefacts in an objective, clinical fashion, but rewrite the story through a series of descriptions (e.g. labelling and guides) and reproductions (e.g. models and explanatory diagrams). Adams explores how audio description invites a particularly close reading or looking and sensory experience. She also considers how this might be redeployed into mainstream visitor experience, and whether there would be a broader benefit – can audio description produce new ways of seeing for all? Museums offer the space for experimentation, dialogue, and the promotion of progressive policies, to practise inclusion rather than just expect disabled people to integrate. The study of disabled people requires consideration of the aids, prostheses, and strategies set in place to compensate for their impairment or even 'normalise' their experience. The results can be fascinating and frustrating in equal measure, and they are certainly fundamental to understanding the full human condition.

Both Draycott and Goggins refer to inspiration porn – that gush of emotion experienced by the non-afflicted when they observe a disabled person being terribly brave in overcoming their obstacles. Many disabled activists have spoken out against this phenomenon. But I feel we should allow ourselves a feeling of pride in the ingeniousness of the human response to explore solutions for the negative impacts of certain impairments and conditions (developed both by and for disabled people). And this speaks well of humanity. In 2020, the global economy received a deliberate, manmade knock, caused by lockdowns to protect the vulnerable and those treating them, rather than allow nature to take its course. At this time of crisis, this was the collective, human response – which leaves the traditional neglect of disability and illness in Humanities disciplines all the more exposed and inexplicable.

Chapter 4

Prostheses in classical antiquity

A taxonomy

Jane Draycott

Abstract

The literary, documentary, archaeological, and bioarchaeological evidence attests that a variety of different types of prosthesis were used by Greeks and Romans to replace their missing body parts, but the ways that these prostheses were described, discussed, and conceptualised could be very different, with some being viewed with considerably more favour than others. In this chapter, I shall examine the discourses surrounding prostheses in classical antiquity in an attempt to determine the place that each type had in ancient culture and society, and the ways in which the type of prosthesis that an individual used could affect their life and lived experience, for better or for worse. I shall explore the extent to which an individual's age, gender, status, or other significant factors about them had an impact upon not only the type of prosthesis they chose to use, but also the ways that they and their prostheses were viewed by their contemporaries. I shall propose that, although prostheses were not necessarily commonplace in classical antiquity, there was something of a recognised taxonomy.

Introduction

Curiously, classical prostheses have not received much in the way of attention from scholars, unlike those of later historical periods (Porter, Walter and Healy 2017; Withey 2016; Kwass 2006; Jones 2017; Hasegawa 2012; Neumann 2010; Ott, Serlin and Mihm 2002; Smith and Morra 2006). Despite the growing interest in the subject of impairment and disability in classical antiquity, discussions of prostheses, prosthesis use, and prosthesis users have so far played a relatively minor role in scholarship undertaken on it. The first monograph devoted to impairment and disability in classical antiquity, Robert Garland's *The Eye of the Beholder: Deformity and Disability in the Graeco-Roman World*, included a brief acknowledgement of the famous story of Hegesistratus of Elis and his wooden foot in a chapter focusing on medical diagnosis and treatment, but simply noted that it was possible for an ancient amputee to use a prosthesis (Garland 1995 [reissued 2010], 126; the story of Hegesistratus appears in Herodotus, *Histories* 9.36–7 and

Plutarch, *On Brotherly Love* 3.1). The second, Martha L. Rose's *The Staff of Oedipus: Transforming Disability in Ancient Greece*, the first attempt to integrate the relatively new discipline of disability studies into Classics, devoted slightly more space to the subject in the opening chapter of the work, an effort to set the scene in advance of a series of studies focused on particular aspects of impairment and disability in the ancient Greek world (Rose 2003 [reissued 2013], 26–7). However, Rose concluded that ancient prostheses would, in all likelihood, only have been cosmetic (Rose 2003, 26). In the years since this work was first published, this notion has been comprehensively disproved through new research on old discoveries, and new discoveries (Finch 2019; Li et al. 2013). The third, Christian Laes's *Beperkt? Gehandicapten in het Romeinse Rijk* (*Restricted? The Handicapped in the Roman Empire*), contains an entire chapter on mobility impairments, but prostheses are mentioned only in passing, and the English translation, a slightly updated version of the original Dutch text, *Disabilities and the Disabled in the Roman World: A Social and Cultural History*, follows suit (Laes 2014, 2018). Discussions of impairment and disability in the classical world are more frequently found in the form of edited volumes, and accordingly one might expect to find rather more discussion of prostheses here in the form of a focused individual chapter or two, but this has unfortunately not been the case; these, likewise, do not devote more than a sentence or two to the subject (Collard and Samama 2010; Breitwieser 2012; Laes, Goodey and Rose 2013; Krötzl, Mustakallio and Kuuliala 2015; Laes 2017).

In 1996, Lawrence Bliquez published what was, even then, a cursory and incomplete survey in *Aufstieg und Niedergang der römischen Welt*, yet, despite the increasing interest in the history and archaeology of medicine in the classical world over the last two decades, to date no more extensive study has appeared (Bliquez 1996; this was inspired by a shorter piece of work, Bliquez 1983). More recently, my research into ancient prostheses has resulted in the edited volume *Prostheses in Antiquity*, the proceedings of a workshop held in 2015 that was funded by the Wellcome Trust, published in 2019 (Draycott 2019a).[1] This comprised eight chapters, each one dealing with a different type of prosthesis or an issue relevant to the subject. However, the subject has been far from comprehensively covered, and I am in the process of writing a monograph that aims to be the definitive treatment of prostheses, prosthesis use, and prosthesis users in classical antiquity (Draycott, in preparation).

The literary, documentary, archaeological, and bioarchaeological evidence that survives from classical antiquity attests that a variety of different types of prosthesis were used by Greeks and Romans to replace various missing body parts, but the ways in which these prostheses were described and discussed by ancient authors likewise varied considerably, with some being viewed significantly more favourably than others by ancient commentators and thus, potentially, ancient society as a whole. So, in this chapter, I shall use the literary references to classical prostheses in conjunction with other types of evidence to examine the discourses surrounding them in order to attempt to determine the place that each type had in ancient culture and society, and the ways in which the type of prosthesis used by an individual could consequently affect their life and lived experience.

Terminology and definitions

First things first: we should define exactly what I mean by the term 'prosthesis'. The term itself is a relatively modern one. Although it is a compound of the Greek terms πρός ('on the side of') and θέσις ('setting' or 'placing'), it is not a term that was readily utilised by ancient authors, and it only entered the English language in 1533. It was initially used in a grammatical capacity to designate the addition of a syllable to the beginning of a word; then, in 1704, it began to be used in a medical capacity to refer to an artificial device that replaces or augments a missing or impaired part of the body, and it was only in the middle of the nineteenth century that it came to mean this almost exclusively (Wills 1995, 218; Davis 2013, 68).

So, today, in the twenty-first century, a prosthesis is some sort of device that is used to replace a missing body part, and each one is designed and assembled according to an individual's appearance and functional needs. A standard prosthesis is usually, but crucially not always, as unobtrusive and as useful as possible so as to maximise the chances of the individual's acceptance of it, as the psychological aspects of coming to terms with needing to use a prosthesis are also important (Gallagher, Desmond and MacLachlan 2008). The missing body part might be absent owing to a congenital or an acquired impairment. However, it is by no means certain that an individual missing a body part for either reason will accept a prosthesis as a substitute (Murray 2005). Refusal of a prosthesis is particularly common in elderly amputees (Massey, personal communication).[2] Embodiment, as well as the phenomenological embodiment of prosthesis use, is an important consideration, and studies have shown that, if an individual both mentally and physically accepts their prosthesis and is satisfied with it, they will be more likely to use it, and it should not come as a surprise that users are more inclined to accept a prosthesis that is aesthetically pleasing to them (Mills 2013; Murray 2008).

The reasons why individuals abandon their prostheses are complex and are as much to do with the individuals themselves (for example, age, sex, gender, ethnicity, level of education, etc.) as the prostheses, but studies have made clear the importance of comfort and functionality in successful prosthesis use (Murray and Fox 2002; Pezzin et al. 2004; Biddiss and Chau 2009). Consequently, considerable effort is expended by the prosthetist to match an individual's skin tone, hair colour, and so on, or to design and create something unusual and truly unique if that is what the individual desires (Massey, personal communication). Users are also more inclined to accept a prosthesis that makes their life easier than one that makes their life harder, and the sooner after the amputation the prosthesis is fitted, the more likely the user is to accept the prosthesis and use it successfully (Pezzin et al. 2004). So, we should consider each contemporary prosthesis as having something of a dual role, one aspect being its form and another being its function, although these aspects can also overlap. The nature of these forms and functions varies from prosthesis to prosthesis. An extremity prosthesis such as a finger, hand, or arm not only resembles the missing finger, hand, or arm but can also restore some, but not all, of its functionality. A facial prosthesis such as an eye or a nose resembles the missing eye or nose and, although it does not restore the lost sense of sight or smell, it does enable the user to 'pass' if that is what they wish to do. A recent study has shown that facial prosthesis users tend to prefer implanted prostheses over adhesive ones; the users of the latter type feel more self-conscious (Wondergem et al. 2016). These are all useful starting points from which to consider classical prostheses.

When the word πρόσθεσις ('application') is used in Greek literature, it tends to indicate the application of an object to the body for a specific purpose, and when it comes to medical practice, this includes the application of a medicinal remedy such as a pessary or a piece of medical equipment such as a cupping vessel (pessary: Hippocrates, *The Affections of Women* 1.11, and *On the Nature of Women* 11; ladder: Thucydides, *History of the Peloponnesian War* 4.135, see also Polybius, *Roman Histories* 5.60.7; cupping vessel: Aristotle, *Rhetoric* 1405b3). Despite this, no surviving ancient Greek or Latin medical treatise mentions prostheses – clearly, the application of a prosthesis to replace a missing body part was not considered a medical remedy. Although this might seem strange to a contemporary reader, accustomed as we are to viewing prostheses and other types of assistive technology as objects that are thoroughly medicalised and provided by the British National Health Service, this makes sense when we consider the way that the author of the Hippocratic treatise *On Joints* feels that they have to explain and justify their decision to include recommendations regarding which type of crutch is best for rehabilitating different types of injury that affect an individual's mobility:

> One might say that such matters are outside the healing art. Why, forsooth, trouble one's mind further about cases which have become incurable? This is far from the right attitude. The investigation of these matters too belongs to the same science; it is impossible to separate them from one another. In curable cases we must contrive ways to prevent their becoming incurable, studying the best means for hindering their advance to incurability; while one must study incurable cases so as to avoid doing harm by useless efforts.
>
> Hippocratic Corpus, *Joints* 58 (trans. E.T. Withington)

The irrevocable loss of a body part is the very definition of an incurable case and was recognised as such; hence, perhaps, the provision of prostheses was not of interest to, or at least not considered relevant by, medical writers, even those who provided step-by-step guides to limb amputation such as Celsus, Heliodorus, Archigenes, or Leonidas. Aristotle differentiated between body parts that, once lost, would grow back and those that would not; he described individuals who experienced the latter type of loss as 'mutilated' (κολοβός; Aristotle, *Metaphysics* 5.27.4).

Whereas in the twenty-first century we tend to refer to prostheses using the noun 'prosthesis' or the adjective 'prosthetic', and, in the National Health Service at least, one prosthetist will make any number of different types of prosthesis, in ancient literature, whatever the type of prosthesis under discussion, when prostheses are referred to, they are not described as 'prosthetic [body part]', they are described using the combination of the substitute body part and the substance from which it is made. Thus, Pelops has a shoulder of ivory (ὦμος ἐλεφάντου or *umerus eburno*), Pythagoras has a thigh of gold (μηρός χρυσοῦν), Hegesistratus has a foot of wood (πούς ξυλίνου), Marcus Sergius Silus has a hand of iron (*manus ferream*), and Statyllius has the hair belonging to another (ἀλλότριος πλόκαμος). This apparent lack of recognition of an overall category of object goes some way towards explaining what can appear to be a certain amount of cognitive dissonance on the part of ancient authors when it comes to their discourse, as we shall see shortly.

Research methodology and data

No umbrella term, such as the adjectives 'prosthetic', 'artificial', or 'false', was used by ancient authors to refer to ancient prostheses. Perhaps the closest ancient authors come to that is referring to prosthetic hair and teeth using the adjective 'purchased'. Consequently, what, exactly, we should include in the category of prosthesis is open for debate. In Lawrence Bliquez's initial study 'Prosthetics in classical antiquity: Greek, Etruscan, and Roman prosthetics', he focused his attention rather selectively:

> The scope of this investigation was confined to those devices attached to the human body which had some practical as well as cosmetic purpose; that is to say, I was interested in dental appliances and false limbs, as opposed to wigs and bodily padding of the sort detailed by comic poets and satirists.
>
> Bliquez (1996, 2641)

I have discussed the issues with Bliquez's differentiation between what he perceived to be practical and impractical prostheses elsewhere (Draycott 2019b, 71–2). Using this rationale, he collated fifteen ancient literary references to prostheses, comprising eleven dental prostheses and four extremity prostheses (three feet, one attached to a leg, and one hand). To date, I have found 102, and these include references to prosthetic hands, shoulders, feet, legs, thighs, eyes, noses, teeth, and hair (see Table 4.1), and, owing to the nature of the search, even this is not necessarily exhaustive. Although these ancient literary references include both factual and fictitious prostheses, and both historical and mythological ones (see Table 4.2), to a degree, bioarchaeological and archaeological evidence supports their veracity, with examples of prosthetic toes, feet, legs, teeth, hair, and a hand having been recovered from tombs and graves around

Table 4.1 Ancient references to prostheses

Body part	*References*	*Total*
Finger		
Hand	Statius, *Thebaid* 94-7 (1); Dio Chrystostom, *Eighth Discourse: On Virtue* 28 (2); Pliny the Elder, *Natural History* 7.29 (1)	4
Arm	Diodorus Siculus, *Historical Library* 3.52 (1?)	1(?)
Shoulder	Pindar, *Olympian* 1.37 (1); Pseudo-Hyginus, *Fabulae* 83 (1); Ovid, *Metamorphoses* 6.405 (1); Martial, *Epigrams* 12.84 (1); Vergil, *Georgics* 3.7 (1); Philostratus, *Imagines* 1.30 (2); Lucian, *The Dance* 54 (1); Tibullus, *Elegies* 63-4 (1); Pliny the Elder, *Natural History* 28.6.24 (1); Nonnus, *Dionysiaca* 15.24-30 (1); Sextus Empiricus, *Against the Professors* 255-6 (1); Pausanias, *Description of Greece* 5.13.4-6 (1); Dio Chryostom, *Eighth Discourse: On Virtue* 28 (1)	14
Toe		
Foot	Herodotus, *Histories* 9.36-7 (1); Plutarch, *Moralia: On Brotherly Love* 3.1 (1); Lucian, *The Ignorant Book Collector* 6 (2); Babylonian Talmud Yebamot 102b-103a (1)	5
Thigh	Aristotle, *On the Pythagoreans* Fr. 191 (1); Porphyry, *Life of Pythagoras* 28 (1); Diogenes Laertius, *Pythagoras* 11 (1); Plutarch, *Numa* 65 (1); Lucian, *Alexander the False Prophet* 40 (1); Aelian, *Historical Miscellany* 4.17 (1); Aelian, *Historical Miscellany* 2.26 (1); Lucian, *Dialogues of the Dead* 416 (1); Ammianus Marcellinus, *Roman History* 22.21 (1)	10
Leg	Erycius, *Greek Anthology* 9.233 (1); Martial, *Epigrams* 10.100 (1); Babylonian Talmud Chagiga 3a (1); Mishnah Shabbat 6.8 (1); Tosefta Shabbat 5:1-2 (1); Talmud Yerushalmi Shabbat 8:8, 8c (1); Babylonian Talmud Yoma 78b (1)	7
Eye	Dio Chrysostom, *Eight Discourse: On Virtue* 8 (2); Palestinian Talmud/Yerushalmi Nedarim 9.8 (1)	3
Nose	Theophanes, *Chronographia* (1)	1
Teeth	Laws of the Twelve Tables 10.8-9 (1); Hippocratic Corpus, *On Joints* 33.9-10 (1); Celsus, *On Medicine* 6.12 (1); Horace, *Satires* 1.8.47-50 (1); Martial, *Epigrams* 14.46 (1); Martial, *Epigrams* 12.23 (1); Martial, *Epigrams* 1.72 (1); Martial, *Epigrams* 9.38 (1); Martial, *Epigrams* 5.43 (1); Lucian, *Professor of Public Speaking* 24 (1); Macedonius the Consul, *Greek Anthology* 11.374 (1); Lucillius, *Greek Anthology* 11.310 (1); Mishnah, Shabbat 6.5 (2); Palestinian Talmud, Shabbat 6.5 (2); Palestinian Talmud/Yerushalmi Nedarim 9.8 (1); Babylonian Talmud Nedarim 66a-b	21

Table 4.1 (Cont.)

Body part	*References*	*Total*
Hair	Horace, *Satires* 1.8.47-50 (1); Martial, *Epigrams* 12.23 (1); Martial, *Epigrams* 9.38 (1); Martial, *Epigrams* 12.45 (1); Martial, *Epigrams* 6.12 (1); Lucillius, *Greek Anthology* 11.310 (1); Lucillius, *Greek Anthology* 11.68 (1); Lucian, *Dialogues of the Courtesans* 11 (4); Avienus, *Fables* 11.7-12 (1); Lucian, *Alexander the False Prophet* (1); Aristophanes, *Women at the Thesmophoria* 258 (1); Suetonius, *Caligula* 11 (1); Suetonius, *Nero* 26 (1); Suetonius, *Otho* 12 (1); Josephus, *Life of Josephus* 47 (1); Juvenal, *Satires* 6.120-2 (1); Herodian, *History of the Empire* 4.7.3 (1); Aelian, *Historical Miscellany* 1.26 (1); Athenaeus, *Learned Banqueters* 10.415a-b (1); Apuleius, *Metamorphoses* 11.8 (1); Xenophon, *Cyropedia* 1.3.2 (1); Ovid, *Metamorphoses* 14.654-60 (1); Dio Cassius, *Roman History* 80.2 (1); Polybius, *Histories* 3.78 (1); Philostratus, *Epistles* 22 (1); Myrinus, *Greek Anthology* 6.254 (1); Petronius, *Satyricon* 110 (2); Mishnah, Shabbat 6.5 (2)	33
Eyebrows	Petronius, *Satyricon* 110 (2); Martial, *Epigrams* 3.38 (1)	3
Total		**102**

Table 4.2 Nature of prosthesis user, real or imaginary

Body part	*Fact*	*Fiction*	*Hypothetical*	*Total*	*Historical figure*	*Mythological Figure*
Finger						
Hand	1	1	2	4	1	1
Arm	1(?)			1(?)	1(?)	
Shoulder		14		14		14
Toe						
Foot	2	2	1	5	2	
Thigh	9	1		10	8	
Leg	1		6	7	1	
Eye				3		
Nose	1			1	1	
Teeth	6	2	13	21		
Hair	18	10	2	33	12	1
Eyebrow	1	2		3		
Total	39	32	24	**102**		

the ancient Mediterranean. Thus, this data set can be used to elucidate a substantial amount of information about prostheses in classical antiquity, and the ways in which they were viewed in ancient culture and society. This information includes the gender of the prosthesis user (see Table 4.3) and the material from which the prosthesis was made (see Table 4.4), and using it I propose to advance a theoretical taxonomy of ancient prostheses.

Discussion

In the discussion that follows, I am going to focus on a representative selection of six specific examples from these works of ancient literature and demonstrate how they can be used to glean more information about prostheses in the classical world than the simple fact of their existence. I have selected these specific examples for several reasons. First, although they are a combination of factual and fictitious examples, they are to all intents and purposes historical rather than mythological examples (two are factual and involve real historical figures, four may or may not be fictitious, yet are very specifically grounded in space and time). Second, they are relatively detailed regarding the prosthesis, the prosthesis user, and their prosthesis use. Third, they can give insights into the lived experiences of the individuals in question and, by implication, other ancient prosthesis users too. Fourth, they contain enough information to enable us to start to consider ancient prostheses in relation to each other rather than in isolation.

Table 4.3 Gender of prosthesis user (if known)

Body part	*Male user*	*Female user*	*Unspecified*	*Total*
Finger				
Hand	4			4
Arm	1(?)			1(?)
Shoulder	14			14
Toe				
Foot	5			5
Thigh	10			10
Leg	4		3	7
Eye	2	1		3
Nose	1			1
Teeth		18	3	21
Hair	16	17		33
Eyebrow	2	1		3
Total	55	37	3	**102**

Table 4.4 Material of ancient prosthesis (if known, and no bronze or textiles known)

Body part	*Gold*	*Silver*	*Iron*	*Wood*	*Ivory*	*Bone*	*Horn*	*Diamond*	*Malachite*	*Leather*	*Hair*	*Unspecified*	*Total*
Finger													
Hand	1		1		2								4
Arm										1(?)			1(?)
Shoulder					14								14
Toe													
Foot				4								1	5
Thigh	9									1			10
Leg				4								3	7
Eye	1							1	1				3
Nose	1												1
Teeth	8	1				1	1					10	21
Hair										1	4	28	33
Eyebrow												2	3
Total	20	1		8	16	1	1	1	1	3	4	44	102

Case study 1: Hegesistratus of Elis, Marcus Sergius Silus, and Lucian's 'Rich Man'

> Hegesistratus of Elis was his diviner, the most notable of the sons of Tellias. This man had been put in prison and doomed to die by the Spartans for the much harm that he had done them. Being in this evil case, inasmuch as he was in peril of his life and like to be very grievously maltreated ere his death, he did a deed well nigh past believing: being made fast in iron-bound stocks, he got an iron weapon that was brought in some wise into his prison, and straightway conceived a plan of such hardihood as we have never known; reckoning how best the rest of it might get free, he cut off his own foot at the instep. This done, he burrowed through the wall out of the way of the guards that kept ward over him, and so escaped to Tegea; all night he journeyed and all day he hid and lay close in the woods, till on the third night he came to Tegea, while all the people of Lacedaemon sought him; and they were greatly amazed, seeing the half of his foot cut off and lying there, but not being able to find the man himself. Thus did he then escape from the Lacedaemonians and take refuge in Tegea, which at that time was unfriendly to Lacedaemon; and after he was healed and had made himself a foot of wood, he declared himself an open enemy of the Lacedaemonians. Yet the enmity that he bore them brought him no good at the last; for they caught him at his divinations in Zacynthus, and slew him.
>
> Herodotus, *Histories* 9.36–7 (trans. A.D. Godley)

> Nobody, in my judgement at all events, can rightly rank any human being above Marcus Sergius, albeit his great-grandson Catiline diminishes the credit of his name. Sergius in his second campaign lost his right hand; in two campaigns he was wounded twenty-three times, with the result that he was crippled in both hands and both feet, only his spirit being intact; yet although disabled, he served in numerous subsequent campaigns. He was twice taken prisoner by Hannibal (for it was with no ordinary foe that he was engaged), and twice escaped from Hannibal's fetters, although he was kept in chains or shackles on every single day for twenty months. He fought four times with only his left hand, having two horses he was riding stabbed under him. He had a right hand of iron made for him and going into action with it tied to his arm, raised the siege of Cremona, saved Piacenza, captured twelve enemy camps in Gaul: all of which exploits are testified by his speech delivered during his praetorship when his colleagues wanted to debar him from the sacrifices as infirm – a man who with a different foe would have accumulated what piles of wreaths! inasmuch as it makes the greatest difference with what period of history a particular man's valour happens to coincide. What civic wreaths were bestowed by

> Trebbia or Ticino or Trasimeno? What crown was won at Cannae, where successful flight was valour's highest exploit? All other victors truly have conquered men, but Sergius vanquished fortune also.
>
> Pliny the Elder, *Natural History* 7.29 (trans. H. Rackham)

> Not long ago there was a rich man in Asia, both of whose feet had been amputated in consequence of an accident; they were frozen, I gather, when he had to make a journey through snow. Well, this of course was pitiable, and to remedy the mischance he had had wooden feet made for him, which he used to lace on, and in that way made shift to walk, leaning upon his servants as he did so. But he did one thing that was ridiculous: he used always to buy very handsome sandals of the latest cut and went to the utmost trouble in regard to them, in order that his timber toes might be adorned with the most beautiful footwear! Now are not you doing just the same thing? Is it not true that although you have a crippled, fig-wood understanding, you are buying gilt buskins which even a normal man could hardly get about in?
>
> Lucian, *The Ignorant Book-Collector* 6 (trans. A.M. Harmon)

Hegesistratus of Elis and Marcus Sergius Silus were, as far as we can tell, real historical figures, whereas Lucian's rich man is likely a fictional character created by Lucian to make his point, although aspects of his portrayal may have been based upon one or more real individuals that Lucian had encountered in the mid to late second century CE. The story of Hegesistratus of Elis comes from Herodotus's *Histories* and can be dated to 479 BCE, but it seems to have been reasonably well known as, over five centuries later, Plutarch refers to it (Plutarch, *Moralia: On Brotherly Love* 3.1). The story of Marcus Sergius Silus is only known from this entry in Book 7 of Pliny the Elder's *Natural History*, in which he is presented as an example to follow and a paragon of virtue (Beagon 2002, 2005, 293–8). Its basic tenets are, however, supported by a reference to his quaestorship by Livy, which can be dated to 197 BCE, and a coin issued by one of his descendants, who bore the same name, in either 116 or 115 BCE that depicts him on horseback holding his sword and the severed head of an defeated enemy in his left hand rather than his right (Livy 32. 27.7; 32. 31.6; 33. 21.9; 33. 24.4; Crawford 1976, 286/1).

It would appear that both Hegesistratus of Elis and Marcus Sergius Silus conform to the 'super crip' stereotype, the 'super crip' being an impaired person who:

> triumph[s] over the tragedy of their condition … who, through astounding personal endeavour overcomes their disability … dramatically, this image is useful to script writers for whom a disabled person's triumph over their impairment is a metaphor for the more general human struggle to overcome life's obstacles.
>
> Harnett (2000, 21; however, see also Schalk 2016)

Other individuals from the classical world can be said to conform to this 'supercrip' stereotype too (Garland 1995 [2010], 31–2). They triumph over several different types of adversity: first, the actual loss of their extremities; second, their imprisonment by their enemies; third, in the case of Marcus Sergius Silus, attempts made by his peers to marginalise him because of his impairment (Beagon 2002). Thus, both could be said to be setting positive examples and potential sources of inspiration for amputees regarding the possibilities of prostheses – the ancient equivalent of the contemporary 'inspiration porn' (Grue 2016). Additionally, for those aware of both of these individuals, the rich man, or any real individual that resembled him, would be compared with them and found wanting in the way that they used their prostheses (both human and extremity). Elsewhere, Dio Chrysostom, writing in the late first century CE, makes the point that, 'as if there were any use in a man having a golden or ivory hand or eyes of diamond or malachite; but the kind of soul he had men did not notice', so perhaps we can take from this that there was a tendency for some individuals to use overly elaborate prostheses, or to make their usage performative, much to the chagrin of onlookers (Dio Chrysostom, *Eighth Discourse: On Virtue* 28, trans. J.W. Cohoon).

Also, notable here is the role that other people played in the daily life of an amputee. The rich man requires the assistance of other people, the enslaved members of his household, to assist him in using his wooden feet to restore his physical mobility, and so we might consider such individuals 'human prostheses' (van Schaik 2019; see Blake 2012, 2016 on the role that the enslaved played in the lives of their enslavers generally). It is likely that Marcus Sergius Silus also utilised the enslaved, and that they assisted him in arming himself and helping him on to his horse, at the very least. Animals of various sorts seem to have been utilised as assistants as well (Draycott, in preparation).

Finally, although certain aspects of these ancient literary accounts might seem highly questionable, there is archaeological and bioarchaeological evidence that supports all three. Regarding the use of wooden feet in classical antiquity, a wooden prosthetic toe, the 'Cairo Toe', from Egypt has been dated to either the 21st or 22nd Dynasty (circa 1065–740 BCE; Finch 2019). Regarding the feasibility of using a prosthetic hand in a historical battle, a weaponised prosthetic hand with a knife attachment from Italy has been dated to the period of the sixth to the eighth centuries CE (Micarelli et al. 2018), and this perhaps offered its wearer a degree of functional advantage in certain situations, such as physical combat.

Case study 2: Galla, Statyllius, and Giton

> You are at home yourself, Galla, but you are made up in the middle of Subura. Your hair is manufactured in your absence. You lay your teeth aside at night as you do your silks, and lie stored in a hundred caskets.

> Your face does not sleep with you. Yet you ogle with an eyebrow that is brought out for you every morning and have no respect for your hoary cunt, which you can now number among your ancestors. However, you promise the earth; but my cock is deaf, and though it be one-eyed, it sees you.
>
> Martial, *Epigrams* 9.38 (trans. D. Shackleton Bailey)

> When Time was about to drag down to Hades pathic Statyllius, the effeminate old stump of Aphrodite, he dedicated in the porch of Priapus his light summer dresses dyed in scarlet and crimson, his false hair greasy with spikenard, his white shoes that shone on his shapely ankles, the chest in which reposed his bombasine frippery, and his flute that breathed sweet music in the revels of the harlot tribe.
>
> Myrinus, *Greek Anthology* 6.254 (trans. W.R. Paton and M.A. Tueller)

> One of Tryphaena's maids took Giton below decks, and ornamented the boy's head with some of her mistress's clustered curls. Further, she also took some eyebrows out of a box, and by cunningly following the lines where he was defaced she restored his proper beauty complete. Tryphaena recognized the true Giton, there was a storm of tears, and she then for the first time gave the boy a kiss with real affection. Of course, I was glad to see him clothed again in his former loveliness, but still I kept hiding my own face continually, for I realized that I was marked with no common ugliness, since not even Lichas considered me fit to speak to. But the same maid came and rescued me from gloom, called me aside, and decked me with equally becoming curls. Indeed, my face shone with a greater glory. My curls were golden!
>
> Petronius, *Satyricon* 110 (trans. M. Heseltine, W.H.D. Rouse, and E.H. Warmington)

It is possible that Gallus and Statyllius were real historical figures whose likenesses were captured in Martial's and Myrinus's satirical epigrams during the late first century CE, whereas Giton and Encolpius are both characters in Petronius's satirical novel *Satyricon*, which dates to the middle of the first century CE. In all three examples, we see individuals, both male and female, wearing wigs, and this seems to have been reflective of a reality in which both men and women wore wigs and hair pieces in ancient Roman society (Draycott 2019b). However, the differences in the ways that works of ancient literature describe men and women wearing wigs and hair pieces are clear. Most men described as wearing wigs do so in order to disguise themselves, usually before doing something nefarious, with only a few described as wearing wigs to cover a deficiency such as premature or temporary hair loss (wigs used as disguise: Ovid, *Metamorphoses* 14.654–60; Suetonius, *Caligula* 11; Suetonius, *Nero* 26; Josephus, *Life of Josephus* 47; Dio Cassius, *Roman History* 80.2; Polybius,

Histories 3.78. Wigs used to cover hair loss: Suetonius, *Otho* 12; Martial, *Epigrams* 12.45; Avienus, *Fables* 11.7–12).

With women, the situation is reversed (wigs used to cover hair loss: Horace, *Satires* 1.8.47–50; Martial, *Epigrams* 6.12, 9.38, 12.23; Macedonius the Consul, *Greek Anthology* 11.374; Lucillius, *Greek Anthology* 11.68, 11.310; Lucian, *Dialogues of the Courtesans* 11.4; wigs used as disguise: Juvenal, *Satires* 6.120–2). The criticisms Martial directs at Galla are typical, and there are traces of these in Myrinus's account of Statyllius, whom he describes as effeminate, too: prosthetic hair is inherently false, and its usage is designed to deceive; it is viewed as a type of luxury like silk and perfume; it is essentially a type of cosmetic. In Petronius's *Satyricon*, we see prosthetic hair and eyebrows belonging to a woman repurposed by two men, and presumably this idea of two men wearing prosthetic hair in a feminine hairstyle was intended to be comedic, part of the joke being that the men themselves did not understand this.

Just as Lucian's rich man required the assistance of enslaved individuals to use his prosthetic feet effectively, so too do Giton and Encolpius require the assistance of an enslaved individual to apply their prosthetic hair and eyebrows effectively, and there are numerous ancient literary references to and artistic depictions of attendants dressing their mistress's hair.

There is also archaeological and bioarchaeological evidence that supports all three literary accounts, as numerous examples of wigs and hair pieces have been recovered from tombs and graves dating to the Roman period from sites around the empire (Draycott 2019b). These range from hair extensions in the form of braids that could be used to supplement existing hair and elaborate upon hair styles to full wigs (for braids, see discoveries from France and Britain, at Audollent 1921, 163; 1923, 311–2, pl. 8, nn. 3–6; Wood 1883, 108; Black 1986, 225; for a full wig that was found in conjunction with a gold hair net and belonged to a woman named Aebutia Quarta, see Legrottaglie 2005 and Benecchi 2005).

Gender

As we have seen in Table 4.3, both men and women are presented as having used prostheses in classical literature. However, there are significant differences not only in the types of prosthesis that they are presented as using, but also in the ways in which these stories are told. Broadly speaking, there are significantly more examples of men using prostheses than women. Why might this be? Is it simply a result of the generally gendered nature of ancient literary sources? Very possibly, for, although it is notable that the references are found in both prose and poetry across a range of genres, certain types of reference are found in specific genres. The references to men using prostheses are found in all literary genres, whereas the references to women using prostheses are concentrated in satirical poetry and prose such as the works of Horace, Juvenal, Martial, Lucillius, Mardonius, and Lucian.[3]

Men are presented as using extremity prostheses (feet, legs, hands), whereas women are presented as using facial prostheses (teeth, hair). Is this indicative of a reality in which men were more likely to lose limbs, and women were more likely to lose facial features? This is possible, as ancient literature attests that there was a considerable range of ways in which an individual could lose a body part. An individual might be born without a body part: phocomelia, the absence of the proximal part of a limb which causes the hands or feet to be directly attached to the torso; meromelia, the congenital absence of specific parts of a limb; hemimelia, the partial absence of terminal parts of the limb; or amelia, the complete absence of the limb. However, this congenital absence of a body part is extremely rare, and relatively few examples survive in the skeletal record from any period of history (Mann, Thomas and Adams 1998, 295). Much more common was an individual experiencing the loss of a body part during life, and this acquired loss of a body part could occur through a variety of different circumstances: traumatic amputation, surgical amputation, martial amputation, judicial amputation, extra-judicial amputation, self-mutilation or mutilation, and the natural ageing process (Draycott, in preparation).

Although, realistically, it is likely that both genders could lose any number of body parts in any number of ways, in literature we do seem to see a focus on men losing their body parts through military or agricultural activity, and women losing their body parts through mutilation or ageing. For men undertaking military activity, the loss of the right hand (the sword hand) and one or both eyes (owing to lack of appropriate protective gear) seems to have been particularly common, whereas, for men undertaking agricultural activity, the feet or legs were at risk from accidents with agricultural tools or bites from venomous creatures.[4] Women seem to have been at risk from facial mutilation that occurred as the result of interpersonal violence and was carried out so as to purposefully spoil their beauty and so make them less attractive to men and, therefore, less valuable, and the natural female ageing process that resulted in the loss of teeth and hair receives much more commentary from ancient writers than the male one, again because of the effect that this had on a woman's beauty, her attractiveness to men, and her intrinsic value.[5] In ancient Jewish literature, facial prostheses are recommended specifically to restore a woman's physical attractiveness and make her a more desirable potential bride (Palestinian Talmud, tractate Nedarim 9.41c; Babylonian Talmud, Nedarim 66b; for discussion, see Lehmhaus 2019, 112–3). But perhaps there was some sort of visible imbalance in ancient society, and this fed into existing stereotypes and bolstered them.

Archaeological and bioarchaeological evidence supports these demarcations. Of the extremity prostheses that have survived from classical antiquity, all those found in situ were found in the tombs and graves of men. These include the third-century BCE 'Capua Limb' and the sixth-century CE 'Hemmaberg Limb'. Of the facial prostheses that have survived from classical antiquity, all of those found in situ were found in the tombs and graves of women, and the size of those that are unprovenanced indicates that they belonged to women too (Becker and Turfa 2017, 113–4).

Material

As we have seen in Table 4.4, the materials utilised to make prostheses varied considerably and included gold, silver, iron, wood, ivory, bone, horn, diamond, malachite, leather, hair, and other types of textile such as linen and plant fibres. Thus, it is not surprising that the technical sophistication and complexity of prostheses should vary too. After all, a prosthesis composed of one material only required one type of artisan, yet a prosthesis composed of two or more types of material required multiple artisans working in collaboration at all stages of the manufacturing process, and so was exponentially more complicated. Why are the literary references so variable, and did this reflect reality? Were some prostheses simple and others complex, and, if so, why? Possibly, it was simply a matter of utilising whatever material one had to hand, and some materials were considered more suitable to certain types of prosthesis than others. The wealthy elite may have been more likely to invest in a technically sophisticated and complex prosthesis, but, if so, why? Possibilities include practicality and usability.

Contemporary prostheses can be problematic for their users, and it is debatable how practical or usable any ancient prosthesis was. We need to consider what a prosthetic limb could offer its user that an alternative type of assistive technology such as a staff, a walking stick, or a crutch could not (Draycott, in preparation 2021). Perhaps we should consider prostheses as 'bodywear' and include them in our discussions of dress and clothing, imagining wealthy and high-status individuals using their prostheses to make specific statements about themselves, just as individuals in subsequent periods of history have done. The ancient Jewish religious teachings debate whether a prosthetic leg or foot should be considered a shoe or a tool, and individual rabbis have different opinions on this. If one's prosthetic leg or foot was classed as a shoe, it did not affect their ability to access the temple or even leave their house on the Shabbat, but, if one's prosthetic leg or foot was classed as a tool, one was subject to the same restrictions about using it as any other piece of equipment, no matter how crucial it was to one's day-to-day life. It would certainly appear that wigs, hair pieces, eyebrows, and teeth were considered to be cosmetic and, as a result, part of the broader category of dress and clothing and, on occasion, even costume. Thus, we can see how, like expensive and beautiful jewellery, for example, a prosthesis might be utilised by its wearer as a means of communicating not just wealth, status, and prestige, but also good taste and even fashion sense, just as bespoke prostheses, such as the ones created by companies such as the Alternative Limb Project, do today.

It should be noted that a number of ancient literary references to prostheses state that the individual acquired their prosthesis 'themselves', and so we can infer that some individuals made their own prostheses, and, presumably, these were absolutely reflective of that individual's taste, but it is important to bear in mind that the process of designing, commissioning, and manufacturing any object is frequently elided in ancient literature. Something that is apparent in the discussions of prosthetic teeth and hair that is not mentioned in discussions of other types is the frequency with which these items are purchased; apparently, in the city of Rome, wigs could be purchased near the Porticus Philippi, in front of the temple of Hercules and the Muses (Ovid, *Art of Love* 3.167–8). This implies that there was enough trade in prosthetic teeth and hair, at least, to allow makers to specialise and potentially even provide ready-made versions rather than made-to-measure ones.

Again, archaeological and bioarchaeological evidence supports these demarcations. Judging from the other grave goods found in the inhumations, cremations, and mummifications that contain prostheses, sophisticated prostheses have been found in the tombs and graves of high-status individuals, both male and female. But it needs to be borne in mind that metal survives where organic materials such as wood and leather do not, and the prostheses of the poor were not necessarily any less technically sophisticated, for all that they may have been made from less prestigious materials (Li et al. 2013).

The most commonly cited material used in the production of prostheses is gold, and there are several reasons why this might have been the case. Gold is, thanks to its colour and shine, instantly recognisable and an indicator of wealth, status, prestige, and luxury. Thus, for members of the social elite, it would be a suitable material for a prosthesis, particularly one that was small yet highly visible, such as an eye, a nose, or a tooth.[6] In turn, individuals who were elite in some way, or who wished to be perceived to be elite in some way, such as Pythagoras and his imitator Alexander the False Prophet, might be expected to have a golden prosthesis as an indicator of that special quality that set them apart from others. There are also practical reasons why gold was a suitable choice for prostheses, particularly those that came into contact with the interior of the body such as the eye socket or the mouth, and that is its purity and resultant harmlessness (Becker and Turfa 2017, 101). It is also a malleable metal, which would make beating or engraving it relatively easy and straightforward.

Also commonly cited are ivory, bone, and horn, and these were likely used in the production of prostheses for similar reasons to gold. There was a mythological antecedent in the tale of Pelops and his ivory shoulder, and so ivory had divine connotations, and, as it was most often associated with foreign creatures such as elephants, it was itself seen as exotic and luxurious and was imported from far-away territories such as Africa and India. Thus, it was a prestige material, and this status is reflected in its use for cult objects such as chryselephantine statues. However, like gold, ivory's qualities also made it suitable for prostheses, particularly false teeth. It came in the right sorts of size and shape, it had the right sort of appearance, and it could be worked with relative ease. However, an additional aspect of using materials such as ivory, bone, and horn to consider is that, unlike metals, they had once belonged to living creatures. In the case of dental appliances, an individual might utilise their own extracted teeth, but, if the reason that their teeth had been extracted in the first place was that they were in some way damaged or defective, as the discarded teeth found during archaeological excavation of facilities such as ancient dental surgeries and bath-houses tend to be (Becker 2014), they would need to repurpose someone or something else's. For example, one ancient Etruscan dental appliance incorporates an animal rather than a human tooth (Becker and Turfa 2017, 110, 209).

What might these teeth, tusks, bones, or horns have signified not only to their users, but also to others who witnessed them being used in this way? What qualities might they have been thought to impart? For example, the user may have been considered, for better or for worse, a human–animal hybrid (Hughes 2010). By way of comparison, one ancient prosthetic leg recently recovered from a grave at Turfan in China (c.300–200 BCE), makes its hybridity explicit. It was made from leather, sheep or goat horn, and the hoof of either a horse or an Asiatic ass. It consisted of a plate that was fastened to the left thigh by leather straps and tapered into a peg-leg (Li et al. 2013, 339). No attempt was made to carve the peg-leg to resemble the human limb that it was supplementing; on the contrary, the peg-leg terminated in a hoof, which may, in fact, have rendered the prosthesis easier to use. The materials and form of the prosthesis can be seen as entirely practical, even utilitarian, a means of stabilising its user as he moved around. But it is also possible that this choice of an animalistic rather than humanoid limb was influenced by his Subeixi culture's interaction with the Pazyryk culture of the Scythian communities in the nearby Altai mountains. There is no evidence that any Greek or Roman prosthesis user was inspired to model their prosthesis after an animal this explicitly, but they may have done so implicitly, by exercising their ability to choose materials for their own specific reasons. Alternatively, they may simply have considered using animal products in their prostheses as being akin to using animal products in their cosmetics, jewellery, or clothing, which brings us back to the idea of prostheses as 'bodywear'.

Although not very many of the ancient literary references to prosthetic hair specifically state that these items were made from human hair, other literary evidence for the hair trade in classical antiquity and archaeological evidence in the form of wigs and hair pieces indicate that this was, in fact, the case. Again, the reasoning that lay behind this was likely owing to the nature of the material itself. As human hair comes in a variety of colours and textures, one can choose: it would appear that blonde hair was particularly popular in imperial Rome, for example (Ovid, *Amores* 1.14.45–6, *Art of Love* 3.163–8, 3.242–50; Martial, *Epigrams* 14.26 refers to 'Teutonic locks' (*teutonicos capillos*); Draycott 2019b). Although wigs and hair pieces made from other types of textile such as leather and plant fibres are attested, these would have been in one fixed style. Wigs and hair pieces made from human hair, on the other hand, had the advantage of being able to be arranged into different styles.

Finally, it is perhaps surprising that so few ancient literary references are to prostheses made of wood, especially considering the archaeological evidence not just from classical antiquity, but from all historical periods up to the twentieth century, indicates that that was the material most commonly utilised for them, particularly extremity prostheses. The ancient references that refer to wooden prostheses – notably legs and feet rather than arms and hands – align with this. Possibly, wood was the material most commonly used for such prostheses, just as it was used for other types of assistive technology, such as staffs, sticks, canes, and crutches; being so common, it did not necessarily rate a mention, unlike the more unusual gold or ivory. After all, with the exception of certain types of rare imported wood such as ebony or citrus, wood was not a prestigious material in the ancient Mediterranean: in the only instance in which the type of wood used for a prosthesis is specified, the wood is olive, which was readily available and a popular material for tools. Wood would have been a good choice of material for an ancient prosthesis: it is readily accessible in most places, as a result of which it is cheap or perhaps even free to acquire, it is relatively easy to work even for someone with rudimentary carpentry skills, and it is strong enough to bear the weight of the prosthesis user while being lighter and more manoeuvrable than metal. Associated with this is another possible explanation, which is related to the users of wooden prostheses. Individuals situated lower down the social hierarchy, with less recourse to expensive and luxurious materials from which to fashion prestigious statement prostheses, were much less likely to rate a mention by the sorts of ancient author who record cases of prosthesis use – after all, in a society where impairment and disability were common, what was noteworthy about an ordinary person using an ordinary prosthesis?

Conclusion

It is clear from the literary, documentary, archaeological, and bioarchaeological evidence that classical prostheses were, if not rare, certainly uncommon. More significantly, it is clear that they were not standardised, even those that sought to replace the same parts of the body, such as the 'Greville Chester Toe' and the 'Cairo Toe', and the 'Capua Limb' and the 'Hemmaberg Limb'. This is to be expected in items that were, in all likelihood, designed, commissioned, and manufactured entirely at an individual's direction and discretion. Yet there does seem to have been some sort of consensus, at least in the literature that survives, regarding the relative merits of different types of prosthesis in ancient society and culture, and this literature allows a partial reconstruction of a taxonomy and a tentative reconstruction of the lived experience of the classical prosthesis user.

Extremity prostheses seem to have been viewed relatively positively, at least in situations where it is clear that they were being utilised as necessities rather than luxuries. They were practical, useful, they empowered their users and facilitated their return to some semblance of normality. There are broad similarities with the way that extremity prostheses were used by veterans in the US Civil War, and the First and Second World Wars, although the restorative effects of these on the individuals themselves and on their societies more broadly were made much more explicit in the way that the prostheses were marketed and advertised (Figg and Farrell-Beck 1993; Hermes 2002; Neumann 2010; Hasegawa 2012). However, facial prostheses seem to have been viewed relatively negatively. Although they may have been, in reality, just as practical, useful, and empowering for their users as extremity prostheses were for theirs, they were dismissed by the individuals writing about them as ridiculous, vainglorious, and fundamentally dishonest and deceptive in a way that extremity prostheses were not. They seem to have been classed as a type of cosmetic rather than a type of assistive technology.

Why the difference? It is possible that these differences are due to the nature of the surviving evidence, coupled with the fact that the individuals recording these examples for posterity were working within pre-existing literary traditions and conventions. However, we should also consider the nature of the prostheses themselves: no matter how technologically sophisticated they could be, an extremity prosthesis was unlikely to be mistaken for the limb that it sought to replace, whereas prosthetic teeth and hair feasibly could be, or at least that seems to be the fear that is expressed by ancient authors in their writings. This leads us to wonder what the purpose of a prosthesis in the classical world was, and how far it differed from the purpose (or purposes) of a prosthesis in the contemporary world. There is far more evidence of all kinds for individuals using other forms of assistive technology that would have been potentially much more effective than a prosthesis to compensate for some sort of physical deficiency, and so prosthesis use was a deliberate and definitive choice, the motivations for which are up to us to continue to try and interpret.

Notes

1 For the conference, see Wellcome Trust Small Grant 108557/Z/15/Z.
2 Ian Massey of the NHS Wales Artificial Limb and Appliance Service.
3 Horace, *Satires* 1.8.47–50; Juvenal, *Satires* 6.120–2; Martial, *Epigrams* 1.72, 5.43, 9.38, 12.23, 12.45, 14.56; Lucillius, *Greek Anthology* 11.68, 11.310; Macedonius, *Greek Anthology* 11.374; Lucian, *Professor of Public Speaking* 24.
4 Loss of the right hand in the course of military activity: Pliny the Elder, *Natural History* 7.29; Plutarch, *Camillus* 142; Lucian, *Friendship* 10, 62; Ammianus Marcellinus, *Roman History* 17.10; Nonnus, *Dionysiaca* 2.427–35, 22.196–202. Loss of one or both eyes through military activity: Dionysius of Halicarnassus, *Roman Antiquities* 5.23.2–25; Plutarch, *Sertorius* 4.2; Caesar, *Civil Wars* 3.53.4; Suetonius, *Caesar* 68.4; Lucan, *Pharsalia* 6.213–6. Loss of the foot or the leg through agricultural activity: Erycius, *Greek Anthology* 9.233.
5 Loss of facial features through mutilation: Plautus, *Pot of Gold* 188–9; Diodorus Siculus, *Library of History* 1.78.4–5; Hermesianax, *Fragments* (*Leontion*) 2.4. Loss of teeth and hair through the natural aging process: Cokayne 2003; Parkin 2003.

6 *Laws of the Twelve Tables* 10.8–9; Hippocratic Corpus, *Joints* 33.9–10; Celsus, *On Medicine* 6.12; Lucian, *The Professor of Public Speaking* 24; Palestinian Talmud, Shabbat 6.5; Babylonian Talmud, Shabbat 65a; Palestinian Talmud, Yerushalmi Nedarim 9.8, 41c; Babylonian Talmud, Nedarim 66a–b.

References

Audollent, Auguste (1921) 'Les tombes des Martres-de-Veryre.' *Man* 21, 161–4.

Audollent, Auguste (1923) 'Les tombes gallo-romaines à inhumation des Martres-de-Veyre (Puy-de-Dôme).' *Mémoires présentés par divers savants à l'Académie des inscriptions et belles-lettres* 13, 275–328.

Beagon, Mary (2002) 'Beyond comparison: M. Sergius Silus, Fortunae Victor.' In Gillian Clark and Tessa Rajak (eds), *Philosophy and Power in the Graeco-Roman World. Essays in Honour of Miriam Griffin.* Oxford: Oxford University Press, 111–32.

Beagon, Mary (2005) *The Elder Pliny on the Human Animal: Natural History Book 7.* Oxford: Clarendon Press.

Becker, Marshall J. (2014) 'Dentistry in ancient Rome: direct evidence based on teeth from excavations at the Temple of Castor and Pollux in the Roman Forum.' *International Journal of Anthropology* 29(4), 209–20.

Becker, Marshall J. and Jean M. Turfa (2017) *The Etruscans and the History of Dentistry: The Golden Smile through the Ages.* London: Routledge.

Benecchi, Francesca (2005) 'Il reticulum.' In Maria P. Rossignani, Marco Sannazaro and Giuseppina Legrottaglie (eds), *La Signora del sarcofago: una sepoltura di rango nella necropoli dell'Università cattolica: ricerche archeologiche nei cortili dell'Università Cattolica.* Milan: Vita e pensiero, 103–16.

Biddiss, Elaine A. and Tom T. Chau (2009) 'Upper limb prosthesis use and abandonment: a survey of the last 25 years.' *Prosthetics and Orthotics International* 31(3), 236–57.

Black, E.W. (1986) 'Romano-British burial customs and religious beliefs in South East England.' *Archaeological Journal* 143, 201–39.

Blake, Sarah (2012) 'Now you see them: slaves and other objects as elements of the Roman master.' *Helios* 39(2), 193–211.

Blake, Sarah (2016) 'In manus: Pliny's Letters and the arts of mastery.' In A. Keith and J. Edmondson (eds), *Roman Literary Cultures: Domestic Politics, Revolutionary Poetics, Civic Spectacle.* Toronto: University of Toronto Press, 89–101.

Bliquez, Lawrence J. (1983) 'Classical prosthetics.' *Archaeology* September/October36, 25–9.

Bliquez, Lawrence J. (1996) 'Prosthetics in classical Antiquity: Greek, Etruscan, and Roman prosthetics.' *Aufstieg und Niedergang der römischen Welt II* 37(3), 2640–76.

Breitwieser, Rupert (ed.) (2012) *Behinderungen und Beeinträchtigungen/Disability and Impairment in Antiquity.* Oxford: Archaeopress.

Cokayne, Karen (2003) *Experiencing Old Age in Ancient Rome.* London: Routledge.

Collard, Franck and Evelyne Samama (eds) (2010) *Handicaps et sociétés dans l'histoire: L'estropié, l'aveugle et le paralytique de l'Antiquité aux temps modernes.* Paris: L'Harmattan.

Crawford, Michael H. (1976) *Roman Republican Coinage.* Cambridge: Cambridge University Press.

Davis, Lennard (2013) *The End of Normal: Identity in a Biocultural Era.* Ann Arbor, MI: University of Michigan Press.

Draycott, Jane (ed.) (2019a) *Prostheses in Antiquity*. London: Routledge.

Draycott, Jane (2019b) 'Prosthetic hair in ancient Rome.' In Jane Draycott (ed.), *Prostheses in Antiquity*. London: Routledge, 71–96.

Draycott, Jane (in preparation 2021) 'Staff or stick? Cane or crutch? Mobility aids in ancient Greece and Rome.' In Isabella Bonati (ed.), *Words of Medicine: Technical Terminology in Material and Textual Evidence from the Graeco-Roman World*. Berlin: De Gruyter.

Draycott, Jane (in preparation) *Prosthetics and Assistive Technology in Ancient Greece and Rome*.

Figg, Laurann and Jane Farrell-Beck (1993) 'Amputation in the Civil War: physical and social dimensions.' *Journal of the History of Medicine and the Allied Sciences* 48, 454–75.

Finch, Jacky (2019) 'The complex aspects of experimental archaeology: the design of working dodels of two ancient Egyptian great toe prostheses.' In Jane Draycott (ed.), *Prostheses in Antiquity*. London: Routledge, 29–48.

Gallagher, Pamela, Deirdre Desmond and Malcolm MacLachlan (eds) (2008) *Psychoprosthetics*. London: Springer-Verlag.

Garland, Robert (1995, 2010) *The Eye of the Beholder: Deformity and Disability in the Graeco-Roman World*. London: Bristol Classical Press.

Grue, Jan (2016) 'The problem with inspiration porn: a tentative definition and a provisional critique.' *Disability & Society* 31(6), 838–49.

Harnett, Alison (2000) 'Escaping the 'evil avenger' and the 'supercrip': images of disability in popular television.' *Irish Communications Review* 8, 21–9.

Hasegawa, Guy R. (2012) *Mending Broken Soldiers: The Union and Confederate Programs to Supply Artificial Limbs*. Carbondale and Edwardsville, IL: Southern Illinois University Press.

Hermes, Lisa (2002) 'Military lower extremity amputee rehabilitation.' *Physical Medicine and Rehabilitation Clinics of North America* 13, 45–66.

Hughes, Jessica (2010) 'Dissecting the classical hybrid.' In Katharina Rebay-Salisbury, Marie Louise Stig Sørensen and Jessica Hughes (eds), *Body Parts and Bodies Whole: Changing Relations and Meanings*. Oxford: Oxbow, 101–10.

Jones, Claire L. (ed.) (2017) *Rethinking Modern Prostheses in Anglo-American Commodity Cultures, 1820–1939*. Manchester: Manchester University Press.

Krötzl, Christian, Katariina Mustakallio and Jenni Kuuliala (eds) (2015) *Infirmity in Antiquity and the Middle Ages: Social and Cultural Approaches to Health, Weakness and Care*. Farnham: Ashgate.

Kwass, Michael (2006) 'Big hair: a wig history of consumption in eighteenth century France.' *American Historical Review* 111(3), 631–59.

Laes, Christian (2014) *Bepurkt? Gehandicapten in het Romeinse rijk*. Leuven: Davisfonds.

Laes, Christian (ed.) (2017) *Disability in Antiquity*. London: Routledge.

Laes, Christian (2018) *Disabilities and the Disabled in the Roman World: A Social and Cultural History*. Cambridge: Cambridge University Press.

Laes, Christian, Chris Goodey and Martha Rose (eds) (2013) *Disabilities in Roman Antiquity: Disparate Bodies* a Capite ad Calcem. Leiden: Brill.

Legrottaglie, Giuseppina (2005) 'Considerazioni sulla pettinatura.' In Maria P. Rossignani, Marco Sannazaro and Giuseppina Legrottaglie (eds) *La Signora del sarcofago:*

una sepoltura di rango nella necropoli dell'Università cattolica: ricerche archeologiche nei cortili dell'Università Cattolica. Milan: Vita e pensiero, 97–102.

Lehmhaus, Lennart (2019) '"An amputee may go out with his wooden aid on the Shabbat": dynamics of prosthesis discourse in Talmudic traditions.' In Jane Draycott (ed.), *Prostheses in Antiquity*. London: Routledge, 97–124.

Li, Xiao, Mayke Wagner, Xiaohong Wu, Pavel Tarasov, Yongbin Zhang, Arno Schmidt, Tomasz Goslar and Julia Gresky (2013) 'Archaeological and palaeopathological study on the Third/Second Century BC grave from Turfan, China: individual health history and regional implications.' *Quaternary International* 290–1, 335–43.

Mann, Robert W., Michael D. Thomas and Bradley J. Adams (1998) 'Congenital absence of the ulna with humeroradial synostosis in a prehistoric skeleton from Moundville, Alabama.' *International Journal of Osteoarchaeology* 8, 295–9.

Micarelli, Ileana, Robert Paine, Caterina Giostra, Mary Anne Tafuri, Antonio Profico, Marco Boggioni, Fabio Di Vincenzo, Danilo Massani, Andrea Papini and Giorgio Manzi (2018) 'Survival to amputation in pre-antibiotic era: a case study from a Longobard Necropolis (6th–8th centuries AD).' *Journal of Anthropological Sciences* 96, 1–16.

Mills, Frederick B. (2013) 'A phenomenological approach to psychoprosthetics.' *Disability and Rehabilitation* 35, 785–91.

Murray, Craig D. (2005) 'The social meanings of prosthesis use.' *Journal of Health Psychology* 10(3), 425–41.

Murray, Craig D. (2008) 'Embodiment and prosthesis use.' In Pamela Gallagher, Deirdre Desmond and Malcolm MacLachlan (eds) *Psychoprosthetics*. London: Springer-Verlag, 119–29.

Murray, Craig D. and J. Fox (2002) 'Body image and prosthesis satisfaction in the lower limb amputee.' *Disability and Rehabilitation* 24(17), 925–31.

Neumann, Boaz (2010) 'Being prosthetic in the First World War and Weimar Germany.' *Body & Society* 16(3), 93–126.

Ott, Katherine, David Serlin and Stephen Mihm (eds) (2002) *Artificial Parts, Practical Lives: Modern Histories of Prosthetics*. New York: New York University Press.

Parkin, Tim (2003) *Old Age in Ancient Rome: A Social and Cultural History*. Baltimore, ML: Johns Hopkins University Press.

Pezzin, Liliana E., Timothy R. Dillingham, Ellen J. MacKenzie, Patti Ephraim and Paddy Rossbach (2004) 'Use and satisfaction with prosthetic limb devices and related services.' *Archives of Physical Medicine and Rehabilitation* 85(5), 723–9.

Porter, Chloe, Katie L. Walter and Margaret Healy (2017) *Prosthesis in Medieval and Early Modern Culture*. London: Routledge.

Rose, Martha (2003, 2013) *The Staff of Oedipus: Transforming Disability in Ancient Greece*. Ann Arbor, MI: University of Michigan Press.

Schalk, Sami (2016) 'Re-evaluating the supercrip.' *Journal of Literary and Cultural Disability Studies* 10(1), 71–86.

Smith, Marquard and Joanne Morra (eds) (2006) *The Prosthetic Impulse: From a Posthuman Present to a Biocultural Future*. Cambridge, MA: MIT Press.

van Schaik, Katherine (2019) 'Living prostheses.' In Jane Draycott (ed.), *Prostheses in Antiquity*. London: Routledge, 140–58.

Wills, David (1995) *Prosthesis*. Stanford, CA: Stanford University Press.

Withey, Alun (2016) *Technology, Self-Fashioning and Politeness in Eighteenth Century Britain: Refined Bodies*. London: Palgrave Macmillan.

Wondergem, Marloes, George Lieben, Shirley Brouman, Michiel W.M. van den Brekel and Peter J.F.M. Lohouis (2016) 'Patients' satisfaction with facial prostheses.' *British Journal of Oral and Maxillofacial Surgery* 54(4), 394–9.

Wood, Humprey (1883) 'Roman urns found near Rainham Creek, on the Medway.' *Archaeologica Cantiana* 15, 108–10.

Chapter 5

Displaying the forgotten other in museums

Prostheses at National Museums Scotland

Sophie Goggins

Abstract

This chapter explores the challenges and opportunities in portraying disability, specifically prosthetics, in a museum context. It presents some of the concerns that curators face in displaying such personal objects, particularly the absence of the user's voice and agency. At times, this exclusion is deliberate; at others, the archival context has been lost. Instead, collectors and donors have lent their name to the object, a process that leans towards the medical model approach to disability. Having presented some examples of exhibitions that have showcased prosthetics, this chapter focuses on the permanent collection at National Museums Scotland.

Inclusion and exclusion of voices

In the past, the inclusion of the voices and experiences of people living with a disability has been sparse in museum collections, permanent galleries and exhibitions (Sandell et al. 2005). This is owing to either intentional exclusion, by choosing not to tell the stories of those living with a disability or acquire objects that represent their stories, or unintentional exclusion, where the information necessary to tell those stories is lacking or separated from objects in collections.

Medical content in museums is often perceived as difficult to exhibit for both the public and museum staff. For the public, objects can be seen as off-putting, or the technology behind the objects can be hard to understand. Museums are aware that visitors may see a medical object behind the glass that they have used either for themselves or a loved one, eliciting a negative emotional response (Bonnell and Simon 2007). Museums are aware that there are many ethical issues concerning informed consent when displaying medical objects, particularly photographs.

This presents an uncomfortable question for museums and curators: does one avoid controversy or unpleasantness in exhibitions and displays in order to avoid a negative response? A curator can refuse to display the darker parts of collections or erase the user's experience from an object's history (Anderson and O'Sullivan 2010). This is intentional exclusion. Unintentional exclusion is a different issue. Disability narratives in museums have been limited to temporary exhibitions and funded projects, with notable exceptions (Goggins, Phillipson and Alberti 2017). Museums have inherited historic medical teaching collections that have not been correctly managed in museological terms, with a lack of staff and resources to modernise outdated displays and collections (Condrau 2013). In some cases, the focus on the preservation of specimens has resulted in the loss of context and provenance, which cannot then be reconstructed for visitors (Huistra 2015). Object labels have limited space, and so either object description or input from the user may be selected for comment. Including user voice can be seen as an unnecessary layer, especially when there is not a direct connection to an object.

Uncatalogued material found in museum collections can result in challenges for interpretation and research, and museums are often hesitant to include unsubstantiated evidence in their labels. Connecting objects back to user experiences once they have been separated takes a tremendous amount of research and, even then, can result in anecdotal connections. Occasionally, research reveals inaccurate associations. For example, the Science Museum's iron artificial arm was originally catalogued as belonging to Gotz von Berlichingen, a German knight, dating from 1560–1600 (Science Museum Group A121449 n.d.). Later research showed this to be highly unlikely, as the individual had lost his right arm, and the prosthetic is for the left one (Wellcome Collection Iron Artificial Arm, Europe 1560–1600 n.d.). This prosthetic is now acknowledged as a possible later copy, although it is still considered to be representative of prosthetics dating from von Berlichingen's time.

In some cases, further research can dispute the original interpretation, as with the case of the 'Lady Pianist's Prosthetic', also at the Science Museum (Science Museum Group 1999-553 n.d.). Acquired from Queen Mary's Hospital in Roehampton, this carved wooden right-arm prosthetic has spread, padded fingers, allowing the user to play a full octave on the piano. Though the object record showed it was made by Mr Rowden, a surgical instrument maker based in Roehampton, the user was unknown. The prosthetic's documentation presented a tantalising piece of information. The arm was recorded as being used by the lady pianist to play at the Royal Albert Hall in 1906. But who was she? Although the collection was acquired earlier, it officially came into the Science Museum collection in 1999. In 2013, the Science Museum posted a blog asking for more information, but no answers were forthcoming (Emmens 2013). Only after a national television appearance and appeal was the prosthetic's owner named as Elizabeth Burton, a music and singing teacher born in the early 1860s. Although further research revealed more information about her family life and how she lost her arm, it did not reveal or confirm if she ever played the piano at Royal Albert Hall (Emmens 2019), and so this original 'fact' is now in doubt.

This crowdsourcing strategy to identify or supplement material is not uncommon and can be particularly useful for regional museums. The Museum of Healthcare in Kingston (Canada) possesses six prosthetic legs but very little documentation about who used them and how they were acquired. The museum knew that a man called Ernest Hanna used two of the prostheses. After a call was placed on its local community Facebook group, Ernest Hanna's niece contacted the museum and related how he lost his leg in 1931 and how the leg had survived and entered the collection (Ryan 2019). These calls to communities can yield rich seams of information and enhance documentation of a collection, but they take resources, time and effort to unearth.

Donors and collections

Objects in science and technology collections are commonly donated by or acquired from creators or makers and are viewed as their legacy. Objects entering collections in this way focus on the work of the creator and often lack the point of view of the user. This can be seen in collections across the globe, and particularly with prosthetic collections. The Smithsonian's collection of material relating to heart disease and artificial hearts began for the exhibition *Telegram from Your Heart*, which opened in 1954. Many of these objects were put on display in the new permanent gallery that opened in 1966. What followed, according to the curator, was an influx of new objects into the collection: 'Objects continued to arrive. Whether in the hope of immortality or from a keen sense of history, many famous individuals without solicitation generously donated artefacts to the national collection' (Chelnick, 2013, 207). This 'hope of immortality' and 'keen sense of history' could contain some hubris on the part of the donor, be it misguided or rightly placed. For example, Robert Jarvick, the inventor of the Jarvick-7, the first artificial heart to be successfully transplanted into a human, offered to donate an example to the Smithsonian Museum. However, Jarvick also demanded that the Smithsonian agree to display it permanently, which the Smithsonian was not able to indulge. The University of Arizona later donated one to the Smithsonian with no strings attached, even if with less prestige than the example offered by the inventor (Chelnick 2013). These demands by donors can result in an added barrier to inclusion of important objects in collections and, by proxy, patient stories.

A large portion of the Science Museum's prosthetics collection came from Queen Mary's Hospital in Roehampton, including the aforementioned lady pianist's arm. Dr Ian Fletcher, a senior medical officer at the hospital, curated the material over time. The only information on the owners and users of these prosthetics came from those who created and stored the prosthetics, not the users themselves. This means that, although personal stories may be held about these objects, they are second-hand, and whether the user consented to their story being recounted in this way is unclear. These stories can often be uncomfortably personal. One of the many prosthetic legs in the Science Museum collection is dated to after the First World War and was patched numerous times at home over the years (Science Museum Group 1999-484 n.d.).

Museum staff do not know why the leg was repeatedly repaired in this way, although standard reasons for the time were concern over loss of work and a reluctance to break in a new limb (Emmens 2019, 48–9). Clearly, any interpretation of this object is purely speculation, highlighting the inherent pitfalls in not recording patient voice at the time of use and/or acquisition.

Impact of the social model in museums and expectation management

The adoption of the social model of disability has had a profound impact on disability activism and empowerment in the United Kingdom. As opposed to the traditional medical model, where physical disability is the disabling factor and something to be fixed, the social model embraces the notion that society itself is the disabling force (Shakespeare and Watson 2002). In order to address the social model, museums have focused primarily on physical access to the museum space for disabled visitors, as opposed to including their experience in displays and exhibitions (Sandell and Dodd 2010). Museums' focus on physical access can overshadow disability inclusion in museum displays and text. Although physical access is undoubtedly important, inclusion of disability narratives and stories is another way of making a museum more accessible.

The introduction of the social model coincided with Annie Delin's research project 'Buried in the Footnotes' (2002), which considered whether the lack of inclusion of disability narratives in museum displays was due to a lack of appropriate material culture. However, she found a wealth of objects that could contribute to meaningful displays on disability. This report encouraged a number of projects across the United Kingdom to address this gap, most notably 'Rethinking Disability Representation'. This group of projects, which ran from 2006 to 2009 in nine different museums across the UK, involved partners from all sectors to improve interpretation for disabled audiences, including those who used prosthetics (Sandell and Dodd 2010). The project shone a light on the challenges and opportunities of including patients' voices in museum spaces. It found the most powerful interpretive approach for visitors was to hear from people in their own words, instead of curators interpreting these voices (Snyder and Mitchell 2006). More recent projects have highlighted one main challenge in this process: expectation management.

Museums have been accused of adhering to the medical model of disability by displaying medical technology used by those who are disabled rather than another aspect of their being (Delin 2002). The challenge to address this becomes even more difficult with historical material. Museums choosing to showcase historical user experience are often left without the opportunity to speak to those who experienced disease and treatment. Although this is possible when working with present-day users of medical technology, it can be challenging to manage the expectations of all partners involved.

In order to introduce patient voice into historic collections, museums have had to think outside of the box. For instance, the Royal London Hospital Archive and Museum collaborated with people who live with similar conditions, such as significant physical deformity, to provide a general idea of this experience. Their project, 'Behind the Shadow of Merrick', created a film about Joseph Merrick, better known to posterity as the Elephant Man. They worked with people who, for different reasons, hide their faces, interacting with artefacts of Merrick and talking about their experience in their own words (Hevey 2010). Although staff at the museum, the filmmaker and the people involved were happy, the public's reaction included some highly emotional responses that museums can find challenging to contend with. Visitor comments questioned why the curator's voice was not included in the film and also the decision to only include voices of people who were disabled in the film. They questioned whether the choice to define people by their disability in the film, instead of using their names, contributed to the view of those who are disabled as a 'freak show' (Dodd et al. 2008, 145).

There are no easy answers to managing expectations. Even when collaboration takes place and people who are disabled speak with their own diverse voices, groups who feel the material also belongs to them can take issue with the way others have chosen to display it. In 2002, The Museum of Sex, based in New York City, was host to *Intimate Encounters: Disability and Sexuality*, an exhibition of photography by the photographer Belinda Mason. Mason's photographs were created collaboratively with her subjects, and each photograph included a personal statement, biography and a line that identified the subject's disability.

Controversy emerged before the exhibition even opened. Local disability groups were angry they had not been included in the planning of the exhibition, and the inclusion of an unfortunate turn of phrase, 'handicapped accessible', on the invitation to the exhibition's private view on opening night meant the museum could face a boycott. There were no external advisors on the project, as the museum could not shoulder the cost. Despite the subjects being happy with their representation, those who felt ownership of a disability found the displays challenging. Visitors to the exhibition, in particular those who represented disabled communities, disagreed with the decision to include a line identifying each subject's disability, even though this detail had been agreed with the photograph's subjects (Murray and Jacobs 2010). This leaves museums in a position where they must accept that they will not make all stakeholders happy.

When a pre-existing relationship is found between patients and museums, there can still be issues with expectation management. The Tyne and Wear Museums, for example, already had established a Museums and Gallery Disabled Access Committee, which had been working with the museum for years to improve physical access to the museum spaces. This committee was at the core of the new consulting group for a 2008 exhibition then in development,

One in Four. The title reflected the fact that one in four people identified as disabled in the Tyne and Wear area, as opposed to the national average of one in five. The group began meeting a full two years before the exhibition opened, and, to begin with, there was a range of different views and opinions on the objects available for display. Crucially, a lack of background knowledge in how museum collections are formed and function made it challenging for some members of the group to work with curators. These problems were only amplified after the consulting group's agreed key messages were edited for clarity at the suggestion of another external think-tank group, which was part of the wider project. In hindsight, staff felt that the power structure could have been better explained to all involved, but it may well have resulted in the same challenges (Little 2008).

The Heritage and Stigma project at the University of Huddersfield was a collaboration between disability charities and the University to help the charities to explore and disseminate their histories. In the team lead's own words, 'co-designing and co-producing outputs allowed individuals the opportunity to represent themselves in their own terms – not just as patients or service users – but as individuals' (Ellis 2017, 95). In addition to this project, the charities decided to produce museum displays. Medical humanities professionals were consulted on how to display the charities' histories appropriately. This negotiation between users, charities, researchers and museums is not uncommon, although museums are often resource-poor, and so a costly collaboration that results in projects that provoke vocal opposition may be challenging (Ellis 2017). However, the appetite for ways to address this work is present in the sector.[1] The final exhibitions took place at the Leeds City Museum (for the charity Leeds Mencap) and Tolson Museum in Huddersfield (for the charity St Anne's). Although the exhibitions were well received, Ellis noted that the process of creating them was likely more important than the exhibitions themselves.

As museums, whose primary currency is objects, we must look to tie together objects with the experience of their owners, enriching the collection and display possibilities (Anderson and O'Sullivan 2010). Although these projects do not relate directly to prosthetics, they highlight the challenges that museums face in working with patient groups and people who identify as disabled. We now turn to our redevelopment project at National Museums Scotland.

Case study: prosthetics at National Museums Scotland

National Museums Scotland's mission is to preserve, interpret and make accessible the past and present of Scotland, other nations and cultures, and the natural world. Its flagship site, the National Museum of Scotland in Edinburgh, has more than 2 million visitors a year, making it the largest visitor attraction in the UK outside London. The collections are split into five curatorial groups: Science and Technology, Art and Design, Natural Sciences, World Cultures and

Scottish History and Archaeology. National Museums Scotland's broad remit can make presenting specialist content a particular challenge, as, unlike visitors to medical museums or galleries, the audience at National Museums Scotland is most often a general one, with varied expectations and interests. Visitors entering the space may be en route to fashion or Scottish history and do not expect to come across prosthetics or medical content.

The following case study looks at the prosthetics collection at National Museums Scotland and the ways in which it has been collected, displayed and interpreted. It showcases some of the opportunities and challenges in collecting, caring for and displaying disability, prosthetics and patient voice as discussed above.

Most prosthetics and objects related to disability in the collection at National Museums Scotland have been donated by the creator rather than the user. Historically, the Science and Technology collections have focused solely on the technological importance of an object. The personal stories of those who used the technology were seen as the remit of our colleagues in Scottish History and Archaeology, who are responsible for the social history collection. This focus on the technological importance skewed curators' interest towards inventors, rather than users. I would estimate more than 90% of the objects in the medical collection were donated or acquired from creators or medical professionals. True numbers are hard to pin down owing to the nature of our documentation and collections management system, but it is the overwhelming majority.

These objects often form the perceived 'legacy' of an inventor or creator. The largest collection of prosthetic limbs at National Museums Scotland stems from the work of one man, David Simpson. He created the Powered Prosthetic Unit in 1963 in response to the impact of thalidomide, creating with his team gas-powered upper limbs for affected children living in Scotland and Ireland.

The collection was split in two as part of his legacy, with his technical papers going to the Lothian Health Service Archive and his entire collection of prosthetics, from prototypes to the finished article, accessioned into the National Museums Scotland collection. Furthermore, it was his son, Allen D.C. Simpson, who happened to be a former curator at National Museums Scotland, who donated this collection. These 146 prosthetics displayed the evolution of David Simpson's design. Supplementary information was provided by David Simpson's successor, David Gow, and his recollection of how the prosthetics were used. Information about patient experience was scarce and only included in the narrative as it related to the technological use of the prosthetics (Goggins, Phillipson and Alberti 2017). As with the Science Museum's prosthetic collection, the information about the users of prosthetics was second or even third hand, and was only included as part of the object record if it referred to the design of the object. For instance, a prosthetic may be described as having control mechanisms at the shoulder owing to the user's mobility, but with no information given on what that mobility issue may be. Also, David Simpson stated that prosthetics must be robust as they were for children, which led to design changes, but there are no official or personal stories of prosthetics damaged by children.

In 2011, prosthetics from this extensive collection were put in a space that focused on the impact of thalidomide and the work of David Simpson. As part of the display, the curator wanted to use a quote that compared the children with deep sea divers, because of the gas canisters that had to be worn in order for the Simpson prosthetics to function. The donor objected and was unhappy with the unflattering comparison, and so the quote was not included in the display. The displays instead focused on the positive impact of the prosthetics on the lives of children affected by thalidomide, but did not include any of their voices. No trace of the user experience was found in the object records and the subsequent interpretation. It is only by pure serendipity that we came to know some of the users of this technology, which allowed us to capture and showcase their voices in our new displays.

In 2014, a member of the visitor experience team was approached by a man who wanted to speak to the display's curator. This man, Allan Shannon, identified himself as the young boy whose image, wearing Simpson's prosthetics, could be found in the display. A friend, who still lived locally in Edinburgh, had let him know his image was on our wall. He was not angry, but he did want the curator to know that the experience portrayed in the museum was not the same as his personal experience. Allan stayed in touch with the museum and even came back to visit with some friends who had also worn some of the prosthetics in our collection. When the new Science and Technology galleries were created, which opened in 2016, Allan and a friend, Yvonne Kavanagh, agreed to tell their stories in the museum, using their own words and chosen images. Their stories are told on a digital screen in front of the display of prosthetics. This allows visitors to hear from Allan and Yvonne directly and without the space limitations of object labels. However, despite the main eye-catching graphics positioned directly above the digital screen, visitors were generally found to instead interact with the cases containing objects on either side and ignored the screen altogether.

Both Allan and Yvonne rejected prosthetics as adults and do not use them now. This has been a source of conversation for many of our visitors, who are surprised to see prosthetics, traditionally celebrated as a solution triumphing over adversity, presented as a force that held users back. Incorporating Alan's and Yvonne's stories and insights into our displays was part of an attempt to redress the balance between the medical and social models. Historically, the museum has displayed prosthetics in the purely medical model, presenting prosthetics as the solution to a problem, without incorporating any user voice. In these new displays, we hoped to show not only the importance of technological advances in prosthetics, but also the pitfalls of their imposed use and the effects of the medical model on real people. This importance of the 'real' voice cannot be underestimated. Visitor feedback reinforces the presumption that it is people's stories that visitors really engage with, despite some visitors' lack of interaction with our digital screens.

We undertook visitor research when the redevelopment of the galleries began. It included a ranking of interest in the new topics covered by the Science and Technology and Art and Design galleries, which were each being refurbished. Galleries spanned from fashion to technology. In the list of those new topics, biomedicine was classed as the 'least interesting'. But, when visitors were presented with actual biomedical objects, including prosthetics, they found them among the most interesting. These findings were echoed in our final visitor evaluation. Visitors seemed unsure about what the word 'biomedicine' meant when asked if they had an interest in the topic. However, when asked as part of visitor research, many said their favourite interactives were the ones that focused on biomedical concepts (ScotInform 2016).

This led to the challenge of displaying biomedicine objects without labelling them 'biomedicine'. The result was that the biomedical content in the new galleries was woven throughout the three floors and did not have its own 'biomedical ghetto'. The prosthetics, for example, are found in the section entitled Technology by Design, which looks at design solutions for technological problems. The gallery posed some practical challenges. It is a Victorian building, and this particular gallery is one of our balcony galleries, with five exit and entry points along the periphery of an atrium space. This layout means that we have no control over where visitors begin their journeys.

Visually, one of the largest draws of the space is the wall of bicycles and motorcycles. The design of the space assumed that visitors may encounter our displays of motorcycles, then bicycles and then wheelchairs, internal implants and prosthetics. The idea is that a visitor interested in the technology of motorcycles would also appreciate the technology of bicycles and wheelchairs. That interest would, in theory, carry them to find out more about the technology of prosthetics. Of course, this approach, and even the gallery title, lends itself more to the medical than social model of disability. Displaying the prosthetics collection in what is an engineering, technology and design gallery once again sets up limb loss as a problem to be solved. The prosthetics are displayed alongside pacemakers and assistive technology, which further reinforces their perceived role as a solution to a problem. Visitors stated that they were pleasantly surprised to find that part of the museum was dedicated to disability, which they have not seen elsewhere.

As part of the displays, there is also an interactive, functioning i-Limb, the first prosthetic hand with individually powered fingers. The hand is set up so that visitors can choose from a selection of five grips and see how the hand moves. The interface was designed so that visitors would choose a grip, watch a video of how that particular grip would be used on the touch screen and then watch the hand in the case move and demonstrate the grip. Immediately, from our initial testing, we found that visitors did not watch the videos on how the hand worked. In fact, they often tried to tap the screen to 'skip' them. The importance to the museum, and the company who created i-Limb, of giving context to what each grip did was not at the forefront of our visitors' experience.

Although Technology by Design is a permanent gallery, and thus unchanging, it does include an update case, intentionally included to showcase contemporary material. These update cases are not common practice in the national museum space. Including them was a commitment to the Wellcome Trust, a part funder of the project, and a nod to contemporary biomedicine. It is important to National Museums Scotland to be seen as somewhere that engages with, collects and showcases cutting-edge science. In order to do so, some spaces needed to be adaptable, which would require ongoing financial and staff support.

The update case sits within the display of wheelchairs. It is a tall, rectangular glass case and originally contained gait prosthetics. When looking at options for the first 'update' of the case, I went back to my original 'wish list' for the new galleries. A contemporary piece that I was unable to acquire during the gallery redevelopment was a bespoke prosthetic limb from the Alternative Limb Project. These prosthetics are designed by Sophie de Oliveira Barata, a London-based prosthetic designer and head of the Alternative Limb Project. These limbs can be practical, but can also be highly stylised art pieces. I was interested in her prosthetics as they combine both form and function, in juxtaposition to many of the prosthetics in our collection.

I had originally discussed acquiring one of these limbs with Sophie when we were working on the galleries before 2016, and so we had a pre-existing relationship. Sophie was aware that I was very interested in acquiring a limb for the collection, but ideally wanted one that had been used. We discussed various options that Sophie had created for display, once again acquiring from the creator of the prosthetic, as opposed to working directly with a user of these prosthetics. This decision was pragmatic. First, as these limbs are both expensive and bespoke, it seemed unlikely that a user would be willing to part with their prosthetic. Second, by having access to the designer and design process, the acquisition of the limb could include both the prosthetic and background information relating to the design process and imagery, which could be used to enhance the display.

We acquired the Vine Arm (Fig. 5.1), a botanical green tentacle covered in flowers and controlled by sensors located in a matching pair of shoes. The model of the limb, Kelly Knox, was heavily involved in its creation. The design of the prosthetic was inspired by Kelly's love of plants, nature and the supernatural. In working with Kelly, we were able to collect her thoughts on the prosthetic's design, prosthetics generally and the Vine Arm specifically. She does not wear prosthetics in her everyday life, but instead wears them to express herself and explore aspects of her personality. As such, the Vine Arm is beautiful but not functional; it can move and curve, but not assist with everyday tasks. This was intentionally meant to juxtapose with the prosthetics on display that were designed with very practical use in mind (National Museums Scotland 2018).

The case has been popular with visitors, but had an unexpected response on the web. The unveiling of the case coincided with a video, posted to YouTube,

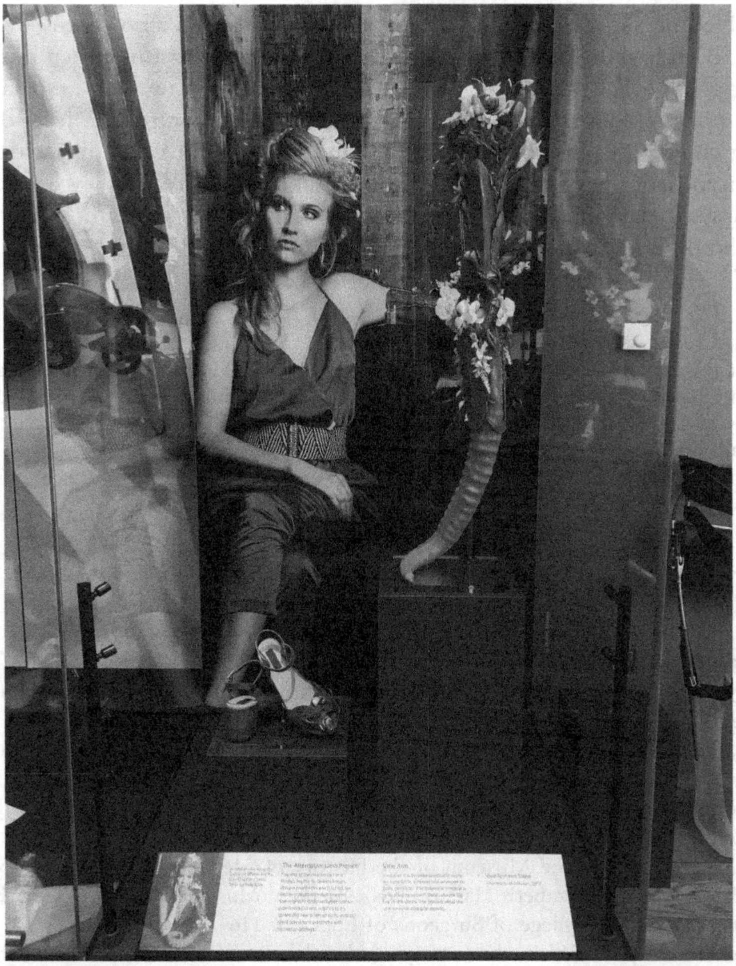

Figure 5.1 **Vine Arm, created by Sophie de Oliveira Barata from the Alternative Limb Project for model and activist Kelly Knox. On temporary display in the Technology by Design gallery at National Museums Scotland. Sourced by author**

of the Vine Arm in use. The video has been popular, with more than 80,000 views, but introduced us to a niche pornographic corner of the internet that we were not expecting or prepared for. As an institution, we were confronted with the concern that, by putting disability and prosthetics on display, we were perpetuating the fetishising of these topics. The comments on the video require a level of moderation to this day.

Museums look to uncover these 'hidden stories' in their collection, but often a person goes 'on display' owing to their prosthetic or disability and not another aspect of their personhood. This is problematic, as it once again frames the disabled person as invisible, which they may well have not been – we just have not been looking. Curators continue to shape the narrative when including user or patient voice. Users who wish to engage with the museum, especially if they are not the donors of the objects, by nature possess a certain level of self-selecting confidence. Empowered people tend to be more vocal and articulate. Our own museum has only captured some user voices because they entered the museum space and made themselves known to members of staff. What about those who do not?

Note

1 Recent projects and events such as the 'Rethinking Disability' symposium hosted in March 2018 at the Museum of Liverpool brought together museum professionals to discuss disability representation in museums and reflect on ways we can tackle this inequality of representation in the future (Niciu 2018).

References

Anderson, Julie and Lisa O'Sullivan (2010) 'Histories of disability and medicine: reconciling historical narratives and contemporary values.' In Richard Sandell, Jocelyn Dodd and Rosemarie Garland-Thomson (eds), *Re-Presenting Disability: Activism and Agency in the Museum*. Abingdon: Routledge, 143–55.

Bonnell, Jennifer and Roger Simon (2007) 'Difficult exhibitions and intimate encounters.' *Museum and Society* 5(2), 65–85.

Chelnick, Judy (2013) 'Collecting medical technology at the Smithsonian Institution's National Museum of American History.' In Samuel J.M.M. Alberti and Elizabeth Hallam (eds), *Medical Museums: Past, Present, Future*. London: The Royal College of Surgeons of England, 200–13.

Condrau, Flurin (2013) 'The Museum of the History of Medicine in Zurich.' In Samuel J.M.M. Alberti and Elizabeth Hallam (eds), *Medical Museums: Past, Present, Future*. London: The Royal College of Surgeons of England, 116–29.

Delin, Annie (2002) 'Buried in the footnotes: the absence of disabled people in the collective imagery of the past.' In Richard Sandell (ed.), *Museums, Society, Inequality*. London: Routledge, 84–97.

Dodd, Jocelyn, Richard Sandell, Debbie Jolly and Ceri Jones (eds) (2008) *Rethinking Disability Representation in Museums and Galleries*. Leicester: RCMG, University of Leicester.

Ellis, Rob (2017) 'Heritage and stigma. Co-producing and communicating the histories of mental health and learning disability.' *Medical Humanities* 43(2), 92–8.

Emmens, Stewart (2013) 'Who was the one-armed lady pianist?' Available at: https://blog.sciencemuseum.org.uk/who-was-that-one-armed-lady-pianist/ (accessed 3 March 2020).

Emmens, Stewart (2019) 'Prostheses at the Science Museum.' In Natasha McEnroe (ed.), *Medicine: An Imperfect Science*. London: Scala Arts & Heritage, 38–65.

Goggins, Sophie, Tacye Phillipson and Samuel J.M.M. Alberti (2017) 'Prosthetic limbs on display: from maker to user.' *Science Museum Group Journal* 2017(8), http://dx.doi.org/10.15180/170806

Hevey, David (2010) 'Behind the shadow of Merrick.' In Richard Sandell, Jocelyn Dodd and Rosemarie Garland-Thomson (eds), *Re-Presenting Disability: Activism and Agency in the Museum*. Abingdon: Routledge, 79–92.

Huistra, Hieke (2015) 'Adieu Albinus: how the preparations in the nineteenth-century Leiden anatomical collections lost their past.' In Rina Knoeff and Robert Zwijnenberg (eds), *The Fate of Anatomical Collections*. New York: Routledge, 113–28.

Little, Kylea (2008) 'One in four.' In Jocelyn Dodd, Richard Sandell, Debbie Jolly and Ceri Jones (eds), *Rethinking Disability Representation in Museums and Galleries*. Leicester: RCMG, University of Leicester, 79–82.

Murray, Elizabeth M.M. and Sarah Jacobs (2010) 'Revealing moments: representation of disability and sexuality.' In Richard Sandell, Jocelyn Dodd and Rosemarie Garland-Thomson (eds), *Re-Presenting Disability: Activism and Agency in the Museum*. Abingdon: Routledge, 155–67.

National Museums Scotland (2018) 'Vine Arm.' Available at: www.nms.ac.uk/explore-our-collections/stories/science-and-technology/vine-arm/ (accessed 20 June 2018).

Niciu, Steph (2018) 'Rethinking disability – time for a change within the museum.' Available at: https://disabilityarts.online/magazine/opinion/rethinking-disability-time-change-within-musem/ (accessed 17 October 2020).

Ryan, Shaelyn (2019) 'Getting a leg up: a brief history of prosthetics through the lens of our collection.' Available at: https://museumofhealthcare.wordpress.com/2019/06/18/getting-a-leg-up-a-brief-history-of-prosthetics-through-the-lens-of-our-collection/ (accessed 3 March 2020).

Sandell, Richard, Annie Delin, Jocelyn Dodd and Jackie Gay (2005) 'In the shadow of the freakshow: the impact of freakshow tradition on the display and understanding of disability history in museums.' *Disability Studies Quarterly* 25(4). Available at: https://dsq-sds.org/article/view/614/791

Sandell, Richard and Jocelyn Dodd (2010) 'Activist practice.' In Richard Sandell, Jocelyn Dodd and Rosemarie Garland-Thomson (eds), *Re-Presenting Disability: Activism and Agency in the Museum*. Abingdon: Routledge, 3–23.

Science Museum Group A12144 (n.d.) 'Iron artificial arm, Europe, 1560–1600.' Available at: https://collection.sciencemuseumgroup.org.uk/objects/co126844/iron-artificial-arm-europe-1560-1600-artificial-arm (accessed 2 September 2020).

Science Museum Group 1999-484 (n.d.) 'Artificial leg with extensive home repairs, England, 1914–1918.' Available at: https://collection.sciencemuseumgroup.org.uk/objects/co476577/artificial-leg-with-extensive-home-repairs-england-1914-1918-artificial-leg (accessed 2 September 2020).

Science Museum Group 1999-553 (n.d.) 'Artificial arm, below-elbow prosthesis.' Available at: https://collection.sciencemuseumgroup.org.uk/objects/co476713/artificial-arm-below-elbow-prosthesis-artificial-arm (accessed 2 September 2020).

ScotInform (2016) 'National Museum of Scotland Summative Evaluation: Visitor Research, Final Report.' Internal NMS report. Unpublished.

Shakespeare, Tom and Nicholas Watson (2002) 'The social model of disability: an outdated ideology?' *Research in Social Science and Disability* 2, 9–28.

Snyder, Sharon L., and David T. Mitchell (2006) *Cultural Locations of Disability*. London: University of Chicago Press.

Wellcome Collection Iron Artificial Arm, Europe, 1560–1600 (n.d.) Available at: https://wellcomecollection.org/works/aebqrxbn (accessed 2 September 2020).

Chapter 6

New light on 'the viewer'

Sensing the Parthenon galleries in the British Museum

Ellen Adams

Abstract

Classicists are beginning to recognise that the traditional template of the ancient viewer is that of an elite, urban, White adult male, and they are attempting to open up the subject to other eyes and voices. But the assumption of 20/20 vision remains, and certain conditions, such as colour blindness or stereoblindness, testify that 'vision' is experienced in a wide range of ways. Furthermore, we all notice, absorb, and remember the world differently. Art appreciation is therefore a personal perception, as is the description of artworks and their impact on us. Intermodal translation of the visual into the verbal has been a long-standing theme in Classics as ekphrasis. This chapter considers what we can learn from engaging with blind people in terms of how we look at, appreciate, and articulate visual art, particularly in terms of audio description (AD). It presents some of the aims, activities, and conclusions of a pilot study conducted in the Department of Greece and Rome and the Parthenon galleries of the British Museum. This involved ADs and touch/handling sessions for a small group of blind or partially sighted people and their companions over a series of four afternoons. A by-product of this approach is to review and reframe the sculptures in innovative ways, including a consideration of how these provisions might benefit sighted people.[1]

Voicing blindness

The blind man (always a man) with cane has been an intriguing philosophical motif since Descartes. He has been fun to think with, although few (such as Diderot: Patterson 2016) are prepared to listen to his actual insights. For example, Merleau-Ponty (2002, 165–6) presents a blind man with cane without engaging with blind and partially sighted people themselves. He did so while promoting phenomenology, which emphasises the empirical, grounded, and first-person view of the world (Adams 2019, 184), therefore setting a striking contradiction. This objectification, with colonial overtones, is beginning to be questioned, as scholars start to draw from personal accounts by ill and disabled people.[2] For example, Emily

Dickinson and Aelius Aristides may inform the modern scholar (Petridou, Chapter 3, this volume), while medical case reports (MCRs) fall in and out of fashion (Flexer and Hurwitz, Chapter 2, this volume). Ancient accounts of blind experiences are rare, but modern ones may still inform and engage, including the history of the discovery of the neurology of vision (Masland 2020).

Helen Keller's voice and perspective are famous, despite her being both deaf and blind. Her plucky and relentlessly positive attitude has generated some resentment among other blind people (Kleege 2006). Keller is a lot to live up to. She provides an extreme example of overcoming adversity (albeit from a position of class privilege), with a superhuman effort to 'beat' the disability and bridge the gap between her natural state and social 'normality'. This commitment to integration was applied to art appreciation:

> I derive genuine pleasure from touching great works of art. As my finger tips trace line and curve, they discover the thought and emotion which the artist has portrayed. I can feel in the faces of gods and heroes hate, courage and love, just as I can detect them in living faces I am permitted to touch. I feel in Diana's posture the grace and freedom of the forest and the spirit that tames the mountain lion and subdues the fiercest passions.
>
> Keller (2005 [1902], 91)

She does not countenance that this alternative access to art might be inferior, and celebrates the subtleties of touch as a kind of Blind Gain.[3]

Oliver Sacks experienced significant sight problems during his life and had a notably poor visual memory. His book *The Mind's Eye* (2010) combines his usual array of case histories (including himself), but also a chapter on various memoires by blind people. These comprise first-hand accounts that can be independently consulted, rather than cases interpreted through the doctor's voice. He explores the unusual experience of John Hull, who came to lose all visual imagery and memory as 'deep blindness', to the extent that the idea of seeing became meaningless (Hull 1990; Sacks 2010, 202–5). This was not a typical response, however. Zoltan Torey became 'able to construct a virtual visual world that seemed as real and intense to him as the perceptual one he had lost – indeed, sometimes more real, more intense' (Sacks 2010, 208–9). Not only do the conditions of impaired vision vary widely (e.g. tunnel vision compared with cataract), but the range of mental responses is also considerable. Oliver Sacks himself had very poor visual imagery but excellent stereoscopy – one does not simply 'see' or not.

There can be considerable variations in sight perception for those with 20/20 vision – colour blindness, for example. Stereoblindness refers to people who experience the world as flat (no depth of field). Depth and distance can still be judged from cues such as relative size (objects becoming smaller as they are further away). Susan Barry did not perceive stereopsis because she had been born with misaligned eyes (a strabismic). Despite having operations to straighten them, her brain did not learn to fuse the images provided by her eyes – instead, it flipped from one to the other in rapid succession. In midlife, Barry, herself a neuroscientist, took vision therapy. She gained stereopsis and two ways of seeing: 'I saw with stereopsis almost all the time, but I could revert to my old strabismic ways under stressful conditions' (Barry 2009, 156). Sight, spatial orientation, movement, and emotional state all shape visual perception. Visits to modern art galleries with stereovision allowed her to 'examine the intriguing pockets of space within each piece of sculpture' (Barry 2009, 162). This rather unusual turn of phrase indicates how she could notice an element of 3D art that someone without such a history may take for granted – to the extent that they did not really 'see' it.

As Classicists, is it anachronistic for us to consider modern accounts by disabled people, or can we weave this strand into a meaningful dialogue? In this chapter, I argue that the process of such engagements can force us to reconsider even the most familiar classical materials. Reference to the ancient world can also be useful to modern disciplines. Jonas Grethlein (2017, 5–6) argued that, 'due to their experimental background, cognitive studies per se lack a historical dimension. Ancient texts are a forceful reminder that there is a history to aesthetic experience, that it loomed large in Greco-Roman antiquity'. In particular, the classical world and the study of it have contributed to visual-verbal translation with the theme of ekphrasis, and it is to this that we now turn.

Visual-verbal intermodal translation: ekphrasis and audio description (AD)

The previous section has indicated how the experience of sight loss or atypical vision is immensely wide-ranging, which would inevitably lead to different experiences. However, the great thinkers on aesthetics, such as Kant, ultimately assume the 'same natural (sighted) standpoint' (Davidson 2008, 144). The 'tyranny of the visual' may be questioned in art appreciation, as, physiologically, 'all the sensory modalities are closely interrelated so that perception is a polysensorial phenomenon' (Bilman 2013, 40). Perhaps ironically, engaging with blind and partially sighted people reiterates this point. Furthermore, cultural framing also shapes what gets noticed and remembered. The viewer applies attention, while drawing from memory to 'make sense' of images and objects. This, then, may be turned into language-sense. Some, like Whistler, may 'prefer to keep words out of painting altogether' (Squire 2009, 90), but most museum visitors wish to be able to communicate at some level about their aesthetic experience. This section will consider and compare two modes of communication that attempt to do just that, ekphratic poetry and AD, drawing from examples based on the Parthenon.

Ekphrasis

Theon provides an ancient definition of ekphrasis as descriptive speech that vividly brings the subject before the eyes (Theon, *Progrymnasmata* 118.7, quoted in Squire 2016, 17–8; see also Squire 2015, 4–5). Ancient Greek ekphrastic poetry suggests how the visual might overpower the other senses – such as how Myron's cow so tricked a real calf that it died of starvation trying to suckle from it, rather than rejecting the feel and taste of the bronze material. But the 36 ancient epigrams that this cow inspired were 'neither descriptive nor informative' in visual terms, instead focusing on 'rhythmic pleasantries' (Goethe's *Myron's Cow* from 1818, quoted in Squire 2010, 589; see Bell 2018, 903–8 for a full translation of this self-published work; see *Palatine Anthology* 9.713–42, 793–8 for the epigrams). As the object in question was long lost when Goethe was writing in the early nineteenth century, his frustration about not being told what it actually looked like is apparent. Squire (2010, 617) argues that the ancient poets had a different pursuit, exploiting 'Myron's sculptural make-believe to interrogate the make-believe of their own epigrammatic response', providing a commentary on the ripples of intermodal simulation. Therefore, the emphasis is on how the *impact* of the visual might be reconstructed in words, rather than the formal description. Regarding the pots used in the Athenian symposium, we have a 'mode of visual and verbal interaction, whereby images were used to do more than "illustrate" a text, just as texts did more than epitomise an image' (Squire 2009, 157).

Modern ekphrasis shares this emphasis on the verbal representation of the visual element of art, particularly poetry and paintings (e.g. Bilman 2013). Stripped down further, ekphrasis is about word and image (Webb 1999), perhaps intertwined (as Simonides had proclaimed that painting is silent poetry and poetry a speaking picture; for sources, see Squire 2009, 147, n. 217). The ekphrastic process articulates the impact and meaning of visual culture: 'The moment we try and "describe" a work of art or make a statement of "fact" about its meaning … we are interpreting the picture, construing its signs and articulating what they signify' (Heffernan 2006, 67). In other words, this is intermodal translation, from one medium (visual mainly, but not only) to another (speech); as such, an element of interpretation and reconstruction is inevitable. Modern ekphrastic poetry based on the Parthenon demonstrates the issues of intermodal translation and senses of space and time,[4] as illustrated by Byron, Hardy, Melville, and Keats.

Byron's attack on Elgin's actions in dismantling, scavenging, and exporting the Parthenon sculptures to London is one of the more famous poetic responses to the monument. 'The Curse of Minerva' (1811) is set not in the British Museum, but on the mutilated Athenian Acropolis. Canto II, stanza XV from *Childe Harold's Pilgrimage* (1812) reiterates this scorn, whereby it is a cold heart or dull eye that fails to be moved by the defaced walls, 'And once again thy hapless bosom gored, / And snatchd thy shrinking Gods to northern climes abhorrd!'. The British government still bought the sculptures shortly after, in 1816. This sense of outrage produces a politically passionate response to the sculptures, with little description of what they actually looked like.

Thomas Hardy's 'Christmas in the Elgin Room' (1905 and 1926) picks up on the considerable climate difference between the Athenian Acropolis and the gloomy, gaunt, cold room in the British Museum. The permanent chill of the Parthenon galleries (particularly noticeable in the winter, as the heating is thinly spread to accommodate the new Great Court) is a distinctive feature of visits to this space. A somewhat sentimental poem, Hardy's Greek gods bewail their new setting and the loss of their religious power to Christianity. In emphasising the distorted and disjointed religious context, Hardy implicitly conveys some of the cathedral atmosphere that great museums possess, whereby the magnificence of the setting frames not the power of a deity, but the achievements and creations of humans. Hardy also draws attention to the fragmentary nature of the sculptures, 'whose limbs were shards beneath some Acropolitan clod'.

A poem that highlights (if implicitly) the stark contrast between the original context and the galleries in the British Museum is Herman Melville's 'The Parthenon' (1891). It is set in Athens, and the reader initially experiences the Parthenon remotely as a landmark, moving in to appreciate the architecture, then viewing the continuous Ionic frieze and, finally, focusing on the last tile placed, which completes the monument. Space is rather fluid in this poem, as the description of the frieze is of that from inside a museum, at eye level, so that the 'airiest touch' of the chisel could be perceived. There is no sense of the rather hidden original context, unreached by direct sunlight (see below). These changes in viewpoints and perspectives reinforce how ekphrastic depiction does not necessarily produce a static description, but easily moves through space and, by extension, time. The poem embraces the fact that the viewer is rarely completely stationary, but moves towards, around and away from that which is viewed – even if the artwork itself is fixed.

Time is more famously the theme of Keats's 'On seeing the Elgin Marbles' (1817), in which the timeless nature of the sculptures is compared with the young man's mortality. Indeed, the poem is remarkably fixed in space, 'incapable of movement', with images 'painfully static' (Scott 1990, 138). Belonging in the genre of ekphrastic poetry, the poem manages to mediate between the two opposing aesthetic responses to the marbles when they first arrived in Britain: wonder at the past perfection, and frustration at the ruined, fragmentary nature of the pieces (Scott 1990). More specifically, Scott argues that, 'the poet provides us with a far greater insight into the mechanism of aesthetic perception than into the artworks themselves' (Scott 1990, 131). This is an interesting angle on ekphrasis, not descriptively or critically focusing on the object, but on the range of reactions (arguably Goethe's 'rhythmic pleasantries' referred to above).

How, then, does the intermodal translation/interpretation of AD compare? A survey of key works on ekphrasis has not revealed any references to AD (e.g. Heffernan 1993; Mitchell 1994; Bartsch and Elsner 2007; Cheeke 2008).[5] Research on AD, however, is prepared to explore the ekphrastic tradition (e.g. Neves 2012; Snyder 2014, 1–2). One aim of the present research is to explore whether a more evenly balanced engagement would be mutually beneficial, such as a comparison of modes of delivery.[6] For example, AD is always dispensed orally, preferably live, unlike the focus on the written word in modern ekphrasis (even in the case of Homer, his oral poetry is studied as a text). In AD, seeing and sensing are achieved through hearing, whereas the ekphrastic tradition has become based on reading.

Audio description (AD)

The formal use of AD to generate access for blind and partially sighted people has only been around since the 1970s. Developed in America, Britain is now the most prolific provider of AD for live performance, film screenings, and DVDs (Snyder 2014, 19–22; Perego 2018). Most scholarship explores AD for film (e.g. Maszerowska, Matamala and Orero 2014; Pérez-González 2014; Fryer 2016; Matamala and Orero 2016; see also guidelines in Ofcom 2000). Museum AD is recognised as a distinct area (Hutchinson and Eardley 2019) and often relies on contributions by in-house staff. Visual art tends to be stationary, removing the requirement to fit the AD into gaps in the dialogue and key sound elements (including the musical score).

Audio describers are aware that 'the visual' is not an objective entity, and that the process of verbalising it is a form of intermodal translation (Fryer 2016). Any translation requires a degree of selection and interpretation. Furthermore, AD is a productive act – to the extent that 'the approach of the AD may be to offer a kind of *transcreation*, the creation of a new artwork, rather than a translation' (Eardley et al. 2017, 201). This is subjective, immersive, and an experience that may be enjoyed by sighted as well as blind and partially sighted people. For example, the AD on the Parthenon frieze's speeding chariot scene includes the evocative and memorable phrase: 'their manes are like flames, blown by the wind; their tails too are flowing' (British Museum n.d.a). This is visually vivid, with a nod to heat, touch, and sound.

It might be assumed that AD serves merely to replace the unseen visual. However, audio describers develop multisensory narratives – despite, or perhaps because, they serve blind people, who are well aware that sight does not work in isolation. The use of words to represent, reproduce, and interpret visual art (which is inevitably material as well) requires an engagement with a multisensory imagination. As such, one definition of ekphrasis as 'a type of speech (logos) that has a certain effect upon an audience' (Webb 1999, 11) may fit AD the best.[7]

In addition to being multisensory, AD need not remain focused solely on description; context and background are part of what we are seeing (when done at length, this becomes 'audio narration'). Background context may be offered not only by the information label, but also by certain visual cues. A general drawing of a Greek temple, for example, has connotations of time, place, and social status that reach well beyond the physical details of the image, at least for a particular demographic (understanding such connotations cannot necessarily be assumed, especially with a global audience with varying cultural backgrounds). These connotations bring us to the realm of 'mental modelling' rather than straightforward 'seeing' (Braun 2007). An experienced audio describer is aware of all of these factors, while alert to the fact that ADs need to be kept succinct.

Many countries have provided guidelines for AD, intended to support good practice (e.g. Ofcom 2000). There is an overwhelming, almost exclusive, use of the present tense and present participles in AD. This generates a sense of vividness, but also timelessness, which is perhaps particularly appropriate for immobile art. Sentences should be succinct, while rich and colourful. Adverbs should not be subjective, and a colourful verb is better than general verb + adverb (e.g. 'Mary rushes in' versus 'Mary enters quickly'). All AD guidelines agree that colour should be mentioned. A blind or partially sighted person may experience or even see some colour, have a good working memory of it, or even simply understand the personal, cultural, and symbolic connotations that colour can have (red = blood = danger). Psycholinguists have explored the cultural variations of colour, and the perception of colour is heavily framed by cultural categorization (Fryer 2017). Visual attributes should not be avoided in the name of tact. Helen Keller (2009 [1908], 16) embraced such vivid, visual vocabulary: 'This hazardous game is half the delight, the frolic, of daily life. I glow as I read of splendours which the eye alone can survey'.

The size of an object should always be described – context that perhaps a sighted person would take for granted and forget to mention. Barry Ginley, access officer at the V&A Museum and blind himself, has set out guidelines for AD in museums (Ginley 2013). He suggests the 'clock method', moving around a painting from 12 o'clock. This is not favoured by audio describers today; one concern is that it imposes an artificial framework on a painting, rather than allowing the artwork to dictate the starting point as a sighted person would experience it. AD is a developing, fluid craft, responding to regular feedback and experimental techniques.

A new programme of AD clips has recently been provided for the British Museum in collaboration with VocalEyes and is publicly available.[8] Perego (2019) has analysed eighteen of these ADs, including two from the Parthenon sculptures. The audios were considered in terms of type–token ratio (lexical variation or diversity in a text), lexical density (the proportion of information or content words in a text), mean word length, and mean sentence length, which enabled an impersonal, quantitative view, while a more qualitative consideration of adjectives was also brought into play. Perego (2019) expected a restricted level of type–token ratio for clarity, a high proportion of lexical density to convey information, a slightly longer mean word length than in standard English due to the use of abstract concepts in art, and a standard average sentence length. Her summary was that these ADs indicated particularly precise, descriptive, and informative texts. Around one-fifth of the overall AD words comprised adjectives with high variability. Emotive adjectives are generally avoided. This is, therefore, a particular style of English, beyond serving a particular function. As such, we might consider whether it could benefit sighted people as well, which could, in turn, produce more integrated and inclusive museum practice.

AD for sighted people

In a survey of blind and partially sighted people, 50% stated that they did not like access events to be segregated, whereas 50% liked the special, separate events (Pereira 2009, 14). There is, therefore, a demand to make mainstream events more inclusive, in addition to providing specific access events. For example, AD can be intertwined with storytelling in theatre, as performed by the blind and partially sighted Extant Theatre Company (Cavallo 2015) or Graeae Theatre productions. This section explores whether, in addition to providing inclusive practice, AD might also benefit sighted people. Some practical advantages have been noted, such as following a television show while engaged in other activities (Snyder 2008, see also Kleege 2016). Remael, Reviers and Vercauteren (2015, 15) list other beneficiaries, such as immigrants and language learners and people with ADHD (see also Incalcaterra McLoughlin 2017; Eardley et al. 2017).[9] But might there also be benefits in terms of art appreciation?

In the museum context, Snyder (2008, 194) argues that, 'using AD techniques for the description of static images and exhibitions not only enhances accessibility, but it also helps develop more expressive, vivid, and imaginative museum tours'. AD can guide sighted people, help them engage with artworks, and increase memorability (Eardley et al. 2017, 195). Cachia (2017, in a paper in *Art Journal*) suggests that AD might become part of visual studies. Ideally, this new approach to inclusivity would closely involve the traditional professions of curators, art historians, archaeologists, heritage experts, and visual culture specialists, and redefine how we think of 'the viewer'. By extension, although it is standard for a sighted person to provide access for blind and partially sighted people, such engagements are mutually beneficial. Sacks quotes Arlene Gordon, who is blind: '"Sighted people enjoy traveling with me," she said. "I ask them questions, then they look and see things they wouldn't otherwise. Too often people with sight don't see anything! It's a reciprocal process – we enrich each other's worlds"' (Sacks 2010, 24). It is one thing to be able to see; it is quite another to know how to look.

Ian Jenkins, when commenting on scholars' theorizing regarding the meaning of the Parthenon frieze, has stated that:

> the only way out of this maze is a return to the first principles of *looking*, and if I have exercised my own capacity to speculate on the meaning of the frieze, it is not with the intention of finding a once-and-for-all solution, but with a view to establishing a common ground founded upon close observation of the sculpture itself.
>
> Jenkins (1994, 7, original italics)

Interestingly, this process of deliberate looking included a major project for blind and partially sighted people, based in the Parthenon galleries.

The British Museum's Tiresias Project responded to the 1995 Disability Discrimination Act, which required public institutions, such as museums, to provide access to disabled people (by making 'reasonable adjustments'). This project, named after the blind seer of Greek myth, culminated in 1998 with the opening of auxiliary rooms 18a and 18b (Fig. 6.1a) and the publication of *Second Sight of the Parthenon Frieze* (Bird, Jenkins and Levi 1998). This is a tactile book with raised line drawings (RLDs) and Braille text alongside the English script. When opened, it sits at over 90 cm wide and 32 cm high. It is accompanied by a detailed (5-hour) AD on tapes, which leads the listener through the raised images of the book. As it is a guide to a tactile experience, it works rather differently from standard audio books that provide background information. Eye, ear, and hand are deployed in combination as fits the individual; the vast majority of blind and partially sighted people have some sight, so many could make out the simplified, contrasting black and white images.

The Tiresias Project entails looking at the sculptures from fresh and original perspectives, as well as in close detail. The process of rendering the sculptures accessible has resulted in certain unexpected insights. For example, particular features on the frieze, such as men's heads, horses' heads, and horses' hooves, create rhythmic wavy lines rising and falling throughout the composition, which themselves generate rhythms. 'These compositional lines are not usually noticed by the ordinary spectator, and have to be pointed out' (Bird, Jenkins and Levi 1998, 8): this is not an unusual feature of art appreciation. Some figures occur in quiet isolation, whereas others clump together in a loud crescendo. Ian Jenkins (1994, 31) has developed a symphonic metaphor for the frieze, from the introductory *adagio* on the west side, which is 'followed on the north and south sides by successive *allegro* movements, the first *moderato*, the second (the chariot race) *molto*, "at full tilt"'. Then the fourth movement, on the east side, comprises a long, solemn *andante*. 'The music culminates in sublime fashion with an *adagio* finale as the procession on the east frieze is brought before the company of the gods' (Jenkins 1994, 31). Presenting the frieze in music to provide access to such rhythmic changes would be a fascinating way to recreate the frieze.

The Tiresias Project produced bird's eye (or god's eye) views of the composition of the procession, which spatially isolates the figures for a clearer understanding of the depth of fields. Figure 6.2 shows the start of the North Frieze,

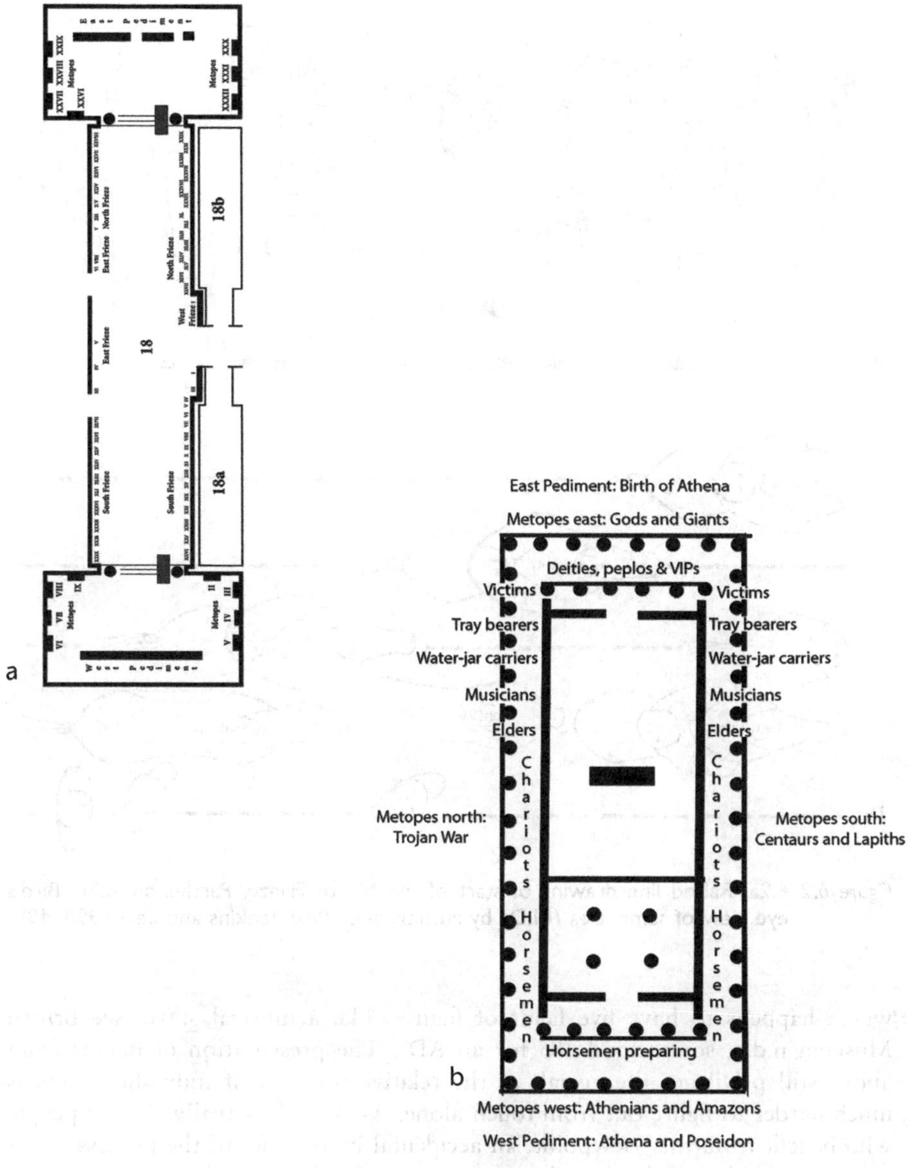

Figure 6.1 6.1a: Current Parthenon Gallery (18), including auxiliary rooms 18a and 18b; 6.1b: original sculptural programme (images by author)

a

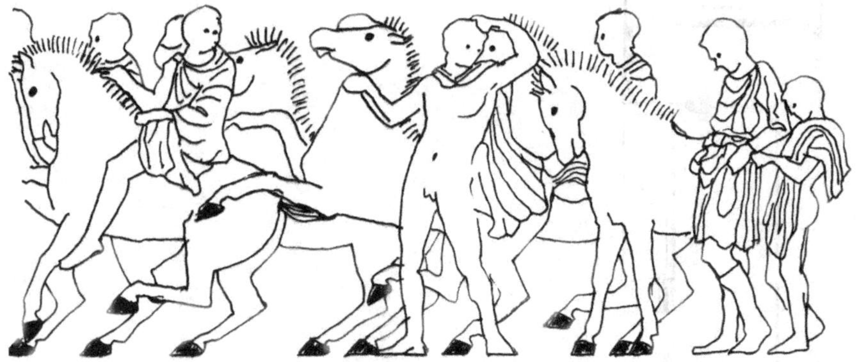

b

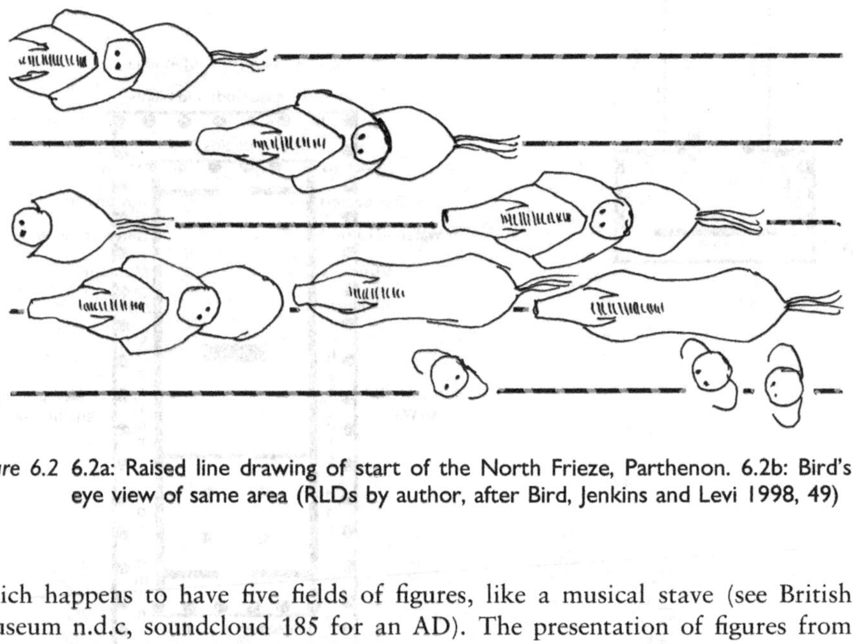

Figure 6.2 **6.2a: Raised line drawing of start of the North Frieze, Parthenon. 6.2b: Bird's eye view of same area (RLDs by author, after Bird, Jenkins and Levi 1998, 49)**

which happens to have five fields of figures, like a musical stave (see British Museum n.d.c, soundcloud 185 for an AD). The presentation of figures from above still privileges the visual, as the relative position of individual units is much harder to figure out from touch alone. As such, it is really sighted people who benefit from this viewpoint, an accidental by-product of the process of re-presenting and repackaging the composition for blind and partially sighted people. It may also be that *only* sighted people benefit from the tactile element of such RLDs. Tracing images while looking at them provides an additional layer of engagement, perhaps similar to the old archaeological adage that, if you really want to look at an object, you should draw it.

Might AD be of merit in teaching art and archaeology to sighted people (as well as blind and partially sighted students)? Visual description provides a translation into a usable format for analysis, through case studies, typologies, and so on (Marcus, Love and Best 2016), and students are often asked to prepare image commentaries. One teaching technique is to set students in pairs, with one describing an image that the other cannot see, who then has to draw what they hear. Another exercise tested the validity for using AD in art modules. I showed a painting (Alma-Tadema's *Phidias Showing the Frieze of the Parthenon to His Friends*, 1868) to nearly 40 university students for 28.63 seconds.[10] After the image was switched off, they were asked to draw an outline of the painting, or describe it in words, noting setting, activities, and figures. They indicated whether they had seen the painting before (as this would impact on their memory of it). After time had been given for this, they were shown the picture again, with an AD. Significant observations were listed as missed during the initial viewing – even by those who stated that they had known the painting before. And the feedback was much more positive than I expected, as I had assumed that an AD would be considered too basic – however, the vast majority welcomed this feature. Extending the target audience for AD warrants future investigation.[11] For now, let us turn in more detail to the Parthenon.

The Parthenon

The Parthenon exemplifies classical Greek architecture and Athenian (or Pericles's) ambition. The building was constructed between 447 and 438 BC, using Pentelic marble, and took a further 7 years to finish. Built mainly in the Doric order, it had eight columns in total on the short sides, and seventeen on the north and south ones. The internal space was divided, with no way through between the larger chamber on the east for the statue of Athena and the smaller west treasury. It rested on a platform nearly 71 by 31 metres. It is famous for having no true horizontal or vertical lines, with architectural refinements that cannot be replicated in a museum setting (Jenkins 2006, 78–9).

The Parthenon's primary function was as home to the colossal chryselephantine (gold and ivory) statue of Athena Parthenos, which loomed 12 metres tall. She wore a peplos, aegis, and an elaborate helmet. A small Nike stood on the palm of her outstretched right hand, and her left grasped a shield resting on the baseline. The outside of this shield showed a fight between Greeks and female Amazons (Amazomachy); the inside portrayed a fight between gods and giants (Gigantomachy). Her sandals were decorated with a fight between northern Greek Lapiths and centaurs (Centauromachy).

These themes, along with the Trojan War, were the subjects selected for the building's metopes (west [14], east [14], south [32] and north [32], respectively: see Fig. 6.1b). The Doric frieze (consisting of metopes and triglyphs) lay on the outside of the building, below the pediments on the shorter east and west sides. At 1.2 metres high and 1.22–1.33 metres wide, the metopes were perfect spaces for compositions involving two figures in a variety of poses. They were sculpted in deep relief. The two pediments, or triangular gables, were decorated with two key events of Athena's life, her birth on the east pediment, sprung fully armed from the head of Zeus and, on the west pediment, her contest with Poseidon for the patronage of Athens. The sculptures are poorly preserved, but those that survive are exemplary examples of free-standing sculptures (carved in the round).

The internal, Ionic frieze was cut in low relief, running 160 metres around the inner band of the building some 12 metres above ground level. The outer colonnade therefore blocked its continuous view. This frieze showed a procession with more than 200 human figures and numerous animals, including a cavalcade, starting out in both directions from the south-west corner. It probably represented an idealised version of the Panathenaic (all-Athenian) procession; 'idealised', as some elements, such as horsemen, did not figure in the real parade. The Olympian gods framed the central scene on the eastern, most important side, the focus being on the folded cloth, probably the peplos given to the venerated ancient wooden statue of Athena. The British Museum possesses around 75 of the 160 metres of the frieze, 15 of the 92 metopes (from the south side), 17 figures from the two pediments, and various other pieces. Around half of the surviving sculptures are now in London.

The auxiliary rooms 18a and 18b

The Parthenon galleries in the British Museum comprise the main Duveen space (18) and two auxiliary areas (18a and 18b) and were purpose built for these artefacts (Fig. 6.1a). The presence of these sculptures in London is extremely controversial in itself (e.g. Beard 2010). Leaving this debate to one side, the British Museum was an innovator in creating a permanent space for blind and partially sighted people in the auxiliary rooms. Following feedback, over winter 2019–20, it revamped the spaces and made changes to the provision.[12]

Both auxiliary rooms (18a and 18b) are around 20 metres long by 4.5 metres wide (in the main section). Funded by generous American sponsors, Lawrence and Barbara Fleischman, they were refurbished in 1998 as part of the Tiresias Project. Room 18b was specifically curated with blind and partially sighted people in mind. The two most distinctive aspects of the room are the touch model of the Parthenon, complete with some Braille on the minimal labelling (e.g. 'west', 'north'), and the modern casts of the West Frieze, derived from Elgin's moulds of 1802. Over the winter of 2019–20, both rooms received an extensive makeover. Although fewer lights are used, the two rooms are now bathed in a stronger, clearer, more accessible light. It was always the intention for visitors to feel free to touch the plaster casts, which, in a museum setting, is highly unusual (see new information board Fig. 6.3, no. 1). Prior to this revamp, there was no notice stating that this was allowed.

Most of the information boards continue the same theme after the renovation, if simplified – so, for example, 'Polychromy: painted decoration' becomes 'Painted decoration', terms such as 'architrave' are removed, and the English

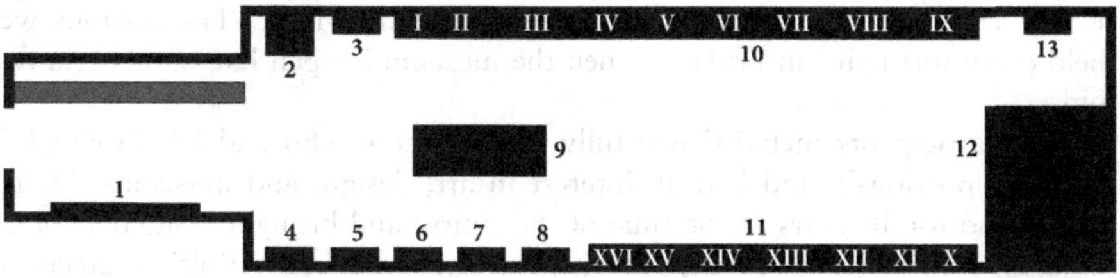

1a: The Parthenon Galleries
2a: Frieze crown
3a: Polychrony painted decoration
4a: The Panathenaic Way
5a: The Acropolis
6a: Plan of Parthenon
7a: The Parthenon Sculptures
8a: West Frieze of Parthenon
9a: Parthenon touch model
10a: Cast of the West Frieze (numbered blocks)
11a: Cast of the West Frieze (numbered blocks)
12a: Column top (with life sized reconstruction)
13a: The Doric Order of the Parthenon

1b: The Parthenon
2b: Frieze crown
3b: Painted decoration
4b: A festival procession
5b: The Acropolis
6b: The Parthenon
7b: The Parthenon Sculptures
8b: The Parthenon frieze
9b: Parthenon touch model
10b: Cast of the West Frieze (numbered blocks)
11b: Cast of the West Frieze (numbered blocks)
12b: Column top (with life sized reconstruction)
13b: The Doric Order of the Parthenon

Figure 6.3 Room 18b. The desk (in grey) by the entrance was removed in the revamp of 2019–20. The key shows the changes in information boards (pre-2020 on left, current on right); all were replaced apart from no. 13 (image by author)

has become more basic. Some visual information is no longer presented, such as the RLD plan of the Parthenon, which is perhaps surprising as the touch model does not allow investigation of the floorplan (the roof cannot be removed). On the original information boards, a Braille script was set beneath or 'behind' the English text; the new versions do not have these. A small proportion of blind and partially sighted people have learned Braille, but it is unclear how it can be used independently when inserted on boards like this (you need to be notified that it is there to be used). The labels for the blocks of casts are broadly similar, comprising a written description of the artwork positioned above. However, the RLD and bird's eye views of the original labels have not been included in the revamp (see, for example, Fig. 6.2). These were deemed unpopular by blind and partially sighted people, who were unable to distinguish the individual figures from the mass of detail, and the rationale for viewing it from above was unclear (see below for further discussion of RLDs).

AD and engaging with blind and partially sighted people

The Parthenon is an excellent case study to explore this chapter's key question – namely, what AD might contribute to art appreciation, with or without RLDs (the related research on touch tours and touch description will be presented elsewhere). A course comprising four afternoon sessions ran over the summer of 2019, and the small number of participants (three plus companions) allowed a very high level of qualitative feedback (and was necessary for access reasons, notably guiding).[13] It was intended to coincide with the revamping of

Room 18b, although this did not happen until the winter. The sessions were held every fortnight on Fridays, when the museum is open late and is relatively quiet.

The participants included one fully blind person, who had been sighted for 60 years previously and had an interest in art, design, and museums. He had been blind for 16 years at the time of the course and brought a sighted companion to each session. Another participant had advanced retinitis pigmentosa, but could perceive light and broad shapes. She was accompanied by a sighted companion. A further visually impaired person joined the group for one of the four sessions, without an access companion. This working-age participant was the only one who could read Braille (contracted Braille preferred – a code used by more experienced readers). This reflects the tendency for Braille users to be blind and partially sighted from a young age.

The first 90 minutes of each session was spent in the Study Room of the Department of Greece and Rome; then, after a break, tours of the galleries were conducted. The broad aims of the course were:

- To deliver an in-depth access course for blind and partially sighted people on the art, architecture, and history of the Parthenon
- To offer a range of speakers and types of audio tour (some delivered with touch tours, some with RLD, some seated in the study room, some in the galleries)
- To provide sessions of handling Greek antiquities, some with RLD to clarify images
- To explore the development of 'touch description' of materials and objects
- To consider how access activities may offer the 'viewer' a new way of seeing, or art appreciation

Following an introduction to the author's research project and the course, the first session introduced the city of Athens, the Panathenaic Festival, the Acropolis and the Parthenon. The author presented ADs with RLDs of the town, Acropolis, and Parthenon (plan and elevation). An RLD of the sculptural programme was also provided, in an attempt to convey the themes and locations of the three main spaces (pediments, metopes, and frieze). For the gallery tour, the group explored Room 18b. In addition to describing the space as a whole, this tour involved handling the touch model of the Parthenon and an AD of the cast of West Frieze Block 7. Participants were able to handle this block both during and after the AD.

In the second session, a professional audio describer presented an AD of Lawrence Alma-Tadema's *Phidias Showing the Frieze of the Parthenon to His Friends* (1868), with an accompanying RLD indicating the main features and selected figures. The session then explored touch description with pots.[14] An RLD was provided for a second AD of the start of the North Frieze in Room 18. This was followed by a tour of the frieze conducted by Ian Jenkins, Senior Curator at the British Museum.

The third session began exploring the tactile book based on the Parthenon frieze (Bird, Jenkins and Levi 1998). The session then focused on the East Frieze, offering RLDs of the figures described by Ian Jenkins in the previous session. The session continued with the development of touch description, noting that the previous sessions had focused on what was represented, rather than the overall feel of the material, size, and shape.[15] Two pots from the previous session were also recalled.[16] Various RLDs were presented with these objects, in order to illustrate the 2D images. A further pot, a Panathenaic amphora, was also handled.[17] A professional audio describer then gave a tour of the East Pediment and Metope XXXI.

The author began the fourth session with an outline of the history of the Parthenon after its initial life as a classical Greek temple. This set the scene for a professional audio describer (same as Session 2) to present an AD of Louis Dupré's painting, *Louis-François-Sébastien Fauvel before the Acropolis* (1819). Two RLDs were provided to accompany the verbal talk, and the depiction of Metope XXXI in the painting created a link to the previous session. The handling session included a revisit of the Panathenaic vase (BM 1849,1122.2), with a variety of accompanying RLDs. This was to check some issues that had arisen the previous session, in terms of the effectiveness of certain types of RLD, and whether the image should be presented as viewed on the pot or rolled out as though it were a standard 2D image. New objects were also handled, including bronze ones.[18] The course ended back in Room 18b, with a touch and audio tour of Blocks 5 and 10 of the West Frieze cast.

AD tours in galleries

The large space of Room 18 is not, at first impression, accessible for blind and partially sighted people. There is no touch opportunity, and the hard surfaces create a noisy, echoey environment. However, AD tours may occur in any museum space. Ian Jenkins, Senior Curator of the Parthenon sculptures, produced a 'real treat' of a tour around the frieze (see comments on musicality above). One of the participants added that 'his insights into the movement of the figures, the Gods and the various elements of the procession all helped to bring it alive'. Another participant added that it was a 'wonderfully engaging and entertaining description, laden with facts and deep knowledge', but added that, 'the lack of touch did inhibit my ability to create a mental image'. The storytelling offered rich insights into the background of the sculptures, beyond giving a simple outline of the visual composition.

A further AD was commissioned for this course for the East Pediment and Metope XXXI. The East Pediment, as so much Greek sculpture, poses problems owing to its fragmentary nature. When the early Christians converted the Parthenon into a church, the central part was completely removed (Beard 2010, 55). Some figures set in the corners survive, and a drawing by J. Carrey from

1674 depicts their slightly better state of preservation. Pausanias (1.24.5) tells us that the subject of this composition was the birth of Athena, who sprang fully armed from the head of Zeus. This topic is rare in classical art, and so there is no stock of comparisons to draw from. Numerous classical archaeologists have attempted to reconstruct the composition (Mostratos 2004).

The audio describer needs to set out sufficient context to empower the listener without sight, but at the same time is required to be highly selective to keep the talk within the recommended limit. What is meant by 'context' here? First, there is display context. How the object is positioned, what it is set next to, how it is lit, background colour, and so on. These factors influence the viewer's experience, whether they are aware of and consciously noting them or not. This contrasts greatly with the original display context of the painted sculptures, 12 metres above ground (e.g. Osborne 1987). Second, there is preservation context and thick visual description of the fragments in their current form (including what is missing), such as the AD on Helios on the East Pediment, where we are invited to imagine what must have once been there.[19] Third, we aim to reconstruct the full composition and identify individuals, establishing the narrative context. The reclining nude on the left is usually identified as Dionysus, for example, through the imagined reconstruction of a raised cup. The process of formulating an AD helps to break down the different levels of reconstruction, or the different layers of identification and interpretation.

The process of setting out an AD also brings home how we can only describe what has survived. In this particular case, visibility plays an unexpected role in preservation. The metopes were badly damaged when the Parthenon was turned into a Christian Church, as the pagan iconography fell out of favour, and the structure needed to be culturally 'cleansed'. But the south side was less visited, being near the edge of the citadel, and less attacked – and so these were the sculptures Lord Elgin decided to take back to England. It seems that the best preserved metopes are such because they were originally the least visible. What is seen and appreciated relies on numerous factors.

During this tour, the audio describer would suddenly pounce upon new observations made on the spot. In discussion afterwards, he commented that the process of describing resulted in fresh insights, however well prepared he had been. Indeed, this was expected and enjoyed by the listeners – all were on a shared journey of discovery. AD is, therefore, a process, rather than a set destination or script. One participant stated that they were able to 'generate a mental image' from the words of the describer. But this description also articulated rich details that could easily be missed by all. Taking Metope XXXI, for example, the detail of the 'tiny indentation' of the centaur's thumb in the Lapith's throat was articulated. How many sighted visitors would perceive this fine feature? The centaur's front legs are vividly and richly described as 'snaked around the Lapith's right leg, intertwined and locked in battle'. The process of noticing and expressing has the potential to engage and inform sighted people as well as those who need AD for access.

Raised line drawings (RLDs) in reconstructions

This course used various kinds of RLDs alongside the spoken information and background context. RLDs used in this way were originally felt, by sighted people, to provide a straightforward replacement for sight. This provision has been described as 'an optical prosthesis in which the experienced hand can extend to read the representation' for blind and partially sighted people (Hetherington 2003, 112), rather than haptic access. In other words, they seek to replace information lost because of the sight impairment, rather than take advantage of and enrich other compensating senses (although, as discussed above, sighted people might enjoy such tactile confirmation of the visual). An understandable reaction against the assumption that the blind can 'see with their hands' has perhaps triggered a pendulum swing to the other extreme and a complete rejection of this format. The course explored whether there remains potential for RLDs with AD on three scales: archaeological (or urban), architectural or sculptural (3D objects), and pictorial (2D images).[20]

The RLDs used for geographical space, namely the Athenian urban area and the layout of the Acropolis, were less successful than those for smaller-scale monuments or paintings. The scale is zoomed so far out that the image has to be extremely simplified, or the mass of detail is too muddled for fingertips to decipher. RLDs in this context may only be used with personalised AD, preferably with hand guidance over the RLD. This means that RLDs offer no gain in independence; the question is whether there is a gain in understanding.[21] In terms of the problem of zooming, one participant stated:

> When I see the big objects such as architecture, things or monuments which contain many parts and each part has different details, I am trying to make the whole image as well. Once I understand the small parts, I'd like to try to connect them to get [the] image closer to the real thing that the sighted see. So I need more time to think of the connection of the parts in relation to each other, of course I'd like to know the detail of each part as well.

Similar feedback was given for the RLD of the Acropolis, containing the Parthenon with other structures.

This comment indicates the main problem with sensing maps via touch alone: the fingers only detect particular sections each time, whereas sight can relate the particulars to the whole in a much more immediate manner. Helen Keller (2009 [1908], 8), who was both deaf and blind, stated something similar:

> My fingers cannot, of course, get the impression of a large whole at a glance; but I feel the parts, and my mind puts them together ... The process reminds me of the building of Solomon's temple, where was neither saw, nor hammer, nor any tool heard while the stones were being laid one upon another. The silent worker is imagination which decrees reality out of chaos.

This 'distal knowledge' at a distance is established by representational practice (Hetherington 2003, 105–6). Perhaps this is particularly appropriate for a monument with numerous architectural refinements to 'correct' certain abnormalities as seen from a distance. But this blind experience also demonstrates the potential that our imagination has in terms of reconstructing the world, and it is unclear whether seeing and the representational have a much closer relationship than touch and the representational (contra Hetherington 2003, 106).

A further limitation of RLDs is that it is difficult to decipher objects with depth of field and overlapping composites, such as the sculptures of the frieze. The distinctive materiality is not represented as it would be when actual objects were touched; haptic engagement with objects allows structural perception of shape and size (Klatzky et al. 2003). An RLD of the centre of the East Frieze, which had the benefit of being a relatively simple composition – at first glance, anyway – was presented to the group. One participant stated that, 'the raised line drawings were a challenge for me, especially with the overlapping images'. For clarification, overlying figures, such as Hermes/Dionysus and Aphrodite/Eros were presented as separated entities. Even this only worked with AD ('I found these raised line drawings very accessible in conjunction with the audio description'), and at times guidance is needed to navigate around the raised image. Although the use of the product may have limitations, the process of setting out this kind of composition as an RLD brings out useful insights – especially with this case study.

The viewing of the Parthenon frieze raises many conundrums. Just how visible was this to the viewer, and how is the spatial arrangement between humans and deities to be understood? Are the gods meant to be positioned among the humans, or overlooking from Olympos? Are they even noticing and appreciating the central focus of the East Frieze, which shows the handing over of the peplos? Dionysus (second from left) is the only deity who is sitting facing the peplos scene (and not the procession), but even he is twisted back to speak with Hermes. Aphrodite actively points out the arriving convoy to Eros, which suggests a lack of interest in the peplos group, and, on the far-left side, Hermes likewise faces the procession. Neils (1999, 12) outlines the 'ingenious explanations' that scholars have offered for this set-up: the gods are invisible, there but not-there; the peplos ceremony is taking place within the monument, and so out of sight; this is not actually Athena's peplos. None of these seems satisfactory, so we should conceive different spatial placements from those set out here (for example, Smith 1908, 68, Fig. 24).

Figure 6.4 represents the scene as imagined in real space, rather than the idealised space of the actual frieze. Rather than interrupting the two sets of gods, the five mortals (with peplos) are placed in front of the row of gods in the background. The gods are arranged in a semicircle, as in a theatre, to oversee all the proceedings – including both procession and peplos scene. However, this is not a perfect semi-circular line. As the British Museum's AD of Zeus and

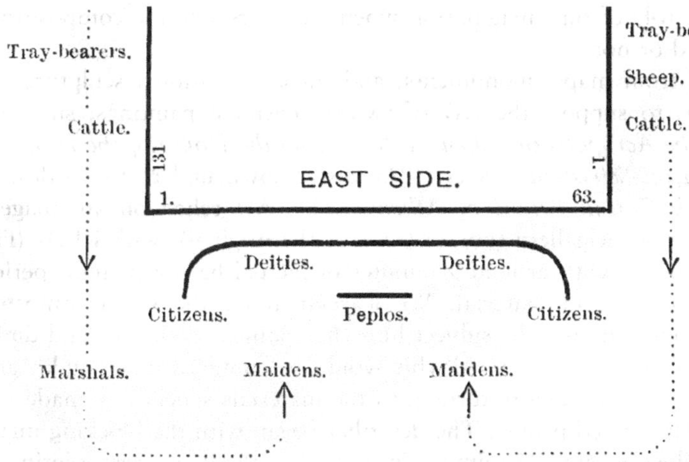

4a

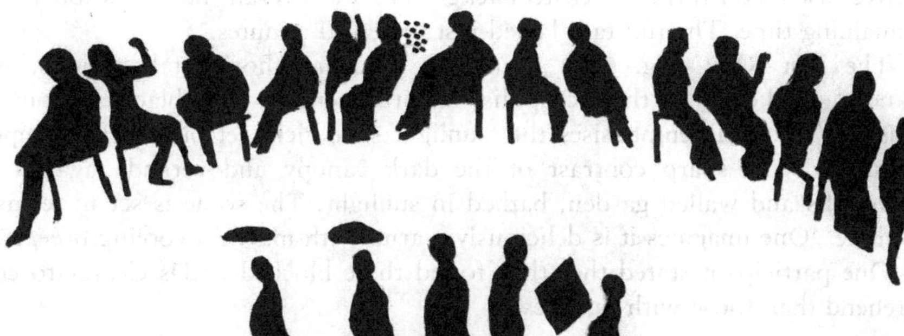

4b

Figure 6.4 Reconstructions of the central part of the East Frieze of the Parthenon. 6.4a: Smith (1908, 68, Fig. 24), followed by Neils (1999). 6.4b: Raised line drawing by author, after Nakamura (2016, 58, Fig. 5 bottom)

Hera points out, Zeus's throne 'is placed nearer to us than Hera's stool, giving the impression that their seats are really side by side' (British Museum n.d.d, Soundcloud 152). This would carry the sense of a train carriage, shunting out in both directions from the centre, rather than a single row of figures. The Parthenon Project Japan further explored the facial expressions and lines of vision between the gods, which suggested narrative dialogues between the figures (Nakamura 2016, 54). This attempt to make conceptual, narrative sense of such a layout shifts some way from the representative sculpture itself. Does it matter? This process certainly raises questions about what we see, how we see it, and the role of our imagination when we appreciate the composition, whether sighted or not.

Moving from maps, monuments, and three-dimensional sculpture, we also used RLDs to support the AD of two-dimensional paintings, such as Louis Dupré's *The Acropolis of Athens as Seen from the House of the French Consul Louis-François-Sébastien Fauvel* (1825; also known under other titles, such as *The French Consul Fauvel at Athens*). This AD relied on an image of the painting (so not a gallery tour in front of the original), with RLDs (Fig. 6.5). The talk opened with around 9 minutes of factual basics: painter, period, title (which version), and material. We learned about the wider atmosphere of French colonialism and the subject himself – painter, collector, and diplomat – and why he was in Athens. All this would be standard in an audio guide for mainstream visitors, before turning to the materials specifically made for blind and partially sighted people. The describer began with the blocking image (Fig. 6.5a) and then, around 17 minutes in, turned to the image representing key figures (Fig. 6.5b). At around 30 minutes, the AD was complete, and the interactive discussion turned back to background and overall interpretation for the remaining time. The full talk lasted just under 40 minutes.

The first RLD (Fig. 6.5a) represents the three horizontal sections, with canopy, backdrop of the Acropolis, and the veranda (the black sections are raised). The RLD emphasises the 'sunlight sandwich' set out in the composition, with the sharp contrast of the dark canopy and veranda against the Acropolis and walled garden, bathed in sunlight. The scene is set in terms of climate: 'One imagines it is deliciously warm, with maybe a cooling breeze ...'.

One participant stated that they found these blocked RLDs clearer to comprehend than those with outlines:

> Where this is done I also find some variations to the surface texture could be helpful in representing different items or materials. Smooth for skin or stone and textured for fur or grass for example. However, this should not be overdone, say no more than 4 to 5 surface finishes in any one drawing and consistency would also be vital.

In this case, the dark/light contrast was clear, but other key distinctions could have been rendered – the hard stone of the veranda with the soft foliage behind, for example. The emphasis on light contrast is natural to a sighted person, but the observations of this individual is a useful reminder that other shades and hues, primarily centred on touch, are also important. Being invited to notice and articulate these kinds of features enhances the sighted person's engagement as well. However, another participant (completely blind, late in life) had trouble visualising anything from RLD touch. He did not feel that other ways of indicating the zones (such as using fabrics of different kinds) would necessarily enhance the experience.

Having laid out the main components of the painting, around 17 minutes in we turn to the second drawing, which has key details and figures outlined or

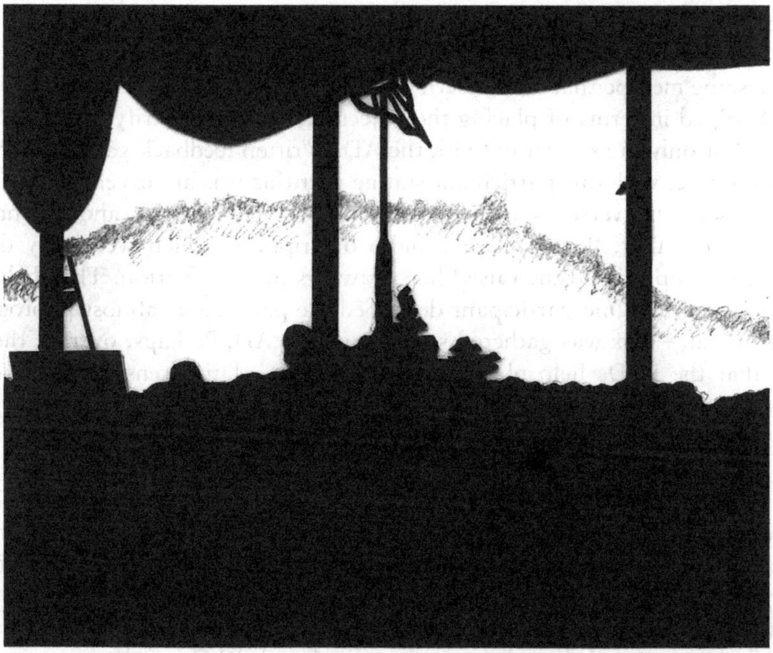

5a

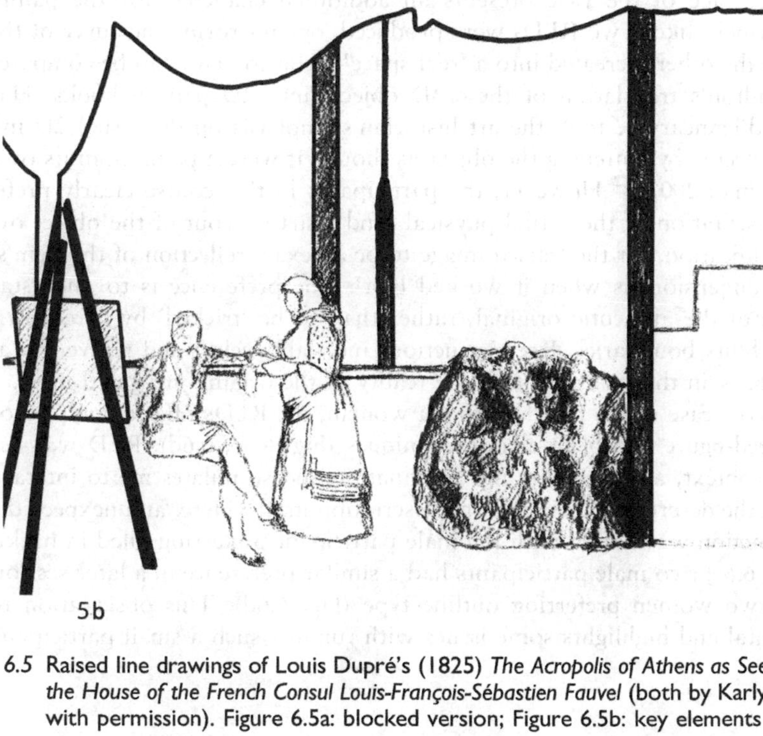

5b

Figure 6.5 Raised line drawings of Louis Dupré's (1825) *The Acropolis of Athens as Seen from the House of the French Consul Louis-François-Sébastien Fauvel* (both by Karly Allen, with permission). Figure 6.5a: blocked version; Figure 6.5b: key elements blocked out (e.g. posts and the tripod legs). Included is Metope XXXI, described as mirroring the two human figures in compositional terms if not tone (this is the same metope that was described in the gallery tour discussed above). This RLD helped in terms of placing the objects in space, or clarifying the composition – but only in association with the AD. Written feedback gathered later was very positive, with one participant stating that this was an 'excellent description and raised line versions assist with scale, image location and orientation'. Another felt that, 'I enjoyed the audio descriptions which were very detailed and really appreciated the raised line drawings in combination. They helped me form a picture.' One participant described the painting as almost photographic in the detail – this was gathered solely from the AD. Perhaps, overall, the sense was that the RLDs help place the features in a relative sense, but the overall sensory experience is mainly drawn out from the AD.

Handling Greek pots: 3D to 2D to 3D

Greek vases are 3D objects with 2D images, and the latter pose a challenge for blind and partially sighted people. One participant stated: 'Amazing to be able to touch these delicate, centuries old pieces, but wouldn't have been able to make out images without audio description'. Several pots were handled initially just as they are, and then they were revisited with RLDs of the image.

One of the vases was a Panathenaic vase (Figs. 6.6a, 6.6b). The curvature of the surface of the vase presents an additional challenge for the painter and describer alike. Two RLDs were produced, one mirroring the curve of the vase, with the other recreated into a 'real space' scenario. This can be compared with Hamilton's translation of these 3D objects into 2D pattern books. Hamilton and d'Hancarville took the art historian's emphasis on the visual 2D image to an extreme by flattening the object as though it were a painting in its own right (Coltman 2001).[22] However, the participants in this course clearly preferred a representation of the actual physical (and visual) layout of the object over this simplification, for the 'raised image to be an exact reflection of the item's shape and dimension, is when it worked best'. The preference is to understand the state of the authentic original, rather than to be 'tricked' by a reconstruction that blurs boundaries. Reconstructions inevitably select and reinvent – and the feedback in this case was that the reality of the original mattered most.

In the case of the pot depicting a woman, the RLDs offer a comparison with the red-figure and black-figure techniques (Fig. 6.6c, 6.6d). RLD was useful in this context, as it 'triggers my imagination and stimulates me to interact more with the described object and the description itself'. Here, an unexpected gender distinction was noted, with the male participant preferring filled-in background (Fig. 6.6c; two male participants had a similar preference in a later session), and the two women preferring outline type (Fig. 6.6d). This observation is coincidental and highlights some issues with running such a small participant base.

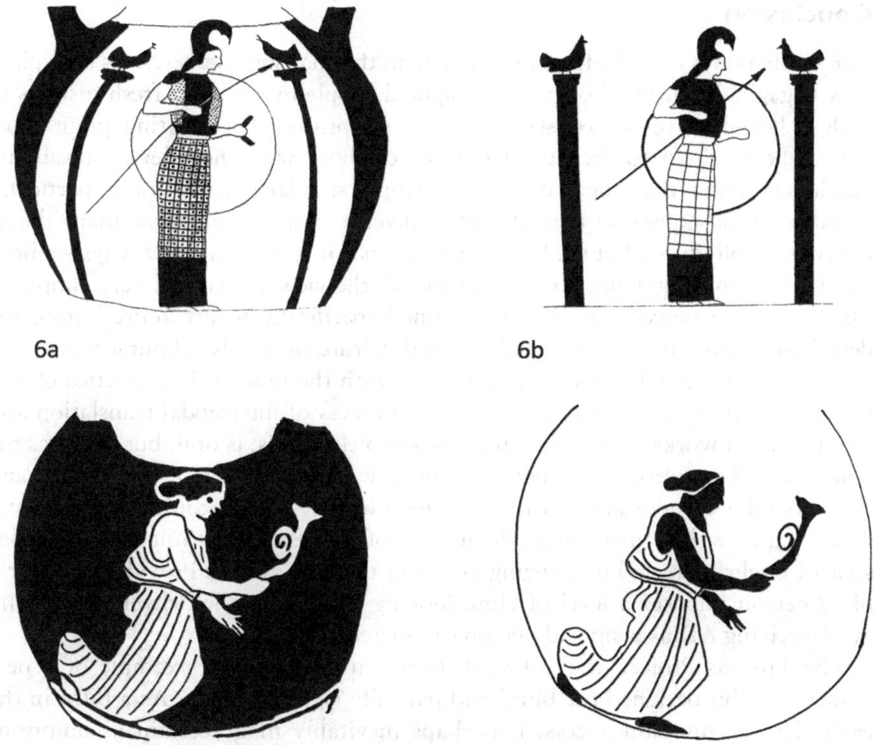

Figure 6.6 Top: Panathenaic black-figure amphora with image of Athena between two columns with cocks, c.550 BC, 35.56-cm high (BM 1849,1122.2). 6.6a: raised line drawing (RLD) as image is perceived on pot. 6.6b: RLD of composition as would be perceived in real space. 6.6c and 6.6d: RLDs of Attic black-figure lekythos with image of girl holding plant, 430–400 BC, 8.89-cm high (BM 1864,1007.1681). Images by author

For all participants, the triangulation of object handling, AD, and RLD combined to create a strong sense of the pot and image; an AD of the image was required simultaneously. One participant (a Braille user) stated:

> I fully enjoyed touching the real pots and tactile images while listening to the description, I could make an image of the pot in my head putting the tactile image on the surface of the pot because I can feel the size and the surface of the pot. But even though I have tactile image, the audio description is essential because it is difficult to interpret the tactile image without description. Thus the best option is touching and listening to the description at the same time.

Conclusion

The Parthenon is a world-famous monument; the challenge set here was to explore how engaging with blind or partially sighted people might bring fresh insights to such a heavily investigated structure and sculptures. The starting point must always be to listen to the personal voice of those with the relevant disability, bearing in mind that there can be no single standard-bearer for a particular impairment, as experiences are always so diverse. Not only are there many different types of blindness, but the brain also responds in a wide range of ways – a brief overview of this highlights that the theme of 'the viewer' masks a very simplistic idea of human perception. We then turned specifically to art appreciation, the description and criticism of visual/material culture in words. Ekphrasis has long been a key theme in Classics, and engaging with the modern live practice of AD provides an innovative angle into how this process of intermodal translation and interpretation works. AD, unlike most modern ekphrasis, is oral, but it shares the tendency to be multisensory (not completely wedded to the visual). Context and background are important to various degrees in AD, as they contribute to mental modelling as well as providing information of interest. Overall, it is a particular style of English directed to bringing artworks to life in words. Providing AD for a blind person imposes a level of close looking that serves the deliverer well, and even receiving AD as a sighted person can increase engagement.

The Tiresias Project at the British Museum offers a rare example of a permanent exhibit designed for blind and partially sighted people. As a pilot in the early days of museum access, it perhaps inevitably made certain assumptions about what this group would want. Most notably, the recent revamp removed the new perspectives such as raised line bird's eye views of the compositions, as these were not working as intended. Indeed, this project's course indicated that RLDs of urban and building plans were too complex to be of use. However, those of paintings (on canvas or pots), presented with an AD, did increase appreciation of the art. The case of the centre of the East Frieze is particularly interesting, as the composition appears to be a slightly abstract rendering of the deities, so that they are the audience of the procession but also central, given their status. The process of describing and reconstructing the figures in other modes (audio and RLD) necessitates a careful consideration of the sculptor's intentions at this point. This multisensory learning has the potential to appeal to blind, partially sighted, and sighted people alike. It is a legal obligation to provide this kind of access, but there may be more scope to adjust mainstream provision rather than segregate all such provision. Collectively, we may reflect on how we appreciate art, and the slippery, subjective nature of vision.

Notes

1 Many thanks to all participants involved in this project based at the British Museum, and to Ian Jenkins, Senior Curator of the Parthenon Galleries, for feedback on this chapter. Ian was committed to opening access to blind people, as his involvement in

the Tiresias Project testifies. I was greatly saddened to learn of his recent death and dedicate this chapter to his memory.

2 Steiner (1982, 1) references the need for analogy, metaphor, and models in science and philosophy, which 'allows a system to be explored in depth or a notion to be followed in all its relations and implications, even if these tend to undermine the original thrust of the iconic formulation'. However, a purely etic approach to establishing this device (i.e. without engaging with disabled people) will only serve to impose assumptions as confirmation bias – such comparisons are ultimately hollow and circular.

3 Borrowed from 'Deaf Gain', this recognises and celebrates the perspective granted from having a sensory impairment – notably the development of sign language by Deaf people, and a more acute sense of touch and other senses by blind people.

4 Much has been made of the difference between poetry and painting, notably Lessing's distinction between the space of paintings and the temporality of linear poetry (e.g. Grethlein 2017; Steiner 1982, 41). Lack of space prevents further discussion here.

5 Mitchell (1994, 161) makes a rare reference to sign languages, however.

6 Observing and drawing from modern activities can be productive; see, for example, Grethlein's (2017, 25–9) discussion of Kendall Walton's consideration of child play and make believe in the process of aesthetic experience.

7 See also her statement (Webb 2016, 213) that powerful ekphrasis does more than describe: it provokes empathy and evokes the other senses.

8 Some 29 ADs of Parthenon sculptures may be found on the British Museum Soundcloud (British Museum n.d.b).

9 They do not mention the sighted companions who often accompany blind and partially sighted people to events and, in fact, enable the visit to happen. One survey on 30 blind and partially sighted people's experiences of museums found that 28 of the respondents (93%) were not confident enough to travel to museums independently, especially on public transport (Pereira 2009, 12). Further research is required to discover what these sighted companions get out of the experience of AD events.

10 This strangely precise time limit was selected as this is the mean average time people look at a painting (and label) in art galleries (Smith, Smith and Tinio 2017).

11 Some museums are opening up to the idea of slow looking. For example, the National Gallery in London runs a 'picture of the month club' and 'a long look' sessions that involve slow explorations of single artworks (with comparisons). It also conducts free talk-and-draw events, whereby people can listen, learn, and reproduce.

12 It has been suggested, without evidence, that 'the British Museum have [sic] chosen to respond to question of access rather than address head on the issue of rightful custodianship' (Hetherington 2003, 110). However, it remains a rare example of a mainstream, permanent space designed for this target audience, and it feels unhelpful and possibly damaging to frame efforts for providing access as cynical virtue signalling.

13 The course was free for all participants, but King's College London provided funding to pay for three AD talks, and a KCL personal research allowance enabled the author to buy a Zyfuse machine and swell paper for RLDs. A KCL research ethics minimal risk form was logged, and participants were sent this chapter to further check consent.

14 BM 1814,0704.484; BM 1922,0512.1; BM 1864,1007.1681.

15 For this reason, the marble lower face of a male head (BM 1927,0214.2) and the limestone lower part of a female standing figure (BM 1886, 0401.1387) were recalled.

16 The Corinthian aryballos (BM 1814,0704.484) and the Squat lekythos (BM 1864,1007.1681).

17 BM 1849,1122.2.

18 BM 1951,0606.9; BM 1867,0508.788; BM 1842,0728.774.

19 'His head is missing, so all that remains of him are his neck, his shoulders, his arms. You might be able to appreciate this better if you are facing the display end on. Helios' hands originally held reins that connected with the horses. We are invited to imagine him and his chariot, drawn by four horses, two of which are shown here, emerging out of the sea ahead of him' (British Museum n.d.e). The describer then refers to the waves on Helios's shoulders, which could never have been seen from the original ground-level context.

20 RLDs are made using swell paper, or microcapsule paper. This has a layer of plastic that contains tiny bubbles of alcohol. The drawing must contain carbon, and the paper is then passed through an infrared heating device. The alcohol bubbles expand under the carbon and so they rise.

21 Canada initiated a tactile mapping programme in 1998, employing audio-tactile maps (Siekierska et al. 2003). Projects have been conducted internationally to aid blind and partially sighted people to navigate unfamiliar space independently. As so few blind and partially sighted people know Braille, audio labels are needed.

22 Josiah Wedgwood was then inspired to transfer these 2D engravings on to 3D neo-classical pots, turning full circle. Hamilton and d'Hancarville were keen to increase the visibility of Greek pots, so often buried in private collections, by dissemination and publication (Coltman 2001, 1). This is another layer of visibility and accessibility that needs to be explored.

References

Adams, Ellen (2019) 'The psychology of prostheses: substitution strategies and notions of normality.' In Jane Draycott (ed.), *Prostheses in Antiquity*. Abingdon and New York: Routledge, 180–208.

Barry, Susan (2009) *Fixing My Gaze: A Scientist's Journey into Seeing in Three Dimensions*. New York: Basic Books.

Bartsch, Shadi and Jaś Elsner (2007) 'Eight ways of looking at an ekphrasis.' *Classical Philology* 102, i–vi.

Beard, Mary (2010) *The Parthenon*. London: Profile Books.

Bell, Matthew (2018) *The Essential Goethe*. Princeton and Oxford: Princeton University Press.

Bilman, Emily (2013) *Modern Ekphrasis*. Bern: Peter Lang.

Bird, Susan, Ian Jenkins and Fabio Levi (1998) *Second Sight of the Parthenon Frieze*. Turin: British Museum Press in association with Silvio Zamorani editore.

Braun, Sabine (2007) 'Audio Description from a discourse perspective: a socially relevant framework for research and training.' *Linguistica Antverpiensia* NS(6), 357–69.

British Museum (n.d.a) Soundcloud 166. https://soundcloud.com/britishmuseum/parthenon-speeding-chariot-audio-description?in=britishmuseum/sets/audio-descriptions (accessed 2 February 2020).

British Museum (n.d.b) Soundcloud. www.soundcloud.com/britishmuseum/sets/audio-descriptions (accessed 2 February 2020).

British Museum (n.d.c) Soundcloud 185. https://soundcloud.com/britishmuseum/parthenon-horseman-audio-description?in=britishmuseum/sets/audio-descriptions (accessed 2 February 2020).

British Museum (n.d.d) Soundcloud 152. https://soundcloud.com/britishmuseum/parthenon-east-frieze-audio-description (accessed 2 February 2020).

British Museum (n.d.e) Soundcloud 183. https://soundcloud.com/britishmuseum/parthenon-helios-audio-description (accessed 2 February 2020).

Cachia, Amanda (2017) 'Curating new openings: rethinking diversity in the gallery.' *Art Journal* 76(3–4), 48–50.

Cavallo, Amelia (2015) 'Seeing the word, hearing the image: the artistic possibilities of audio description in theatrical performance.' *RiDE: The Journal of Applied Theatre and Performance* 20, 125–34.

Cheeke, Stephen (2008) *Writing for Art: The Aesthetics of Ekphrasis*. Manchester: Manchester University Press.

Coltman, Viccy (2001) 'Sir William Hamilton's vase publications (1766–1776): a case study in the reproduction and dissemination of antiquity.' *Journal of Design History* 14, 1–16.

Davidson, Michael (2008) *Concerto for the Left Hand: Disability and the Defamiliar Body*. Ann Arbor: University of Michigan Press.

Eardley, Alison, Louise Fryer, Rachel Hutchinson, Matthew Cock, Peter Ride and Joselia Neves (2017) 'Enriched audio description: working towards an inclusive museum experience.' In Santoshi Halder and Lori Czop Assaf (eds), *Inclusion, Disability and Culture: An Ethnographic Perspective Traversing Abilities and Challenges*. Cham, Switzerland: Springer, 195–207.

Fryer, Louise (2016) *An Introduction to Audio Description: A Practical Guide*. Abingdon and New York: Routledge.

Fryer, Louise (2017) 'Psycholinguistics and perception in audiovisual translation.' In Luis Pérez-González (ed.), *The Routledge Handbook of Audiovisual Translation*. London and New York: Routledge. https://www.taylorfrancis.com/chapters/psycholinguistics-perception-audiovisual-translation-louise-fryer/e/10.4324/9781315717166-14

Ginley, Barry (2013) 'Museums: a whole new world for visually impaired people.' *Disability Studies Quarterly* 33, https://dsq-sds.org/article/view/3761/0

Grethlein, Jonas (2017) *Aesthetic Experiences and Classical Antiquity: The Significance of Form in Narratives and Pictures*. Cambridge: Cambridge University Press.

Heffernan, James (1993) *Museum of Words: The Poetics of Ekphrasis from Homer to Ashbery*. Chicago: Chicago University Press.

Heffernan, James (2006) *Cultivating Picturacy: Visual Art and Verbal Interventions*. Waco, TX: Baylor University Press.

Hetherington, Kevin (2003) 'Accountability and disposal: visual impairment and the museum.' *Museum and Society* 1(2), 104–15.

Hull, John (1990) *Touching the Rock: An Experience of Blindness*. London: Society for Promoting Christian Knowledge.

Hutchinson, Rachel and Alison Eardley (2019) 'Museum audio description: the problem of textual fidelity.' *Perspectives* 27, 42–57.

Incalcaterra McLoughlin, Laura (2017) 'Audiovisual translation in language teaching and learning.' In Luis Pérez-González (ed.), *The Routledge Handbook of Audiovisual Translation*. London and New York: Routledge. https://www.taylorfrancis.com/chapters/audiovisual-translation-language-teaching-learning-laura-incalcaterra-mcloughlin/e/10.4324/9781315717166-3

Jenkins, Ian (1994) *The Parthenon Frieze*. London: British Museum Press.

Jenkins, Ian (2006) *Greek Architecture and its Sculpture*. Cambridge, MA: Harvard University Press.

Keller, Helen (2005 [1902]) *The Story of My Life*. New York: Bantam Dell.

Keller, Helen (2009 [1908]) *The World I Live In*. Cabin John, MD: Wideside Press.

Klatzky, Roberta, Jack Loomis, Susan Lederman, Hiromi Wake and Naofumi Fujita (2003) 'Haptic identification of objects and their depictions.' *Perception and Psychophysics* 54, 170–8.

Kleege, Georgina (2006) *Letters to Helen Keller*. Washington, DC: Gallaudet University Press.

Kleege, Georgina (2016) 'Audio description described: current standards, future innovations, larger implications.' *Representations* 135, 89–101.

Marcus, Sharon, Heather Love and Stephen Best (2016) 'Building a better description.' *Representations* 135, 1–21.

Masland, Richard (2020) *We Know It When We See It: What the Neurobiology of Vision Tells Us About How We Think*. New York: Basic Books.

Maszerowska, Anna, Anna Matamala and Pilar Orero (eds) (2014) *Audio Description: New Perspectives Illustrated*. Amsterdam and Philadelphia: John Benjamins.

Matamala, Anna and Pilar Orero (eds) (2016) *Researching Audio Description: New Approaches*. London: Palgrave Macmillan.

Merleau-Ponty, Maurice (2002) *Phenomenology of Perception*. Translated by Colin Smith. London and New York: Routledge.

Mitchell, William J.T. (1994) *Picture Theory*. Chicago: Chicago University Press.

Mostratos, Georgios (2004) 'A reconstruction of the Parthenon's East Pediment.' In Michael Cosmopoulos (ed.), *The Parthenon and Its Sculptures*. Cambridge: Cambridge University Press, 114–49.

Nakamura, Rui (2016) 'A 3-D recreation of the gods on the Parthenon Frieze: the bodies and space of the "invisibles".' In Toshihiro Osada (ed.), *The Parthenon Frieze: The Ritual Communication between the Goddess and the Polis*. Vienna: Phoibos, 49–59.

Neils, Jenifer (1999) 'Configuring the gods in the Parthenon frieze.' *The Art Bulletin* 81, 6–20.

Neves, Josélia (2012) 'Multi-sensory approaches to (audio) describing the visual arts.' *Monografías de Traducción e InterpretaciónI* 4, 277–93.

Ofcom (2000) 'ITC guidance on standards for audio description.' http://audiodescription.co.uk/uploads/general/itcguide_sds_audio_desc_word3.pdf

Osborne, Robin (1987) 'The viewing and obscuring of the Parthenon frieze.' *Journal of Hellenic Studies* 107, 98–105.

Patterson, Mark (2016) *Seeing with the Hands: Blindness, Vision, and Touch after Descartes*. Edinburgh: Edinburgh University Press.

Perego, Elisa (2018) 'Audio description: evolving recommendations for usable, effective and enjoyable practices.' In Luis Pérez-González (ed.), *The Routledge Handbook of Audiovisual Translation*. London and New York: Routledge, 114–29.

Perego, Elisa (2019) 'Into the language of museum audio descriptions: a corpus-based study.' *Perspectives* 27, 333–49.

Pereira, Eulalia (2009) 'Feasibility study into the potential contribution of VocalEyes' services for museums, galleries and heritage sites.' http://www.culturehive.co.uk/wp-content/uploads/2013/05/VocalEyes_-_Visual_Arts_Research_Study_1-2.pdf (accessed 16 April 2019).

Pérez-González, Luis (2014) *Audiovisual Translation: Theories, Methods and Issues*. London and New York: Routledge.

Remael, Aline, Nina Reviers and Gert Vercauteren (2015) 'Introduction: basic audio description concepts.' In Aline Remael, Nina Reviers and Gert Vercauteren (eds),

Pictures Painted in Words: ADLAB Audio Description Guidelines. Trieste: Trieste University, 9–18.

Sacks, Oliver (2010) *The Mind's Eye*. London: Picador.

Scott, Grant F. (1990) 'Beautiful ruins: the Elgin Marbles sonnet in its historical and generic contexts.' *Keats-Shelley Journal* 39, 123–50.

Siekierska, Eva, Richard Labelle, Louis Brunet, Bill McCurdy, Peter Pulsifer, Monika Rieger and Linda O'Neil (2003) 'Enhancing spatial learning and mobility training of visually impaired people – a technical paper on the internet-based tactile and audio-tactile mapping.' *The Canadian Geographer* 47, 480–93.

Smith, Arthur (1908) *A Guild to the Sculptures of the Parthenon in the British Museum*. London: British Museum Press.

Smith, Lisa, Jeffrey Smith and Pablo Tinio (2017) 'Time spent viewing art and reading labels.' *Psychology of Aesthetics, Creativity and the Arts* 11, 77–85.

Snyder, Joel (2008) 'Audio description: the visual made verbal.' In Jorge Díaz-Cintas (ed.), *The Didactics of Audiovisual Translation*. Amsterdam and Philadelphia: John Benjamins, 191–8.

Snyder, Joel (2014) *The Visual Made Verbal. A Comprehensive Training Manual and Guide to the History and Applications of Audio Descriptions*. Arlington, VA: American Council of the Blind.

Squire, Michael (2009) *Image and Text in Graeco-Roman Antiquity*. Cambridge: Cambridge University Press.

Squire, Michael (2010) 'Making Myron's cow moo? Ecphrastic epigram and the poetics of simulation.' *American Journal of Philology* 131, 589–634.

Squire, Michael (2015) *Ecphrasis: Visual and Verbal Interactions in Greek and Latin Literature*. Oxford Handbooks Online. https://www.oxfordhandbooks.com/view/10.1093/oxfordhb/9780199935390.001.0001/oxfordhb-9780199935390-e-58

Squire, Michael (2016) 'Introductory reflections: making sense of ancient sight.' In Michael Squire (ed.), *Sight and the Ancient Senses*. London and New York: Routledge, 1–35.

Steiner, Wendy (1982) *The Colors of Rhetoric: Problems in the Relation between Modern Language and Painting*. Chicago and London: Chicago University Press.

Webb, Ruth (1999) 'Ekphrasis ancient and modern: the invention of a genre.' *Word and Image* 15, 7–18.

Webb, Ruth (2016) 'Sight and insight: theorizing vision, emotion and imagination in ancient rhetoric.' In Michael Squire (ed.), *Sight and the Ancient Senses*. London and New York: Routledge, 205–19.

[illegible] Revisited in Wonder. [illegible] [illegible] [illegible]

Sassoon, [illegible] (20[illegible]) The [illegible]. London: [illegible].

[illegible] (19[illegible]) [illegible] and the Elgin Marbles [illegible]. [illegible] 29: 12[illegible]–30.

[illegible], [illegible] Laurence, Louis [illegible], [illegible] McCurdy, Peter Poloing, Alenka [illegible] and Linda O'Neil (2013) 'Unfinished [illegible] [illegible] mapping [illegible] [illegible] The Canadian Geographer [illegible]

Smith, [illegible] (19[illegible]) Guide to the [illegible] [illegible]. London: British School at Rome.

Smith, [illegible] Smith and [illegible] (20[illegible]) [illegible] and reading [illegible] [illegible] [illegible] [illegible]

[illegible], [illegible] (20[illegible]) '[illegible] [illegible] [illegible] [illegible] [illegible]' in [illegible] and [illegible] [illegible] [illegible] [illegible] Press.

[illegible] [illegible]

[illegible] (20[illegible]) [illegible] [illegible] [illegible] [illegible] bridge University Press.

Squire, Michael (20[illegible]) '[illegible] [illegible] [illegible] of [illegible]' [illegible] 131: [illegible]–631.

Squire, Michael (20[illegible]) [illegible] and Verbal [illegible] [illegible] [illegible] Books [illegible]

Squire, Michael (20[illegible]) [illegible] [illegible] [illegible] [illegible] [illegible] London and New York: [illegible]

[illegible] (19[illegible]) The [illegible] of [illegible] Problem [illegible] [illegible] and [illegible] [illegible] [illegible] [illegible]

[illegible], Ruth (20[illegible]) [illegible] [illegible]

[illegible], Ruth (20[illegible]) '[illegible] sight and [illegible] the [illegible] [illegible] and [illegible] in [illegible]' in [illegible] [illegible] and the Ancient Senses. London and New York: Routledge, [illegible]

Part 3

Real bodies and retrieving senses: Disability in the ritual record

Ellen Adams

Part 3 follows the museum context of Chapters 5 and 6 and considers archaeology's distinctive data set, acknowledging its different trajectory from mainstream Classics. The following two chapters consider ritual engagements at a Roman sanctuary and unusual burial practices across a wide temporal span in the Greek world. Both also draw from literary sources where appropriate, following the interdisciplinary nature of classical archaeology. The comparisons do not end there.

Both chapters explore the ritual sphere, otherwise separate from everyday life (insofar as they were demarcated). Graham analyses a sanctuary as the locale for pilgrimage, worship, sacrifice, contemplation, and 'time out' from routine bustle. Baker and Francis explore the other world of death and burial, conceptually and spatially distinct from residential and work areas. This follows Draycott's examination of bodily prostheses in Part 2, Chapter 4, which were presumably part of regular life (even if examples were discovered in burials). Encounters with other worlds, whether divine or mortuary, offer the space to think through what it means to be human and the diversity within this, and a contrasting backdrop against which to consider bodily and cultural norms. Disability and illness have a key part to play in the context of healing sanctuaries, while often presenting the reason for death and burial. Furthermore, the polluting element of burial is comparable to the stigma of disability and monstering of this other. As particular burial practices could be deployed as punishment for failing to fit the prescribed norm, so might impairments be perceived as deserved, divine punishment for character flaws. Therefore, these contexts should be of great interest in the pursuit of classical disability studies.

Both chapters engage with the tension between the medical and social models. Graham is explicit, noting how evidence for the medical (artefactual or bioarchaeological) may be used to consider how people were integrated into the wider community and social contexts. Likewise, Baker and Francis place bioarchaeological, medical evidence into the wider social framework, including social groupings and modes of exclusion. In a sense, this attempts medical diagnosis through archaeological typology, which is then meshed into a wider spatial, legal, and social context. Thus, both approaches are able to consider the body itself, how it was treated, and the social environment drawn from literary, legal, and philosophical texts. Graham also cross-cuts these 'medical' and 'social' constructions with the etic–emic tension. She links this to the nature of the sources and the history of the discipline – textual sources rarely give the perspective of the disabled person, and these sources (occasionally with visual ones) form the foundation of classical social history. This allows us to reconstruct the treatment and social position of disabled people, but, in order to explore their lived experience, a different approach is needed, namely that of sensory studies.

The very real, physical nature of archaeological evidence is set against interpretative challenges in both chapters. Baker and Francis push the evidence to its explanatory limits, given the small number of examples cast over a wide timeframe. However, by placing this within more familiar Aristotelian areas of Greek thought and attitudes, we are presented with a persuasive reading of the treatment and experience of these adults, one of whom clearly had head injuries and likely subsequent cognitive issues. That these figures have previously been interpreted as social deviants, implying dubious moral character, suggests that disability had not been a consideration. To categorize such people as children has resonance for those familiar with more modern histories of people with significant learning or mental health issues – whether to allow them agency and decision-making powers is contested in legal and educational battlefields.

Both chapters highlight not just the desire for interdisciplinary approaches, but also the need for them. Graham further notes some peculiar contrasts between classical sensory studies and disability studies:

> It is genuinely incongruous that one subdiscipline of Classical Studies should focus explicitly on identifying and interpreting ancient lived experience while another, which has the varied somatic capacities of human being at its very heart, should only rarely attempt to do so.

It is not uncommon for disciplines with shared interests to move in complete isolation, such as the lack of awareness in studies of ekphrasis of audio description (Adams, Chapter 6, this volume).

Likewise, sensory studies must bear a certain amount of interpretive uncertainty – especially as it has tended to recreate a homogeneous perspective, inevitably based on the male, elite, able-bodied 'norm'. Aristotle epitomises this view: a child is incomplete and has a poor memory, as do people with dwarfism, owing to the strain of the weight of their upper bodies upon the organ of consciousness (Baker and Francis, Chapter 8), a woman is a deformed man, and so on. Such is the power of 'the norm'; we assume we can reach that in history, but no other status or identity. The ableism in sensory studies has been striking, as Graham notes. Furthermore, she emphasises that reconstructing the experiences of disabled people does not just signal political correctness, but also lends a positive contribution. We should not simply add disabled people and stir; the existence and experiences of disabled people bring interpretive importance. For example, the field of disability studies highlights just how wide-ranging people's perceptions and visual experiences may be, even if these differences do not qualify as a formal 'disability' (e.g. Adams, Chapter 6, this volume). This apparent lack or impairment of one sense, such as sight, also led to a focus on other senses, therefore potentially enriching that strand of enquiry. This attention on the replacement or representation, rather than the absence or impairment, takes material form with anatomical votives. Similarly, in Draycott, Chapter 4, in this volume, the focus was on the prosthetic replacement, rather than the missing function.

Archaeology can bring great insights into bodily treatment and experience, including that of the disabled person, and these two chapters have demonstrated this by deploying very different approaches. This introduction was written while Covid-19 gripped the world, and social isolation at home and social distancing in all public and private spaces presented an uncomfortable new norm. This alien, deliberate way of life provoked a re-evaluation of social space, human interaction, and spatial contamination. It also highlighted the various ways in which humans move and interact, strongly supporting Graham's argument that sensory studies needs to appreciate human diversity, including experiences of those with a disability (or fear of illness). Reports of patients dying isolated from family, to be buried with few or no mourners in attendance, served to intensify the distress and fear of contracting the virus. As Baker and Francis note, where and how you are buried matters a great deal when you are alive; if disabled in life, you may be further stigmatised in death.

Chapter 7

Interactional sensibilities

Bringing ancient disability studies to its archaeological senses

Emma-Jayne Graham

Abstract

This chapter presents an argument for the closer integration of ancient disability studies with sensory archaeologies, proposing that, in order to understand the lived complexities of being an embodied human in the ancient world, it is crucial to combine the perspectives offered by both areas of research. More specifically, it spotlights how these approaches might be used in the context of interactional theory to characterise the ancient experiential realities of both sensory perception and disability or impairment. This is explored with reference to a case study concerning ritualised movement at the Roman sanctuary of Fortuna Primigenia at Praeneste (Palestrina), which reveals how greater awareness of the lived experiences of visual and mobility impairments can provide new ways of understanding the sensescapes of ancient religious place and, equally, ancient lived experiences of both religion and disability.

Introduction

In terms of significant new advances in method and theory concerning the identification and interpretation of past lived experiences, sensory archaeologies and ancient disability studies have much in common. Critical evaluation of the complexities of sensory experiences, including the extent to which these underpinned ancient lived identities and ways of being in the world, has flourished in recent years. Over the course of much the same period of time, ancient disability studies research, with its corresponding focus on somatic and sensory impairments and the ways in which these impacted on social attitudes, identities, and perceptions of the world, has begun to redress a significant imbalance in our appreciation of the diversity of ancient experiences. However, their apparent compatibility and shared concerns notwithstanding, scholarship concerning ancient disability (including work that directly addresses sensory impairments) remains remarkably sense-less in terms of its approach and theoretical framing. At the same time, many of the interpretations advanced through the lens of sensory archaeologies continue, in essence, to be inherently ableist, despite ambitions to offer alternative, more holistic and inclusive perspectives on the ancient world. Sensorial-driven investigations of sight, sound, and movement, for instance, frequently presume a somatic norm in which everyone could see, hear, and move in more or less equal ways, whereas studies that identify the varied ways in which the people of antiquity might encounter impaired bodies and minds continue to privilege the socially and legally disabling implications of these circumstances over the ways in which they were felt and lived.

It is my aim in this chapter to draw much-needed critical attention to this paradox. More specifically, I intend to demonstrate quite how far this state of affairs is responsible for actively impoverishing both strands of research, and in particular how it has significant implications for the ongoing characterisation of disability in antiquity as a social 'problem'. Having reviewed these issues, I will argue that, in order to come close to understanding the lived complexities of being an embodied human in the ancient world, it is crucial that ancient disability studies and sensory archaeologies interact constructively with one another, rather than continuing to be treated as essentially independent areas of research. The groundwork laid by this discussion anticipates my second and potentially more significant endeavour, which is to show through example how a collaborative approach to the sensory lived experience of ancient disability and impairment can be realistically achieved via the lens of interactional theory, underscoring the important new perspectives it can bring. To do this, I employ as an illustrative case study the example of ritualised encounters with the first century BCE sanctuary of Fortuna Primigenia at Praeneste (modern Palestrina, Italy). This reveals how understandings of the lived experience of ancient disability and impairment, and the lived experience of a multisensory world of things, can be significantly enhanced when these approaches join forces. In short, I propose that, in order to fulfil its potential, disability studies must be brought quite literally to its senses, and sensory archaeologies must be prepared to disable themselves.

Making sense of antiquity

Both ancient disability studies and ancient sensory archaeologies have emerged comparatively recently as discrete areas of interest within the broad field of Classical Studies. That is not to say that past research never drew attention to the sensory aspects of life in antiquity, such as the likely 'stench' of the ancient city (usually a Roman one such as Pompeii or Rome: Classen, Howes and Synnott 1994; Bradley 2002; Toner 2009; Koloski-Ostrow 2015) and the pervasive presence of sounds, including music, within Roman lives (Horsfall 2003). However, it is only recently that questions have begun to be asked about the nuances of the experiences produced by these sensory encounters and their more complex consequences. Importantly, these new questions extend existing appreciations of the significance of sensory perception beyond rather essentializing reconstructions of what something, somewhere, or someone looked, smelled, or sounded like (for an overview see Betts 2017a; also Betts 2011; Day 2013; Hamilakis 2013; Haug and Kreuz 2016; Skeates and Day 2019). Probing questions are now much more consistently asked – for instance, not about whether something smelled but about exactly *what* scents were associated with particular locations, activities, and routes of movement, how they worked together or against one another, and why it mattered (Betts 2011; Platts 2019); about *how* the senses actively affected certain forms of knowledge (particularly religious knowledge: Weddle 2013; Graham 2017a; 2018; forthcoming; Harvey and Hughes 2018); about *why it might matter* whether one location and not another was marked out by a distinctive scent, or even the lack of one (compare Bradley 2002 with Flohr 2017); and about *how* detectable sensescapes varied across the seasons and even throughout the day (Betts 2017b; Graham 2018). At the same time, queries are more routinely posed about the power of sensory perception to contribute to the dynamic construction of particular identities (Toner 2009) or places (Derrick 2017; Veitch 2017), and how the experience of different participants in the same activities varied because of their discrete encounters with the specific sensory stimuli of material things (Graham forthcoming). Finally, research has begun to identify ways to ensure that these studies are as multisensory in nature as evidence will allow, continuing to question how the human sensorium might work as a coherent collective as well as how the material world might occasionally present a person with dissonant or competing affordances (Betts 2017b; Flohr 2017; Graham 2017a). These primarily archaeological studies draw overtly on theoretical approaches derived from phenomenology, inspired especially by the work of Merleau Ponty (1968), and are implicitly – sometimes explicitly – intent on surfacing and understanding sensory modalities that afforded different ways of being in the world. As a result, many archaeological sensory studies dedicate themselves to recentring the sensorium and sensory perception within our understanding of ancient lived experiences.

At the same time, another strand of ancient sensory research has approached the human sensorium via textual allusions to sensory stimuli and culturally conditioned responses to them. Exemplified by many of the contributions to the Routledge Senses in Antiquity series (Bradley and Butler 2014–2018), which includes volumes on synaesthesia, sight, sound, smell, touch, and taste, scholars of ancient literature, drama, philosophy, philology, and medicine have begun to pursue questions about how the senses were employed in, or made to act within, different communicative genres, as well as how they offered a means of ordering cultural knowledge both within and about the ancient world. The written word not only reinforces the presence of the rich multisensory world posited by archaeological studies, but also some of the ways in which it was comprehended and actively manipulated by ancient writers. Sensory allusions might, for instance, be intentionally adduced, even purposefully complicated or inverted, in order to evoke, affirm, or construct shared cultural ideas (Toner 2009; Butler and Purves 2013). Sources show, then, that Greek and Roman individuals frequently employed shared knowledge of the potential meanings and metaphorical power of the sensory world in relation to their own concerns and areas of expertise. In other words, it is not just modern scholars who seek to notice the ancient sensorium: ancient people were also deeply aware of its possibilities.

Major proponents of ancient sensory archaeologies, among them Eleanor Betts (2017a, 2–3), point out that, rather than being a theory in itself, this is 'a way of broadening our perspective on the past by recognising that by focusing on the visual we have neglected a vast body of data and interpretative tools for understanding ancient societies'. Indeed, of uppermost concern within many (but not all) of these studies is the desire to escape what is regularly described as 'the tyranny of the visual'. This essentially means seeking to incorporate a deeper understanding of the complex multisensory worlds in which humans have always lived and the role these play in how we order, understand, and share knowledge of those worlds (Betts 2011, 118–9). In particular, multisensory approaches to the ancient world reach beyond the canonical five senses to incorporate other forms of perception, such as kinaesthesia, proprioception, interoception, pain (sometimes described as a tactile or broadly haptic sense), even other 'senses of' (e.g. time, place, the uncanny, and humour: Harvey 2018, viii–ix). This set of approaches offers the chance to capture a much wider set of ancient perceptions and experiences and to explore some of the persistent gaps in traditional sources. That is to say that sensory archaeologies present us with constant reminders that there were many more Greeks and Romans than those who happened to write things down, and by implication even more undoubtedly diverse lived experiences.

Although their thoughts may no longer be fully accessible, the potential lived experiences of the non-elite, women, children, non-citizens, enslaved people, and, of course, those with impairments and/or those whom ancient society may have deemed disabled, need not be completely lost when we begin our explorations of ancient lives with a consideration of the relationship between the human sensorium and the real-world material contexts in which those lives were lived. In fact, it becomes possible to ask questions about a much more inclusive range of potential emotions, feelings, thoughts, identities, and other types of experience that the perceivable sensory properties of a location, an assemblage of objects, or a set of activities may have worked to produce in conjunction with those historically contingent sensing human bodies (Kjellström 2010, 54–5; Betts 2017a, 3–4; 2017b, 25). These are, therefore, 'approaches which recognise the diversity of human bodies and experiences, collective as well as individual identities, and the significance of the body in habituated spaces (often taking an insider rather than an outsider perspective)' (Betts 2017a, 2).

Ableist sensibilities?

Integrating a greater awareness of sensory experiences into existing research concerning ancient identities, activities, and ontologies continues to strengthen the discipline of Classical Studies, making it possible to assess the potential experiences of a much wider group of people than can ever be accessed by close focus on a sample of sources composed by a small section of society. It also positively encourages original investigations concerning the experiences of underrepresented individuals and groups, those who do not always leave durable traces in traditional sources: enslaved people in the mines, children participating in religious festivals, workers in *fullonicae*, and the elderly. This is a list to which should certainly be added the disabled and impaired. Indeed, several proponents of sensory approaches have argued that their value lies precisely in their potential to be embedded within existing and long-standing research questions concerning ancient society and culture, rather than something that runs parallel to them (Hamilakis 2013; Betts 2017a). Nevertheless, by regularly bypassing questions of impairment, ancient sensory studies continue to promote an ableist approach to, and understanding of, the past lived experiences they seek to spotlight. Although exceptions do exist, this broad situation persists despite studies of ancient disability establishing that the communities of the ancient world were composed of people with varying ability to see, hear, move, and – although this has received far less attention – perhaps also to smell, taste, and touch (Graham 2013; Zakrzewski 2014; 2015; Lovell 2016). A typical example – chosen because of its relevance to the religious context explored in the latter part of this chapter, not because it is in any way more significant than any other – can be found in a recent account of the likely phenomenological experience of processions in Classical Athens: 'While individual emotional experiences during a festival or deeply personal responses to particular symbols were not necessarily shared, the spectators of a procession saw, heard, or smelled roughly the same sensory symbols' (Warford 2019, 26).

This is not to say that questions about the sensory experience of the impaired and disabled have not been raised – Eleanor Betts (2011, 118) specifically queries, 'how would a blind person find their way around the ancient city?' – it is simply that few have sought either to answer them (despite having posed the question, Betts does not return to it) or to more systematically place people with impairments at the forefront of their analysis. In many cases, this seems to come about because researchers have tended not to consider whether everyone in a particular ancient community will actually see, hear, taste, smell, touch, and move in equal ways, as illustrated by the quote cited above. Additional examples can be found in studies of ancient sound (e.g. Veitch 2017), which, although securely grounded in acoustic principles and rigorous knowledge of the biological capacities of the human ear to detect an audible spectrum of frequencies at particular distances or in specific architectural settings, overlook the fact that, physics aside, within any community there will always be people with a wide range of permanent or temporary forms of deafness or hearing loss (see Laes 2011; 2018; Adams 2020). Omissions of this nature can also lead to rather sweeping generalisations: 'The noise of the non-elite urban environment, though probably lower than the modern level, startled contemporaries' (Toner

2009, 130). The same is true for many investigations that involve aesthetic appreciation or knowledge that is acquired visually, or that rely on the presumed existence of more or less equal visual capacities (e.g. chapters in Squire 2015, with the exception of Coo 2015).

This inherently ableist perspective stands in stark contrast to the fact that researchers engaged in sensory projects remain unerringly alert to the impact of cultural contexts on the interpretation of the experiences that they identify and evaluate, regularly emphasising that interpretations of sensory stimuli are always subjective and culturally or socially constrained, and how essential it is that researchers do not assume that contemporary responses can be decoded in the same way as they would have been by ancient people (Betts 2017b, 24). As Jerry Toner (2009, 123) observes,

> The Roman sensory experience was very different from ours. We cannot hope to re-create their experience in its entirety, but we can establish some of the different cultural meanings that the senses held for them. Above all, Roman sensory experience was related to social status.

Surprisingly, then, the broad range of somatic differences associated with impairment that were inherent *within* all ancient cultural groupings remains largely unacknowledged (the reader might note, for instance, Toner's description of a very singular 'Roman' sensory experience). Of course, compared with other approaches and frameworks for analysis, such as gender theory, sensory studies remains in its comparative infancy, and inevitably it has not yet established methods that allow researchers to convincingly incorporate the potentially limitless variety of humankind without resorting to high-level descriptive accounts or unhelpful banalities. Nor do contemporary publishing constraints support the sort of multifaceted, wide-angled, open-ended perspective that would be needed to successfully encourage this.

These caveats aside, the extent to which it remains excusable to overlook the reality that humans, past and present, will always encounter the world via bodies that diverge significantly from those of others in terms of their sensory and mobility capacities must be called into question, not least because of its consequences. By working on the basis of a broad biological norm that supposes that all people could hear, see, move, or speak more or less equally, sensory studies risks undermining its own project by promoting a homogeneous world in which the sensory experiences that come to the fore are more likely to be nuanced by whether someone is Greek or Roman, rich or poor, than by whether they have a sensory impairment.

I propose, then, that, in order for archaeological sensory studies to flourish, they need to enter into a more constructive dialogue with research concerning the very bodily disparity of the people whose embodied experiences they seek to investigate, and that this dialogue should not be about merely slotting disability or forms of impairment into sensory studies contexts. Instead, the real value of uniting ancient sensory and disability studies lies in adopting a more comprehensive awareness of the multilayered facets of ancient lived experience. Indeed, I would argue that a sensory approach that actively seeks to consider how the physical and social world was experienced, interpreted, and negotiated via the body by foregrounding impaired bodies from the very start, makes it possible to adopt the type of interactional approach that has been developed within contemporary disability studies.

Interactional theory and sensory-disability studies (or why we should be more sensible about disability)

In the context of the current volume, it is unnecessary to balance the overview of ancient sensory studies presented above with an equally comprehensive summary of the development of ancient disability studies (for the relevant scholarly background, see Chapter 1). However, it is necessary to reflect briefly, and in a critical manner, on some aspects of its development as a subdiscipline of Classical Studies and, in particular, to draw attention to how ancient disability studies might benefit from a sensory-driven approach with the capacity to broaden its horizons. Indeed, unlike sensory archaeologies, which place the search for lived experience and its significance at the forefront of their endeavours, some studies of ancient disability assert that it simply is not possible to explore the lived experiences of impairment and disability in the past (e.g. Trentin 2013, 92; Boutin and Porter 2014, 121). In part, this is a consequence of how this area of research has developed within ancient historical traditions reliant on textual (and some visual) sources. As most ancient historians will acknowledge, such sources will never provide the fullest and most inclusive picture: 'The "ordinary", "everyday" life of the visually disabled', notes Christian Laes (2018, 103), 'was seldom worth mentioning' (see also Pestilli 2005, 86 on the absence of mobility impaired people in ancient art). Instead, established social and medical models provide the theoretical frame through which understandings have emerged of how disability was recognised, described, and categorised, and how certain disabling circumstances affected a person's social and legal rights and expectations, if not their actual lived experience (e.g. Edwards [Rose] 1997; Rose 2003; Laes 2018).

Correspondingly, and for good reason, efforts have gone into 'finding' as many of the disabled people of antiquity as possible within the margins and between the lines of these sources, in order to determine how they were treated in both life and death, what that might reveal about how disability was defined by ancient societies and, crucially, by legal systems, as well as what the consequences of those definitions may have been for the rights and level of integration of impaired people within a given society (Laes, Goodey and Rose 2013). Evidence for the circumstances surrounding impairments and attitudes towards them has increasingly been identified in less familiar and non-traditional sources. It has been revealed, for example, hidden in the shadows of texts that do not directly address the existence of people with impairments (Laes 2018 represents a successful example of this type of approach) and through the use of bioarchaeological evidence bringing to light individuals who once experienced a range of impairments and potentially disabling conditions (Graham 2013; Southwell-Wright 2014; Zakrzewski 2014; Baker and Francis, Chapter 8, this volume).

Ancient disability studies has, therefore, succeeded in pinpointing some of the social and cultural attitudes towards disabled and impaired people that may have been prevalent at certain moments or in specific places within the ancient world, as well as broader patterns of social and legal behaviours that demonstrate the varying extent to which, and different contexts in which, these people were treated similarly to, or differently from, their peers. These observations have in turn been employed to establish where, when, and how ancient communities responded to particular bodily or cognitive differences. However, because written sources, especially legal ones, tend to report what society had determined should happen when someone presented with a particular impairment that *marked them out* from those without one, this can occasionally result in ancient people with impairments being framed in unfortunately negative ways, as something of a problem that ancient society was 'confronted with' and ultimately 'coped with' (Laes 2018, 87). Relatedly, even recent works persist in problematically describing ancient people as 'suffering from' a particular condition or impairment (Laes 2018, 16; also 18: 'a man who suffered from gigantism'). Attempts to counter this tendency to begin from an implicitly negative standpoint have emphasised the wide spectrum of bodily disparity in antiquity and the large numbers of people who would have experienced some form of (potentially temporary) disabling circumstances (Graham 2013; Zakrzewski 2014; 2015; Pudsey 2017; Graham 2020). Nonetheless, and in contrast to the favouring of increasingly emic perspectives in sensory studies, the origins of ancient disability studies within ancient social histories has resulted in a favouring of what can be considered broadly etic perspectives, certainly when it comes to considering lived *experiences* of impairment, even if these perspectives are still grounded in the broadly emic sources of a specific social or cultural context. Put differently, the emic experiences of those with disabilities remain under-explored in favour of investigations into how their experiences were mediated by interaction with their peers.

It is genuinely incongruous that one subdiscipline of Classical Studies should focus explicitly on identifying and interpreting ancient lived experience while another, which has the varied somatic capacities of human beings at its very heart, should only rarely attempt to do so. This is even more striking when we consider that accounts of lived experience and the agency of the disabled are increasingly considered indispensable within contemporary disability studies (see Chapter 1, this volume; Sharples 2019 debates some of the pros and cons of this for ancient disability studies). In previous work, I have attempted to address what I consider to be the etic bias of ancient disability studies prompted by an emphasis on the social and medical models by considering mobility impairment through the lens of interactional theory as it has been developed for contemporary disability studies (Graham 2017b; 2020). The ideas associated with interactional theory presented by Tom Shakespeare (2006) and Christopher Riddle (2013a; 2013b) might, however, also offer a way to bridge the gap between ancient disability and sensory studies. In particular, I suggest that this is possible because of the emphasis it places on seeking to understand *experiences of impairment* that arise as a consequence of a complex interweaving of an underlying physical impairment and the world in which a person lives, or the social and cultural context in which that condition was experienced. After all, at its core, interactional theory acknowledges that, 'impairment has both physical and social dimensions' (Riddle 2013a, 32). In other words, interactional studies of disability seek to uncover the lived experience of a physical impairment – something that might be achieved for the ancient world by adopting the sort of perspectives offered by sensory archaeologies – at the same time as it situates its interpretation of these experiences within the relevant social (or cultural) world in which they are lived – the sort of world that has been has been meaningfully constructed by ancient disability studies making use of social models.

The question arises, then, as to whether ancient disability might actually be better understood by actively combining the experiential insights offered by sensory archaeologies and the social ones provided by existing work in disability studies. As Christopher Riddle (2013a, 27) has argued for the contemporary world, 'If what we seek is a model to characterize the reality of the experience of disability, I submit that the social model is not it.' Inevitably, true interactionality will always be more easily achievable for contemporary contexts that allow researchers to gather first-hand accounts from individuals about their lived experiences or of which the researchers themselves have personal experience. In these contexts, the definitions of disability that interactional theory allows to emerge also have direct and hugely significant consequences for contemporary disability rights (Riddle 2013a, 23, 27). However, making use of the sorts of analytical and theoretical perspectives adopted by ancient sensory studies to detect and evaluate embodied lived experience means that an interactional approach to disability may be more attainable for the ancient world than scholars have allowed.

In previous projects, I have aligned the two aspects of interactional theory with the medical and social models more familiar to ancient disability studies, in order to create a productive interactional dialogue between the two. This has entailed finding ways for bioarchaeological and artefactual evidence for the presence of underlying physical impairments (i.e. the 'medical') to be employed in addressing questions about the ways in which people with particular impairments were integrated into wider community contexts (i.e. the 'social'), revealing that, instead of remaining fixed, any resulting social disability might vary in terms of its physical temporality (Graham 2017b; 2020). Interaction between the physical and contextual dimensions of ancient disability or, as noted above, the weaving together of information concerning underlying physical impairments with what is known about the world in which they were experienced, can, however, also be achieved by adopting the more comprehensive understanding of the latter offered by sensory archaeologies. After all, the worlds in which impairments were experienced extended beyond the societal expectations and attitudes presented in ancient textual discourses to incorporate the rich multisensory material and physical worlds in which people actually lived.

Drawing on sensory archaeologies consequently makes it possible to situate the impaired bodies of antiquity in a complex social *and* sensory world of personal lived experience. It allows us to explore not only how impairments affected the extent to which a person was able to participate in social and cultural life, and how that impacted on the ways in which other people identified and categorised them, but also *what it was like* for them to physically live in that world, *how it felt* when their bodies participated in it, and *what those lived experiences meant* for their own personal identities and the ongoing construction of that social world itself. Interactional theory, therefore, encourages increasingly nuanced explorations of the relationship between lived experiences and the determination of both personal identities and wider social attitudes. This, in turn, requires that traditional investigations of ancient impairment and disability become integrated into studies of ancient ways of being in the world that are driven by a greater awareness of experiential (i.e. sensory) factors in the creation of those worlds.

At the same time, relating the personal and social identities of the disabled to the sensory and physical experiences that gave rise to them offers the chance to effectively empower the impaired individuals of antiquity to play a more active role in determining how those sensory worlds should be recognised and interpreted today. It also compels new questions about ancient lived experience that are driven by deeper understandings of ancient impairment, rather than researchers simply attempting to slot impaired bodies into existing interpretations or models retrospectively, essentially succeeding only in highlighting sensory or embodied experiences from which they were potentially excluded. That is to say, instead of writing off the splendour of the view that greeted a person upon reaching the summit of the sanctuary of Fortuna Primigenia at Praeneste as an experience unavailable to a blind or visually impaired visitor (Fig. 7.1), this approach makes it possible to flip those expectations and to actively, and more positively, investigate what the sensory and embodied experience of a visually impaired individual actually may have been. For example, downplaying, but not entirely removing, the potential for visual affordances helps to draw attention to other potential sensory experiences, such as changing levels of light, sounds, smells, or temperature as a person entered the open space from an enclosed staircase, or more broadly haptic experiences of moving into an exposed area on which the sun might beat down, where the wind might move

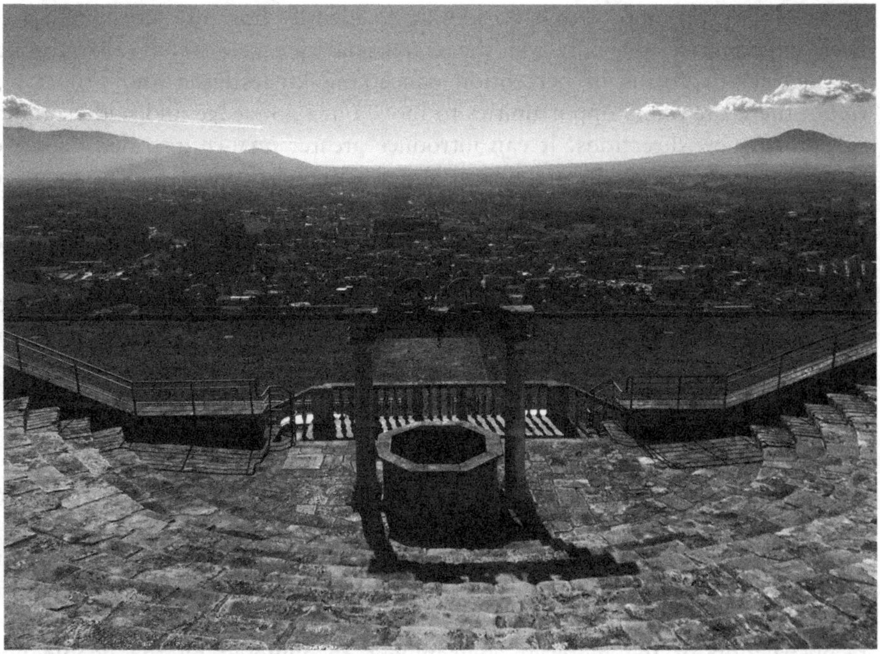

Figure 7.1 View from the *piazza della cortina* (Terrace VI) of the sanctuary of Fortuna Primigenia, Praeneste (Photo by Liana Brent, with permission)

more freely, or where people stand further away from one another. In other words, it encourages a focus on what *was* potentially experienced, instead of what was not.

This then raises questions about whether the wide range of potential affordances offered by the physical environment were also sensed and experienced via the bodies of all visitors, and whether the view really was the only significant aspect of their experience of the piazza. As a result, this more positive perspective on the lived experience of impairment as reconstructed via potential sensory encounters with the material world also supports a wider research agenda – in this case, the quest to understand the role of the sanctuary's architecture in the production of particular ways of being in the world, which in this example involves ways of being that relate to ritual activities and religious forms of knowledge (Graham 2021). At the same time, it makes it possible to identify experiences that were closer to the lived realities of ancient impairment as they were actually felt by different individuals and to understand them on their own terms, rather than as a diminished version of those of their abled peers.

Combining the available evidence for the presence of impairments in the ancient world with the ways of exploring lived experience that sensory archaeologies promote – that is, seeking to identify how the world may have been experienced not only via the traditional five senses but also through broader haptic forms of perception concerning kinaesthesia and proprioception – therefore offers opportunities to move our knowledge and understanding of both in new directions. It can introduce greater nuance into discussions of sensory experience, while enabling a deeper acknowledgement of the impact of impairments on the lives of the impaired and disabled as they were actually lived. The following case study picks up where we left off with the sanctuary of Fortuna Primigenia and puts these ideas into practice, exploring how understandings of the lived experience of a particular location might be changed by foregrounding not merely the presence of impaired and disabled individuals, but their specific responses to the sensory affordances of that location.

Disability, impairment, and religion in Roman Italy

Major sanctuary sites of Republican Italy, such the sanctuary of Fortuna Primigenia at Praeneste, provide a practical context in which to test an interactional approach to ancient lived experience that blends sensory and disability perspectives. In part this is because many of these sanctuaries offer well-preserved, or at least well-documented, archaeological evidence that enables a reconstruction of the material environment encountered by the people who made use of them for ritual purposes. This evidence makes it possible to identify potential activity locations and routes of movement through and around a defined location with a known function. A wealth of existing knowledge concerning Roman ritual practices, especially what these required people in particular roles to do, and the abundance of identifiable potential sensory affordances associated with the material things that these activities caused people to physically engage with (e.g. objects, incense, animals, clothing, flames, liquids, foodstuffs, etc.) can subsequently be combined with this knowledge of the material landscape (the bibliography on Roman ritual is too substantial to list here, but see, for example, Rüpke 2007; Schultz and Harvey 2006; Raja and Rüpke 2015; Moser 2019; Graham 2021). Together, these facilitate an assessment of the potential lived experiences that might arise from ritualised performances at a particular sanctuary.

During the Republican period, sanctuaries across central Italy were also frequently associated with votive practices that appear in many instances to have had a connection with perceptions of healing. Evidence for this appears in the form of hundreds, and sometimes thousands, of anatomical votives: clay or metal offerings shaped into models of body parts (Draycott and Graham 2017; Hughes 2017). These offerings most probably had a connection with requests for divine intervention concerning the bodies and well-being of humans. This large quantity of artefactual evidence consequently attests the presence at sanctuary sites of real individuals with sensory and mobility impairments, even if the precise nature of their circumstances must necessarily remain speculative

(Graham 2017b). Anatomical votives connected with both external and internal human anatomy also highlight very clearly the wide spectrum of bodily disparity that was prevalent within ancient communities, aligning with comparable evidence for physical impairments derived from bioarchaeological studies (Graham 2013; 2017b; 2020). A connection between sanctuaries and the treatment of potentially disabling impairments is also sometimes evidenced by their topographical correlation with thermo-mineral water sources that had demonstrative therapeutic qualities (Bassani 2014; 2019). Sanctuaries at these watery sites also attracted considerable numbers of visitors, and once again this ritual community most probably included people whose somatic experiences were at least temporarily impaired.

Even when circumstances mean that many of the offerings and other portable objects left at sanctuaries have been destroyed, cleared away, looted, or simply lost through later repurposing of the site (as is the case with the example of the sanctuary of Fortuna Primigenia discussed here), it can be asserted with some confidence that people with a host of different impairments would once have visited these locations. This is not only because votive cult was 'probably the "core business" of cult places' (Rous 2010, 23), attracting a diverse community of visitors including those with impairments who might wish to seek divine assistance with their personal well-being, but because of the importance of religious activities to Roman social and cultural ways of being. To date, studies of disability in the Roman world have not been able to demonstrate that people with impairments were systematically excluded from participating in religious rituals, and the evidence for and against the extent of their involvement is often contradictory and highly situational. For instance, although sources indicate that 'speech disorders accompanied by decreased hearing or any other physical defilement were regarded as sufficient reason to reject young girls between the ages of six and ten as Vestal Virgins' (Laes 2018, 139; Gellius, *Attic Nights* 1.12.3), there is also evidence from 14 BCE that attests a blind Vestal (Dio Cassius, *Roman History* 54.24; Laes 2018, 101). The proscription against impairment for new members of the Vestal order was probably connected with the ritual expectations of their discrete and hugely significant public role, whereas the apparently contradictory case of the blind Vestal no doubt arose as a result of a sensory impairment that developed later in life but was not considered significant enough to remove the experienced woman from her role (see DiLuzio 2016, 123).

The Vestals were, however, hardly typical of most people's experiences, and these restrictions on participation cannot be applied more generally. Indeed, the many thousands of anatomical votives that survive from the Republican period surely counter any suggestion that ordinary people with sensory and mobility impairments were routinely excluded from religious places or activities, even if certain impairments may have prevented individuals from holding positions of responsibility within major cults (Laes 2018, 180; for contrasting evidence from Greece, see Dillon 2017, 169–70). Given the cultural importance of maintaining the *pax deorum*, it is difficult to imagine that potentially large numbers of

Roman people were prevented from participating in fairly ordinary religious rituals, such as personal votive cult or attending public sacrifices and festivals, on the grounds of impairment or physical imperfection, as that would almost certainly have ruled out much of the population (see Pudsey 2017, 14).

Multisensory lived experiences at the sanctuary of Fortuna Primigenia

Like other sanctuaries, the monumental complex dedicated to Fortuna Primigenia at Praeneste, about 35 kilometres to the east of Rome, was almost certainly frequented by people with a range of impairments. The monumental sanctuary itself was constructed around the end of the second century BCE (c.110–100 BCE), overlooking the urban area of the city of Praeneste and the hills beyond. Incorporating the naturally steep topography, the sanctuary comprises a series of narrow linear terraces (numbered I–V) accessed via ramps and staircases that led the visitor up to a wide-open space bounded by a three-sided portico (Terrace VI, the so-called *piazza della cortina*), with a further terrace (VII) supporting a theatre *cavea* and a curved portico located in front of a circular temple or *tholos* at the very summit of the structure (Fig. 7.2). Given the small size of the *tholos* and the orientation of the *cavea*, the *piazza della cortina* was most probably the setting for major public rituals. Terrace IV, known as the *terrazza degli emicicli* (the terrace of the hemicycles), was divided into two parts by the sanctuary's central staircase, with what appears to have been an area dedicated to animal sacrifice located on its western side, and an oracular shrine on the eastern platform (mentioned by Cicero, *On Divination* 2.41–2). These must also have hosted specific groups of people engaged in associated ritualised activities, although the restricted space made these gatherings smaller than those in the large piazza. Given the complexity of the site, and its multiplicity of differently arranged open and enclosed spaces, I intend to focus here on the main access route into (and possibly out of) the sanctuary, as this encapsulates a number of potential sensescapes and opportunities for differently lived experiences for those who came to the sanctuary in order to participate in its range of ritualised activities.

Access to the various terraces was facilitated by a succession of ramps and staircases (including the steps of the *cavea*). These structures are commonly interpreted as a means of controlling or directing ritual movement upward, around, and through the sanctuary, primarily through the manipulation of sightlines and a steady increase in elevation. Filippo Coarelli (1987, 43–7, Fig. 14), for example, demonstrated that, as a visitor to the sanctuary ascended, the series of terraces acted to periodically reveal or obscure key monumental components (Fig. 7.3). This visual experience was accompanied by a progressive reduction and then final expansion of space as the visitor emerged from the enclosed ramps and restrictive axial staircase into the *piazza della cortina*, where they were struck by spectacular views of the landscape that had been

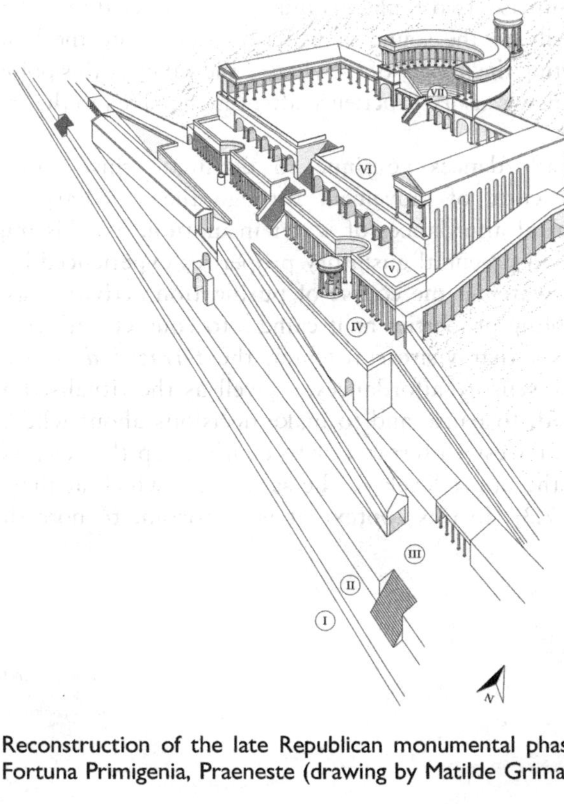

Figure 7.2 Reconstruction of the late Republican monumental phase of the sanctuary of Fortuna Primigenia, Praeneste (drawing by Matilde Grimaldi, with permission)

only briefly glimpsed once before, through a narrower gap at the top of the two main (covered) access ramps. Coarelli (1987, 55) suggested that this view, framed by the wings of the triple portico that also aligned with the peaks of the Monti Lepini and the Colli Albani, was crucial for the message that the sanctuary officials wanted to convey: that is, it visually represented the subordination of the landscape (nature) to architecture (culture).

Benjamin Rous (2010, 105–6) has argued more recently that, at key points along the main access route through the sanctuary, the attention of the visitor was also drawn by other sensory cues, which actively aided navigation and caused the visitor to pause:

> Fountains were placed at the very beginning of the route, at the bottom of the lateral ramps, where pilgrims could ritually cleanse themselves. They were then guided up these ramps by the placement of great fountains placed in niches built into the great substructions walls of the *terrazza degli emicicli*. At the crucial nodal point at the top of the access ramps, water again may have

> influenced the decision of which path should be followed. Placed at the sides of the axial staircase, two fountains must have attracted the attention of the visitors primarily by the sound of water splashing into the basins, thereby partially offsetting the impact of the view of the valley at this point, or at least constituting a new sensory experience after having taken in the scenery.

Although visual affordances continue to dominate this more sensorially informed reconstruction of movement through the sanctuary, Rous draws attention to the aural affordances of water in motion. To this might also be added the tactile and potential gustatory properties experienced by those who engaged with this water in the course of purification activities, as well as its broadly haptic cooling properties as it came into contact with the skin. Rous (2010, 106) suggests that visitors reaching the *terrazza degli emicicli* were compelled by these sensory affordances, as well as the ritualised actions that the water prompted, to pause and to make decisions about whether to enter either the eastern or western terrace, or to continue up the steep central axial staircase towards the upper levels of the sanctuary (which at that point were out of sight: Fig. 7.3). In this context, it is important to note that the two

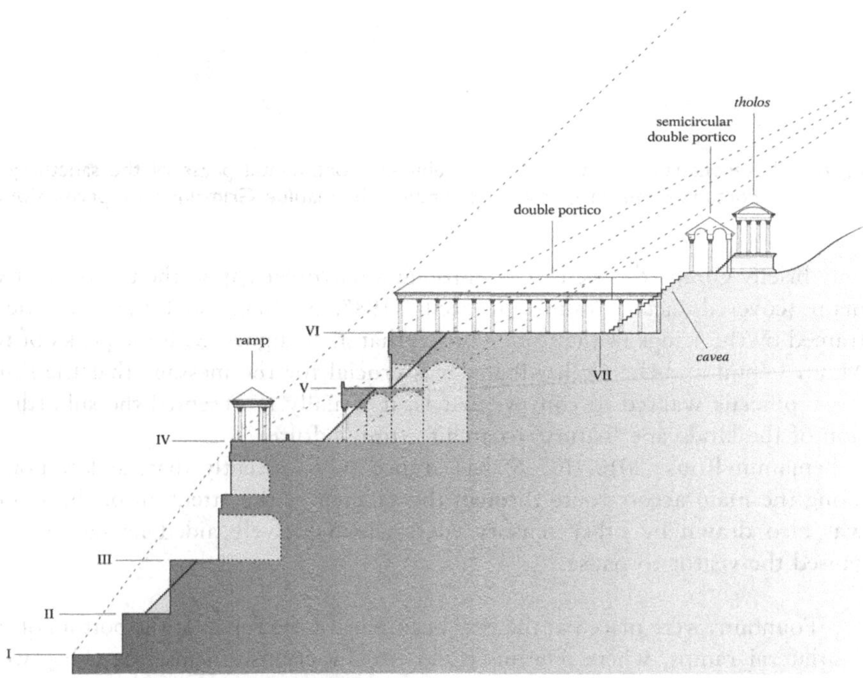

Figure 7.3 Cross-section of the sanctuary of Fortuna Primigenia at Praeneste showing possible upwards sightlines (drawing by Matilde Grimaldi after Coarelli 1987, Fig. 14, with permission)

parts of the *terrazza degli emicicli* may also have prompted different multisensory experiences, as 'the observation of a ground plan alone does not necessarily tell the whole story when talking about itineraries through the complex' (Rous 2010, 6).

The eastern platform housed an oracle, comprising a pit (7.5 metres deep) marked by a tall stone *tholos*, whereas the western side featured a circular altar with associated evidence of burning (Coarelli 1987, 50). The latter appears to have been the primary location within the sanctuary for the performance of animal sacrifices, with access for quadruped victims provided by the additional lateral ramp that led directly up to this part of the terrace in parallel to the main façade ramp. Given the absence of an (identifiable) altar elsewhere in the sanctuary, the incredibly steep architecture of the complex, and with access to the large *piazza della cortina* requiring the negotiation of a narrow flight of steps, it is very possible that large animals were only ever sacrificed in this one part of the sanctuary (Graham 2021). As a result, the sights, smells, sounds, and potential tastes of animal sacrifice may have been especially concentrated on the western terrace, presenting visitors with a sensescape that was markedly different from that on the eastern terrace, where rituals occurred that were connected with the oracle. Nevertheless, these differences would have begun to be detectable from the small area at the top of the main ramps from which these two terraces could be accessed. 'Sound and odour are no respecters of visually or kinaesthetically discrete places', notes Eleanor Betts (2011, 121), and at Praeneste there certainly appears to have been little in the way of architectural impediment to the flow of sounds and smells between the two parts of the terrace and this axial entry point at the summit of the main access ramps.

Although the addition of other sensory affordances to these reconstructions of the experience of moving around the sanctuary prompts an understanding of lived experiences that move away from traditional sight-dominated interpretations, this remains in essence an ableist account of the experiences connected with accessing particular parts of the sanctuary and engaging in specific ritual activities. It assumes, for instance, that every visitor was able to see, hear, and move in equal ways around this architectural configuration, and that, when a person reached the top of the ramps, that they could see, hear, or otherwise assess the possibilities for further movement that were presented to them. Yet, as established in the first part of this chapter, at least some participants in the ritual activities performed at the sanctuary will have experienced physical and/or sensory impairments that combined with this sensescape to produce alternative experiences.

What is more, the aim of interactional approaches to 'characterize the reality of the [ancient] experience of disability' (Riddle 2013a, 27) prompts us to remember that it is insufficient merely to note that not everyone would have seen the suddenly revealed panorama from the top of the ramps or staircase, heard the gentle splashing of the water, or been able to distinguish between the different soundscapes of the eastern and western terraces, or indeed have been able to climb the axial staircase to the higher levels (at least, not without assistance). Although these observations are undoubtedly accurate, they do not provide any particularly valuable insights concerning the lived experience of the sanctuary of Fortuna Primigenia for people with impairments or disabilities. All that can be concluded is that certain aspects of that experience may have been diminished, absent, or experienced differently by some people. In this way, such observations focus unduly on the subtraction of identifiable aspects of experience from a presumed able-bodied 'norm', paring down the experience of disabled people to what is effectively a much less complex lived reality. That is to say that they do nothing but emphasise which aspects of an experience a person with particular impairments may *not* have had, rather than foregrounding the experiences that they *may have had*. So, let's begin again, this time exploring access to the *terrazza degli emicicli* and the *piazza della cortina* from the potential perspectives of people who had varying degrees of mobility and sensory impairments, in order to assess what their experiences may have entailed.

Visual impairment

The sanctuary's two primary access ramps ran for a length of approximately 67.31 metres and were around 5 metres in width (Fasolo and Gullini 1953, 88). The architectural arrangement of each effectively enclosed all visitors within a linear space, with a high wall and the monumental substructure of the *terrazza degli emicicli* cutting them off in multisensory terms from the affective properties of the surrounding landscape on both sides. This must have had the effect of focusing the senses inwards on the unidirectional in-the-moment experience of upwards (or downwards) motion. The ramps also comprised two discrete pathways: one ran against the outside wall and was covered by a roofed colonnade of narrow Doric columns that separated it from the other, unroofed, pathway closest to the terrace substructures (see Fig. 7.2). The width of each side allowed ample space for the use of walking sticks and other mobility aids, and for more than one person to walk abreast, and, despite the absence of handrails, the columns located along its route would have provided regular supports and rest stops for those who required them. Whether the two distinct pathways had clearly defined functions remains uncertain, as does the extent to which their use was formally regulated. It can be argued, nonetheless, that lived sensory experiences of ascending the steep ramps at Praeneste were important for the production of discrete understandings of the sanctuary as religious place (Graham 2021). If worshippers used one 'carriageway' for ascending and the other for descending, for example, then the ramp clearly demarcated different communities of worshippers: those who had, and those who were yet to, participate in certain religious performances. There might also be a host of other things that distinguished the users of the two sides of the ramps: social status, gender, official processions contrasted with casual visitors, those who intended to divert onto one of the discrete activity platforms of the *terrazza degli emicicli* or to continue to a higher point within the sanctuary, and so forth. Regulations may also have varied according to the time of day or in relation to particular festival occasions.

Regardless, the architectural form of the ramps points towards two groups of moving people who were physically separated by the colonnade. People with visual impairments using either side most probably experienced a sense of enclosure, communicated to those who retained some visual perception by lower levels of light caused by the high walls or roof, haptic experiences of the cooler shade of the colonnade, and the acoustic properties of the partially enclosed space through which they moved. The movement of their fellow ritual participants, and the ways in which it related to their own movement, might also be sensed through the slap of leather footwear or striking of hobnails on the stone paving, and the subtle effect on the volume or pitch of voices as people moved by, possibly also through temperature sensitivity and other tactile affordances brought about as walking caused them to move past columns and potentially in and out of the sun, rain, or wind.

These sensory affordances, in turn, continued to allow the people on either side to be aware of the presence of the other group, with multisensory perception actively drawing attention to how their own particular place in the world was signified by their potentially differential movement. This, however, also draws attention to the experiences of other visitors, who similarly had their vision manipulated by the long colonnaded passageway and who not only saw, but also sensed via altered acoustic properties an enclosing wall blocking out the wider world. Everyone ascending the steep ramp via a shaded, dimly lit colonnade, with their perspective largely restricted to what was directly ahead of them, their own regular steps mimicking the repetitive columns, may also have experienced a feeling of heightened anticipation afforded by the physical setting through which they moved. Importantly, then, all of these sensory affordances were available to individuals without visual impairments, but their significance crystallises in new ways when it is visually impaired people who first populate our sensory reconstructions, rather than those who are assumed to be able to see, hear, and feel everything.

Mobility impairment

The material properties of the primary access ramps on the façade of the sanctuary were most probably involved in producing a particularly acute embodied experience for the mobility impaired – that is, for people who experienced the material world with reference to limited or painful independent physical movement of the body, especially in terms of ambulatory motion or circumstances that affected stamina. Most significantly, the ramps were long and very steep: in fact, the 22-degree gradient of the slope of each ramp (Fasolo and Gullini 1953, 88) is actually steeper than is comfortable for the human ankle's angle of flexion when the body is ascending, something that would have resulted in the distortion of normal gait (Hollinshead 2015, 20–1, who notes that a pitch of 5–15 degrees is recommended by modern architectural standards in the USA). Ascending the ramp was consequently not easy and will have been an uncomfortable experience for the bodies of all visitors, but one that was probably even more accentuated for those with mobility impairments that already affected gait, movement, balance, and stamina.

This can be compared with experiences of negotiating the axial staircase that led from the top of the ramps on the *terrazza degli emicicli* to the *piazza della cortina*. With risers of around 0.23 metres and a run (depth of tread) of around 0.39 metres, the staircase appears to have remained close to the ideal dimensions proposed by Vitruvius, whose calculations Mary Hollinshead suggests would have favoured steps 0.22 metres high and a run 0.44 metres deep (Fasolo and Gullini 1953, 118; Hollinshead 2015, 19; Vitruvius, *On Architecture* 3.4.4). This is a height that is slightly above the recommendations of modern design norms of 0.15–0.18 metres, but towards the lower level of the dimensions of the ancient Greek steps connected with religious sites assessed by Hollinshead (2015, 20–1). The poor preservation of the steps has made it difficult to determine their gradient or pitch, although the dimensions proposed by Fasolo and Gullini (1953, 123) of a total rise of approximately 7.85 metres made up of 32–3 steps, and a length from top to bottom step of 12.80–13.20 metres, suggests around 30 degrees. This is also in alignment with the optimum dimensions of 30–35 degrees, and the permissible 30–50 degrees, for the pitch of modern staircases (Hollinshead 2015, 20). However, at Praeneste, the large number of steps in a single flight, combined with the absence of a handrail or other support, required an extended period of difficult climbing that is likely to have presented a challenge for some visitors with mobility impairments (a UK government planning document notes that long flights of steps are problematic in the context of impaired mobility, and that 'the maximum number of risers in a flight should be 12'; Inclusive mobility, n.d.).

Ascending the staircase may, therefore, have represented a physical barrier for some individuals, at the same time as the typical form and characteristic dimensions of the steps would have drawn upon familiar and established muscle memory for others who were able to ascend, albeit with some difficulty, replicating a motion that was experienced in other places such as domestic settings or public entertainment venues. The ramp also required sustained and potentially uncomfortable movement, but, when combined with the wider architectural context, the unfamiliarity of such prolonged, purely linear movement, and the intended ritualised purpose of the ascent, this was likely to have marked this experience out as especially distinctive. As Hollinshead (2015, 20–1) notes, ramps with a pitch of more than 20 degrees are less energy efficient for humans than steps, and 'their gradual path requires approximately five times the area of stairs in achieving a comparable elevation'. As a consequence, even though people will have been familiar with negotiating inclines and slopes within the local environment, it is unlikely that semi-enclosed artificial ramps on the scale of those associated with access to the sanctuary of Fortuna Primigenia were encountered as part of daily life. They were an almost unique part of the experience of visiting the sanctuary in order to witness or participate in particular and potentially special or deeply personal ritual activities. In this way, the experience of ascent differed subtly from the more familiar challenges of the staircase.

Although nobody, impaired or otherwise, approached Fortuna Primigenia in an entirely comfortable manner, this is likely to have been exacerbated for those whose experiences of impaired mobility made movement difficult or painful. As noted in a previous study, pain causes distances to become warped and space to take on new meanings as a person's spatial world is defined with direct reference to the painful body at its heart (Graham 2017b, 259). For people with impaired mobility who encountered the sanctuary of Fortuna Primigenia, the ascent of its ramps may have taken a considerable amount of time and had the potential to be especially physically demanding (perhaps also, of course, for the bodies of anyone assisting them). For people undertaking a pilgrimage to the oracle, or participating in a particular annual festival, this kinaesthetic experience contributed to the production of highly situational and personal forms of knowledge concerning religious ways of being in the world (Graham 2021). In other words, the ramps (and perhaps eventually the steps) were not merely a challenge to be overcome in order for mobility-impaired individuals to participate in the same ritual activities as other members of their community; they were also a core part of the lived experience of that religious activity itself. This was an experience that began long before participants could engage in activities on the upper terraces, being initiated at ground-level as they took their first steps into the sacred built landscape of the sanctuary and as they engaged with preparatory purification rituals at the fountains associated with the ramps. These fountains provided moments in which the visitor could begin to communicate with or adjust their bodies to the divine world that the sanctuary made available, cleansing themselves appropriately.

This suggests that ascending the ramps was more than a practical means of entering the sanctuary; it was instead a multisensory and kinaesthetic act that directly engaged people in the ritualised activities that they had come to perform, even if these would culminate elsewhere in the sanctuary complex. In this way, the ramps began to incorporate their bodies into the religious ways of being that were required of them. Moreover, the ramps were a means through which people could produce and sustain their highly personal or proximal understanding of the religious world of the sanctuary via their own bodily experiences of living it. The ways in which the materiality of the ramps affected the sensing bodies that ascended their pathways indicate that this process involved more than the preparation of a purely cognitive understanding of what it meant to engage in religion, or the readying of a person for what they might encounter when they reached the top. It was, instead, an action that began to situate that religious knowledge in the very body that was living it and that would continue to live it until they departed the sanctuary, as well as during future activities where embodied memories of this experience were evoked. This, therefore, highlights how the situational production of knowledge might differ in subtle ways from body to body, and from person to person, rather than being a singular form of knowledge shared by all (for more examples of this, see Graham 2021).

Assessing the experience of ascending the ramps from the perspective of people with limited or impaired mobility and related conditions reveals that, for some people, approaching the gods was inherently difficult, a challenge that once overcome might produce rich rewards, not necessarily in the form of personal healing or a positive oracular consultation, but in terms of producing understandings related to ways of being in the world that brought together both shared knowledge of ritualised activities and their own personal experiences of living them. It was a part of the production of lived religion itself. Of course, negotiating an ascent via the ramps at Praeneste afforded a lived experience of religion that was also felt in the bodies of all visitors, whether able-bodied or disabled, and the materiality of the ramps compelled everyone to move in an unusual and potentially uncomfortable manner. However, until we foreground the physical experience of those whose bodily experiences of movement were already affected by impaired mobility, as I have done here, these observations tend to go unnoticed in favour of interpretations that focus on sight and that assume that the ramps played a primarily practical purpose in providing (presumed easy) access to the sanctuary.

The discussion presented here, nevertheless, begins to demonstrate how an interactional approach that seeks to foreground the lived experience of impairment can have implications beyond the study of ancient disability itself. In short, the observations that it prompts are relevant for broader understandings of how the sanctuary of Fortuna Primigenia was experienced as a religious place across the whole somatic spectrum, and consequently how religious place contributed to discrete forms of personal religious knowledge. Lived experience of the sanctuary and of the ritualised activities that were performed in relation to it was constituted differently because of the bodies that lived it. This suggests that experiences of impairment certainly will have textured the knowledge that was produced by a visit to the sanctuary, but that these did not necessarily leave impaired individuals with a diminished understanding of religion compared with their non-impaired companions. By incorporating impairment as a potential factor in the ways in which the sensescape of the sanctuary should be analysed, it can be argued even more convincingly that religious experiences and the knowledge that arose from engagement in ritualised practices incorporating engagement with the material world were deeply personalised. As there could be no single experience of accessing the sanctuary of Fortuna Primigenia, interactional theory not only makes it possible to better understand some of the lived realities of ancient impairment, it also allows that knowledge to be incorporated into wider debates concerning ancient social and cultural ways of being.

Conclusions

This chapter has sought to demonstrate that it is both possible and desirable to adopt an interactional approach to ancient disability, and that doing so has the potential to allow both sensory archaeologies and ancient disability studies to flourish in new and exciting ways. Not least among these is the encouragement it brings to foreground the diversity of potential ancient lived experiences of being in the physical material world and the ways in which these, in turn, encourage novel ways of approaching much broader and more long-standing areas of scholarship concerning ancient cultural forms and practices, such as religious experience. At the same time, the perspectives offered by sensory archaeologies make it possible to begin identifying and thinking more critically about how those people with disabilities and impairments encountered and experienced particular places and activities, rather than just how those people themselves were encountered and experienced by society. Indeed, the example of the sanctuary of Fortuna Primigenia, and the approach that I have taken to it, has revealed as much about the similarities of abled and disabled experiences of the sanctuary as it has highlighted the differences, supporting the conclusions of Christian Laes (2018, 173) who has argued that, for Roman society, 'the involvement of people with disabilities was perfectly normal'.

As both texts and archaeology lead us to this same conclusion, it is time to give their experiences equal weight in our analysis of the worlds in which these people lived. Doing so means that it is necessary to start considering how the lived experience of being disabled may have varied across the somatic spectrum of difference, not merely in order to gain a wider and more diverse perspective on the communities of antiquity, but because asking such questions logically leads to more nuanced understandings of ways of being within those communities themselves. I have argued that ancient sanctuaries offer a valuable testing ground for this approach, because evidence attests the uncontested presence at such locations of people with differing mobility and sensory impairments, and the brief case study presented here seeks to capitalise on existing knowledge of these sites. However, the potential disabled and impaired people whose experiences I have highlighted did much more with their lives than just visit sanctuaries. The next challenge is to identify other situations, other places, other activities, in which we might apply the same approach. Doing so will mean that our sensory reconstructions become significantly enhanced, nuanced, and inevitably more complicated in line with the complex realities of real human lived experiences, at the same time as our understanding develops of the real-world agency of those with bodily and sensory impairments in the shaping of their social and cultural worlds.

References

Adams, Ellen (2020) 'Deafness: sensory impairment as communication disability, past and present.' In Christian Laes (ed.), *A Cultural History of Disability in Antiquity*. London: Bloomsbury, 85–100.

Bassani, Maddalena (2014) 'I santuari e i luoghi di culto presso le sorgenti termominerali.' In Matteo Annibaletto, Maddalena Bassani, and Francesca Ghedini (eds), *Cura, preghiera e benessere: le stazioni curative termominerali nell'Italia Romana*. Padua: Padova University Press, 143–60.

Bassani, Maddalena (2019) 'Shrines and healing waters in ancient Italy. Buildings, cults, deities.' In Maddalena Bassani, Marion Bolder-Boos and Ugo Fusco (eds), *Rethinking the Concept of 'Healing Settlements': Water, Cults, Constructions and Contexts in the Ancient World*. Oxford: Archaeopress Roman Archaeology, 9–20.

Betts, Eleanor (2011) 'Towards a multisensory experience of movement in the city of Rome.' In Ray Laurence and David Newsome (eds), *Rome, Ostia and Pompeii: Movement and Space*. Oxford: Oxford University Press, 118–32.

Betts, Eleanor (2017a) 'Senses of empire.' In Eleanor Betts (ed.), *Senses of the Empire: Multisensory Approaches to Roman Culture*. London: Routledge, 1–12.

Betts, Eleanor (2017b) 'The multivalency of sensory artefacts in the city of Rome.' In Eleanor Betts (ed.), *Senses of the Empire: Multisensory Approaches to Roman Culture*. London: Routledge, 23–38.

Boutin, Alexis T. and Benjamin W. Porter (2014) 'Commemorating disability in early Dilmun: ancient and contemporary tales from the Peter B. Cornwall Collection.' In Benjamin W. Porter (ed.), *Remembering the Dead in the Near East: Recent Contributions from Bioarchaeology and Mortuary Archaeology*. Colorado: University Press of Colorado, 97–132.

Bradley, Mark (2002) '"It all comes out in the wash": looking harder at the Roman fullonica.' *Journal of Roman Archaeology* 15, 21–44.

Bradley, Mark and Shane Butler (eds) (2014–2018) The *Senses in Antiquity* book series. London: Routledge.

Butler, Shane and Alex Purves (eds) (2013) *Synaesthesia and the Ancient Senses*. London: Routledge.

Classen, Constance, David Howes and Anthony Synnott (1994) *Aroma: The Cultural History of Smell*. London: Routledge.

Coarelli, Filippo (1987) *I santuari del Lazio in età Repubblicana*. Rome: La Nuova Italia Scientifica.

Coo, Lyndsay (2015) 'Sight and blindness: the mask of Thamyris.' In Michael Squire (ed.), *Sight and the Ancient Senses*. London: Routledge, 237–48.

Day, Jo (ed.) (2013) *Making Senses of the Past: Toward a Sensory Archaeology*. Carbondale: Southern Illinois University.

Derrick, Thomas J. (2017) 'Sensory archaeologies: a Vindolanda smellscape.' In Eleanor Betts (ed.), *Senses of the Empire: Multisensory Approaches to Roman Culture*. London: Routledge, 71–85.

Dillon, Matthew (2017) 'Legal (and customary?) approaches to the disabled in ancient Greece.' In Christian Laes (ed.), *Disabilities in Antiquity*. London: Routledge, 167–181.

DiLuzio, Megan J. (2016) *A Place at the Altar: Priestesses in Republican Rome*. Princeton: Princeton University Press.

Draycott, Jane and Emma-Jayne Graham (eds) (2017) *Bodies of Evidence: Ancient Anatomical Votives Past, Present and Future*. London: Routledge.

Edwards, Martha Lynn [= Rose, Martha Lynn] (1997) 'Constructions of physical disability in the ancient Greek world: the community concept.' In David T. Mitchell and Sharon L. Snyder (eds), *The Body and Physical Difference: Discourses of Disability*. Ann Arbor: University of Michigan Press, 35–50.

Fasolo, Furio and Giorgio Gullini (1953) *Il santuario della Fortuna Primigenia a Palestrina*. Rome: Istituto di Archeologia, Università di Roma.

Flohr, Miko (2017) 'Beyond smell: the sensory landscape of the Roman fullonica.' In Eleanor Betts (ed.), *Senses of the Empire: Multisensory Approaches to Roman Culture*. London: Routledge, 39–53.

Graham, Emma-Jayne (2013) 'Disparate lives or disparate deaths? Post-mortem treatment of the body and the articulation of difference.' In Christian Laes, Chris F. Goodey and M. Lynn Rose (eds), *Disabilities in Roman Antiquity. Disparate Bodies* A Capite ad Calcem. Leiden: Brill, 249–74.

Graham, Emma-Jayne (2017a) 'Holding the baby? Sensory dissonance and the ambiguities of votive objects.' In Eleanor Betts (ed.), *Senses of the Empire: Multisensory Approaches to Roman Culture*. London: Routledge, 122–38.

Graham, Emma-Jayne (2017b) 'Mobility impairment in the sanctuaries of early Roman Italy.' In Christian Laes (ed.), *Disabilities in Antiquity*. London: Routledge, 248–66.

Graham, Emma-Jayne (2018) '"There buds the laurel": nature, temporality, and the making of place in the cemeteries of Roman Italy.' *Theoretical Roman Archaeology Journal* 1(1), 3. http://doi.org/10.16995/traj.147

Graham, Emma-Jayne (2020) 'Mobility impairment: identifying lived experiences in Roman Italy.' In Christian Laes (ed.), *A Cultural History of Disability in Antiquity*. London: Bloomsbury, 31–45.

Graham, Emma-Jayne (2021) *Reassembling Religion in Roman Italy*. London: Routledge.

Graham, Emma-Jayne (forthcoming) 'The haptic production of religious knowledge among the Vestal Virgins: a hands-on approach to Roman ritual.' In Abigail Graham and Blanka Misic (eds), *Sensory and Cognitive Approaches to Roman Religious Rituals*. Cambridge: Cambridge University Press.

Hamilakis, Yannis (2013) *Archaeology and the Senses: Human Experience, Memory and Affect*. Cambridge: Cambridge University Press.

Harvey, Graham (2018) 'Series foreword.' In Graham Harvey and Jessica Hughes (eds), *Sensual Religion: Religion and the Five Senses*. Sheffield: Equinox, vii–ix.

Harvey, Graham and Jessica Hughes (eds) (2018) *Sensual Religion: Religion and the Five Senses*. Sheffield: Equinox.

Haug, Annette and Patric-Alexander Kreuz (eds) (2016) *Stadterfahrung als Sinneserfahrung in Der Romischen Kaiserzeit*. Turnhout: Brepol.

Hollinshead, Mary B. (2015) *Shaping Ceremony: Monumental Steps and Greek Architecture*. Madison: University of Wisconsin Press.

Horsfall, Nicholas (2003) *The Culture of the Roman Plebs*. London: Duckworth.

Hughes, Jessica (2017) *Votive Body Parts in Greek and Roman Religion*. Cambridge: Cambridge University Press.

Inclusive mobility (n.d.) Inclusive mobility. Available at: https://assets.publishing.service.gov.uk/government/uploads/system/uploads/attachment_data/file/3695/inclusive-mobility.pdf (accessed 21 October 2019).

Kjellström, Anna (2010) 'Tracing pain: identifying suffering in skeletal remains.' In Fredrik Fahlander and Anna Kjellström (eds), *Making Sense of Things: Archaeologies of Sensory Perception*. Stockholm: Stockholm Studies in Archaeology 53, 51–67.

Koloski-Ostrow, Ann O. (2015) 'Roman urban smells: the archaeological evidence.' In Mark Bradley (ed.) *Smell and the Ancient Senses*. London: Routledge, 90–109.

Laes, Christian (2011) 'Silent witnesses: deaf-mutes in Greco-Roman antiquity.' *Classical World* 104(4), 451–73.

Laes, Christian (2018) *Disabilities and the Disabled in the Roman World: A Social and Cultural History*. Cambridge: Cambridge University Press.

Laes, Christian, Chris F. Goodey and M. Lynn Rose (2013) 'Approaching disabilities *a capite ad calcem*: hidden themes in Roman antiquity.' In Christian Laes, Chris F. Goodey and M. Lynn Rose (eds), *Disabilities in Roman Antiquity. Disparate Bodies* a Capite ad Calcem. Leiden: Brill, 1–15.

Lovell, Nancy (2016) 'Tiptoeing through the rest of his life: a functional adaptation to a leg shortened by femoral neck fracture.' *International Journal of Paleopathology* 13, 91–5.

Merleau-Ponty, Maurice (1968) *The Visible and the Invisible: Followed by Working Notes*. Translated by Alphonso Lingis. Evanston: Northwestern University Press.

Moser, Claudia (2019) *The Altars of Republican Rome and Latium: Sacrifice and the Materiality of Roman Religion*. Cambridge: Cambridge University Press.

Pestilli, Livio (2005) 'Disabled bodies: the (mis)representation of the lame in Antiquity and their reappearance in early Christian and Medieval art.' In Andrew Hopkins and Maria Wyke (eds), *Roman Bodies: Antiquity to the Eighteenth Century*. London: The British School at Rome, 85–97.

Platts, Hannah (2019) *Multisensory Living in Ancient Rome: Power and Space in Roman Houses*. London: Bloomsbury.

Pudsey, April (2017) 'Disability and infirmitas in the ancient world: demographic and biological facts in the longue durée.' In Christian Laes (ed.), *Disability in Antiquity*. London: Routledge, 22–34.

Raja, Rubina and Jörg Rüpke (eds) (2015) *A Companion to the Archaeology of Religion in the Ancient World*. Malden: Wiley-Blackwell.

Riddle, Christopher A. (2013a) 'The ontology of impairment: rethinking how we define disability.' In Matthew Wappett and Katrina Arndt (eds), *Emerging Perspectives on Disability Studies*. New York: Palgrave, 23–39.

Riddle, Christopher A. (2013b) 'Defining disability: metaphysical not political.' *Medical Health Care and Philosophy* 16, 377–84.

Rose, M. Lynn (2003) *The Staff of Oedipus. Transforming Disability in Ancient Greece*. Ann Arbor: Michigan University Press.

Rous, Benjamin D. (2010) 'Triumphs of Compromise: An Analysis of the Monumentalisation of Sanctuaries in Latium in the Late Republican Period (Second and First Centuries BC).' Unpublished thesis, University of Amsterdam. Available at: http://hdl.handle.net/11245/1.327031 (accessed 3 September 2018).

Rüpke, Jörg (2007) *Religion of the Romans*. Cambridge: Polity Press.

Schultz, Celia E. and Paul B. Harvey (2006) *Religion in Republican Italy*. Cambridge: Cambridge University Press.

Shakespeare, Tom (2006) *Disability Rights and Wrongs*. London: Routledge.

Sharples, Annie (2019) Disabling ableism in Classics. Available at: https://eidolon.pub/disabling-ableism-in-classics-4fd28d02c628 (accessed 21 October 2019).

Skeates, Robin and Jo Day (eds) (2019) *The Routledge Handbook of Sensory Archaeology*. London: Routledge.

Southwell-Wright, William (2014) 'Perceptions of infant disability in Roman Britain.' In Maureen Carroll and Emma-Jayne Graham (eds), *Infant Health and Death in Roman Italy and Beyond*. Ann Arbor: Journal of Roman Archaeology Supplementary Series 96, 111–30.

Squire, Michael (ed.) (2015) *Sight and the Ancient Senses*. London: Routledge.

Toner, Jerry (2009) *Popular Culture in Ancient Rome*. Cambridge: Polity Press.

Trentin. Lisa (2013) 'Exploring visual impairment in Roman antiquity.' In Christian Laes, Chris F. Goodey and M. Lynn Rose (eds), *Disabilities in Roman Antiquity. Disparate Bodies a Capite ad Calcem*. Leiden: Brill, 89–114.

Veitch, Jeffrey (2017) 'Soundscape of the street: architectural acoustics in Ostia.' In Eleanor Betts (ed.), *Senses of the Empire: Multisensory Approaches to Roman Culture*. London: Routledge, 54–70.

Warford, Erin (2019) 'Performing piety: a phenomenological approach to Athenian processions.' In Wiebke Friese, Søren Handberg and Troels M. Kristensen (eds), *Ascending and Descending the Acropolis: Movement in Athenian Religion*. Athens: Monographs of the Danish Institute at Athens 23, 23–41.

Weddle, Candace (2013) 'The sensory experience of blood sacrifice in the Roman imperial cult.' In Jo Day (ed.), *Making Senses of the Past: Toward a Sensory Archaeology*. Carbondale: Southern Illinois University, 137–59.

Zakrzewski, Sonia (2014) 'Palaeopathology, disability and bodily impairments.' In Ryan Metcalfe, Jenefer Cockitt and Rosalie David (eds), *Palaeopathology in Egypt and Nubia: A Century in Review*. Oxford: Archaeopress, 57–68.

Zakrzewski, Sonia (2015) '"Behind every mask there is a face, and behind that a story." Egyptian bioarchaeology and ancient identities.' In Salima Ikram, Jessica Kaiser and Roxie Walker (eds), *Egyptian Bioarchaeology: Humans, Animals, and the Environment*. Leiden: Sidestone Press, 157–67.

Chapter 8

Rational capacity and incomplete adults

The mentally impaired in classical antiquity

Patricia Baker and Sarah Francis

Abstract

The skeletal remains of an adult male were found buried in a well on the slopes of the Athenian Acropolis and the Iron Age necropolis. The remains indicated that the male had survived cranial damage that would have caused irreversible brain injury and mental impairment. Yet, rather than being buried in the manner of an adult, this person was inhumed with a pottery cup, a practice common to children at the time. This interment invited us to question how people with mental impairments were classified and treated in Ancient Greece. By comparing the limited archaeological evidence of adults buried both with and in the manner of children with the philosophical works of Aristotle, we argue that those with mental impairments were perceived as childlike and held the status of children. In his discussions on the nature of children, Aristotle describes them as incomplete humans because they fall short of being fully formed adults capable of reasoning. Therefore, the category of mental disability did not have the medical definition we see today, but one based on ideas for capacities to reason.

Introduction

Greek and Roman period interments of infants and children have been the subject of much archaeological consideration. The manner and locations of their burials commonly differ from those of adults. Archaeologists argue that the different burial practices are an indicator of the social status of children (e.g. Carroll 2018, 15–25, 147–77; Houby-Nielsen, 2000; Laubenheimer, 2004; Mays 2000; Scott 1991). In particular, neonates, infants, and sometimes toddlers were interred in out-of-use wells and pits. On rare occasions, adults were buried with and/or in the same manner as children. Papadopoulos (2000) studied these exceptional well burials of adults and noted that, although unusual, evidence for the practice extended over a long period of time – from the Greek Bronze Age to the Hellenistic period. He maintained that those placed in these positions were considered to be unworthy of the standard rites associated with burial practices for adults because these individuals were branded social deviants, meaning someone who stood outside the norms of their society. The term social deviant, however, has derogatory connotations that might not be appropriate for someone who received a burial, albeit unusual. Evidence from two burials of adult males catalogued by Papadopoulos indicates that their marginal status might not have been as socially aberrant as he argued. One male was interred in the manner of a child, and the other with children. Their remains show signs of physical problems that indicate they required assistance to ensure their survival, similar to the care that infants and children would have received during the course of their formative years. Thus, rather than being a social deviant, we question if people with certain impairments were deemed to be children or held the same status as children in ancient Greece and, hence, were interred according to their status.

The archaeological remains provide an intriguing glimpse into how certain categories of impairment might have been defined, but evidence is limited. Moreover, the two burials date roughly seven to eight hundred years apart from each other, and attitudes and definitions were likely to have changed. Thus, to find new insights into archaeological interpretations for these unusual burials and access possible attitudes and understandings towards those with incapacities, we move beyond strict disciplinary boundaries. We compare the remains with fifth-/fourth-century Greek philosophical discussions concerning conceptions and definitions of infants, children, and adults with impairments. As the two forms of evidence corroborated each other, the implication is that adults with a diminished mental capacity and/or limiting physical impairment were analogous to infants and children in ancient Greek thought. It seems likely that this perception was common across Athens, if not wider Greek society, over an extended period.

Archaeological method

Skeletal remains are generally examined for the condition of the bones to determine the health of the individual. If a condition is found, it is also possible to determine whether it was congenital or caused by a trauma. Certain congenital conditions are easily detected, such as achondroplasia, anencephaly, spina bifida, cleft pallet, and clubfoot. Non-congenital conditions such as trauma, joint disease, and certain infectious diseases such as leprosy are also apparent on bones (Roberts and Manchester 1995).

Even when a condition is detected, it is difficult to state how the individual with it was classified at the time they were living. Therefore, consideration must be given to the archaeological context of the body. When remains are studied along with their provenance and manner of deposition, they can illuminate intangible rules and ideas held by particular societies that may not have been expressed verbally (e.g. Hill 1995; Hodder 1982; Moore 1982). Numerous archaeological studies concerning people living in different periods and geographical regions have found that men, women, and children were often treated differently in burials, which may be a reflection of their social positions while they were alive (e.g. Meskell 1994; Parker-Pearson 1999; Sourvinou-Inwood 1996). The correlation between burials and social status can be considered for interments of those with perceived mental and bodily differences as well. However, it cannot be assumed that such differences were signs of disparity in social status. Bodily norms were different from those of today (Cross 1999; 2007; Molleson 1999). Thus, the skeletal remains of someone found to have a form of disability must be studied along with the burial context.

The burials

Two adult males, one dating to the Greek Iron Age (c.900–850 BC) and the other the Hellenistic period prior to 150 BC, were found interred in Athenian wells (Papadopoulos 2000, 104–5, 110–1; Liston and Rotroff 2013; Liston, Rotroff and Snyder 2018, 26–9). The skeletal remains of the Iron Age male were intact and showed that the individual had two fractures to his skull (Fig. 8.1). The one on the left side was a 'massive compound depression fracture', and that on his right was a shallow elliptical depression fracture. The paleopathological report states that such severe injuries to the head would have caused some form of brain damage. Blows to the left hemisphere of the brain can cause seizures and aphasia, which affects speaking, writing, and/or signing. Seizures to the temporal lobe can result in involuntary speech or movement, uncontrolled anger or fear, and motor or psychic disturbances. In addition to the trauma to the head, he also had compression fractures on his first and third lumbar vertebrae. Such injuries would have been life-threatening. However, there was bone regrowth on the skull, indicating that the man had lived for quite some time after his accident (Little and Papadopoulos 1998, 374–81, 385–92; Papadopoulos 2000, 104–5). Yet, the injuries would have left him requiring the help of others to enable his survival. Though who cared for him and how the care was offered are indeterminate.

The archaeological context of the burial and associated artefact lends further support that this individual was provided with care. In Iron Age Athens, cremation rather than inhumation was the standard rite for adults. The cremation urns were buried in necropoleis. Children, on the other hand, were inhumed in trenches and pits (Kurz and Boardman 1971, 36; Snodgrass 1971, 143–59; Whitley 2001, 94–6). In Greece, necropoleis were commonly placed on the outside of settlement boundaries, usually along roadsides, indicating that there were certain taboos associated with death and the dead. The Iron Age male was deliberately and carefully buried in a crouched position in a well located on the northern slopes of the Athenian Acropolis, and he was buried with a small cup. The well where he was placed lay between the known Iron Age necropoleis located in the grounds surrounding the Acropolis and the settlement located on the top of the Acropolis (Little and Papadopoulos 1998, 376, n. 6). Thus, the

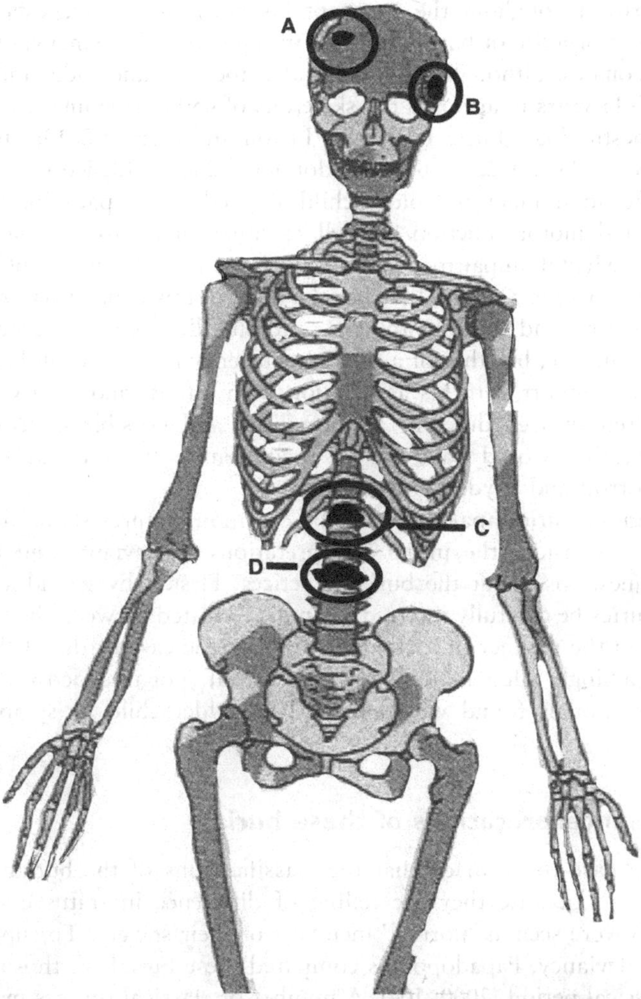

Figure 8.1 Skeletal remains of the male located on the Athenian Acropolis. A = shallow elliptical depression skull fracture; B = massive compound skull fracture; C and D = compression fractures on the first and third lumbar vertebrae. After Little and Papadopoulos 1998, Fig. 1. Drawing by Paula Fisher (with permission)

care given to the burial suggests that this was someone deemed worthy of interment, but he was buried similarly to an infant or child, in a location away from adults.

The second curious interment was found in a well (number G5:3) located at Kolonos Agoraios in the western area of the Agora. This area was abandoned in the Hellenistic period. After it had fallen out of use, the well was reused as a spot for infant burials. Contained within it was an adult male with severe osteoarthritis throughout the joints of his body, which suggests degenerative joint disease or a life of hard labour. With him were the remains of 450 infants, mainly neonates, although there were also foetuses and older infants; a child roughly 8–11 years in age; and the skeletons of 450 plus animals, most of which were domestic dogs (Little 1999, 284; Liston and Rotroff 2013; Liston, Rotroff and Snyder 2018, 30–2, 53–64; Papadopoulos 2000, 110; Rotroff 1999; Snyder 1999). The adult male and older child showed severe pathologies that could have affected motor function as well as other functions (Liston and Rotroff 2013, 67). Mental impairments, however, are not always visible on skeletal remains, so there is a possibility that the male in this context had some form of impairment beyond motor abilities. Admittedly, other interpretations are equally applicable, but that of a mental deficiency is no less valid and may even find further support with his association with infants and even with the dogs. The children showed different abnormalities and possible infections, such as meningitis, that would have led to their demise (Liston and Rotroff 2013; Liston, Rotroff and Snyder 2018, 32–62).

Although centuries apart in date, the common features shared by both were reason to reconsider the initial interpretations of deviants and to ask some detailed questions about the burial practices. First, why would an adult with severe injuries be carefully interred in an area located between the living and the dead and in the manner of a child? Second, in the case of the Hellenistic male, why was a single adult male placed in a burial spot intended for infants, and might the animals found with him and the older child be symbolic of their status?

Previous interpretations of these burials

There is a case to be made that the classifications of the burials in question were unusual because they are telling of difference in status compared with those who were seen as 'normal' members of their society. To support his case for social deviancy, Papadopoulos compared these burials to those of criminals in the classical period (2000, 104). A number of classical sources make reference to the fact that criminals guilty of murder were not permitted a proper burial as a form of punishment for their crimes. According to Greek belief, the soul of someone who had not been afforded appropriate burial rites was condemned to dwell between the earth and the home of the dead. Kurz and Boardman say that criminals were cast into pits, quarries, and the sea, but no references or evidence are provided to support their statement (1971, 198). There are, however, indications that certain criminals might have had their bodies cast out of city boundaries without a burial. Plato advocated such customs in his *Laws* (874b; 909b–c). In this work, he explained which criminals should be punished in this manner: those who had murdered their parents, siblings, or children should be executed, and their naked bodies should be taken to a crossroads outside the city boundaries where each magistrate was to throw a rock at their heads in atonement for the whole state. Then the body was to be taken to the borders of the land and cast out without burial.

In addition, those who were involved with forms of necromancy used to wreck families and states for money were to be imprisoned, and, if they died in prison, the same punishment was suggested (Plato *Leg.* 909b–c). Similarly, Xenophon said that anyone who was found guilty of wronging the people of Athens was executed by being cast into the *barathron*, a pit or cleft, supposedly located beyond the Acropolis (*Hel.* 1.7, 20). Herodotus (7.133) makes reference to people being cast into wells for their crimes, but here the well is specifically used in accompaniment to the *barathron* in order to add to the dark humour of the command given by the Athenians and Spartans to heralds sent by Darius:

> Xerxes did not send heralds to Athens and Sparta for the following reason: when Darius had previously sent them for the same purpose, those who had asked [at Athens] were thrown into a pit (*barathron*) and those [at Sparta] into a well and were ordered to take earth and water from these to their king.

Consequently, the literary evidence, although later in date than the Iron Age, suggests that those classed as deviants were not given any form of burial, which is at odds with our argument put forth about the Iron Age man's social status, as he was carefully interred with an offering. Moreover, although damage to the brain may have led to erratic behaviour, it cannot be assumed that this was vicious behaviour. As for the man buried with infants, again the interpretation of social deviant is questionable. If there were rules against harming the family, this interment would seem inappropriate.

Precedents for unusual burials

In both the Greek and Roman periods, it was common for necropoleis to be placed on the outside of settlement boundaries, along roadsides. Being located outside boundaries and away from dwelling areas indicates that there were certain taboos associated with death and the dead, as mentioned above. Death was polluting, and rituals were set in place to purify both the house in which a person died and the people who came into contact with it (Parker 1996, 35). In spite of these practices and prohibitions, unusual burials are still found throughout the Greco-Roman world, suggesting that the person held a different status to those buried in more conventional locations. Indications of 'disability' status and identity are found in the unusual burial location and manner of skeletal remains with signs of bodily differences, such as in wells, shafts, and boundaries (Molleson 1999, 69).

Boundaries demarcate zones of inclusion and exclusion that create a concept of 'otherness' (Garland 1985, 77–89; Hubert 2000, 5–8; Whittaker 1994, 12–26).

Greeks and Romans marked sacred spaces, building entrances, and land borders with buildings, elaborate entrances, and statues of the head of Janus, for example. Offerings were also made to chthonic deities in boundary zones, most likely to appease the gods and to solicit protection (Whittaker 1994, 24; Livy *History* 1.44; Varro *On the Latin Language* 5.143). In association with these ideas, sometimes skeletal remains were deliberately placed within boundary ditches rather than in cemeteries in other areas and periods. It seems to have been a problem in Republican Rome, indicated by the existence of two decrees recorded on the Esquiline Hill that no one should throw a corpse within boundary zones (CIL 6.31614–15).

Another explanation for the location of peripheral burials can be found in classical mythology. Monsters and people with divergent body types were frequently described as living in isolated areas on the edges of the world (Romm 1992). In the *Nicomachean Ethics*, Aristotle describes certain 'tales' of brutish behaviour, such as the woman who rips open pregnant women and eats their children and various abhorrent pleasures of those who live around the Black Sea (*EN* 1148b19–24). This idea is representative of the general attitude of the time, which may have been reflected in the placement of burial locations that were separated from both the living and the dead.

One example that demonstrates how disability status can be identified in a contextual archaeological study is a child's burial (PC 1114) found in Poundbury, Dorset (Farwell and Molleson 1993, 21, 187, 272). This Romano-British burial dates to the fourth century AD and was one of seven individuals interred in a prone position. The child was roughly 6 years of age at death and was found on the outer edge of the eastern periphery of the cemetery. Both the prone position and the place of burial intimate some form of marginal status. The cranial evidence may offer a reason for this location and manner of burial. The child was deaf in its right ear. The auditory canal did not develop properly and was covered with bone. Unfortunately, the left side is not present in the archaeological record, so it cannot be determined if this child was profoundly or partially deaf. As the skull is incomplete, both possibilities are considered. The child may have been born with a congenital condition known today as microtia. In some cases, this condition affects both ears, but, in most, only one ear is afflicted. Those born with this congenital condition have an underdeveloped outer ear, and, in some cases, no outer ear exists. As for the ear canal, this is blocked, leaving the child deaf in the affected ear (González-del Angel 1999, 120–4). The deafness and possible malformation of the outer ear(s) could explain the prone position.

Artefacts buried with the dead are sometimes indicators of a person's social status, as has been shown with finds of weapons, large amounts of grave goods, and pottery and jewellery, for example. It is not unusual to find puppies and dogs buried with infants in the Roman and Greek world. One suggestion for their deposition is that they were used to ward off evil (Soren and Soren 1998, 619–27). Dogs were associated with chthonic deities such as Hecate and

Asclepius, whose powers might have been invoked in certain rituals related to the dead. However, there might also be a correlation between the status of the child/infant and the status of the dogs and puppies. The remains of the animals in the Hellenistic well ranged in age from foetal stages to older dogs that were showing signs of arthritis and were missing teeth. They also have a clear association with the human remains in the well (Snyder 1999, 284). There is also a correlation with Hecate as a goddess of birth and death, and dogs are associated with pollution and childbirth (see an overview in Liston and Rotroff 2013, 67–9).

It is also striking that Aristotle considered dogs as 'not perfected' when they were puppies. In *Generation of Animals*, he mentions that the canine young are the most peculiar of all animal formations because they are born in an 'incomplete' state (*GA* 742a8–10; *GA* 774b13–6). Aristotle says that polydactylous quadrupeds, such as dogs, lions, wolves, foxes, and jackals, all give birth to blind young, as the eyelid does not divide until after birth, a quality that earns them a place in his description of 'monstrosities' among animals (*GA* 770a35–b2). He goes on to note here that the offspring of some birds are also born 'imperfect' (*atelês*) and blind. This is common, he says, among animals that produce many offspring, and the offspring of this type of animal (such as the dog) are 'not born perfected' (*ou teleiogona*) but born blind. Therefore, Aristotle might provide a key insight explaining the significance of puppies and dogs found in children's burials in Athens. Even if canines were not part of a ritual, they might have still been interred on account of their association with an incomplete state of being.

The archaeological remains of the two men provide an intriguing possibility that those with diminished mental capacities might have been buried in the manner of and with infants on account of the way their condition was defined and understood during the time in which they lived. Although the archaeological evidence may be interpreted in this manner, without further remains showing clear signs of head trauma, such an interpretation cannot be substantiated, but, in comparison with philosophical texts, there seem to have been parallels in thought.

Studies concerned with disability in the past that focus on evidence from ancient literature indicate that the terms used to describe those with bodily differences were vague, such as 'incomplete' (*atelês*), 'lame' (*khôlos*), and 'disfigured' (*anapêros*), and did not indicate strict classifications similar to what we have today (Garland 1995, 8–9; Rose 2003, 11–3). In spite of the imprecise terms, to make distinctions between types of disability, scholars resort to modern typologies, which may be incomparable with how the Greeks perceived people who were considered to be outside the social norm in terms of their mental and bodily conditions. It is more likely, in some cases, that the Greeks categorised people in relation to their philosophies on bodily development and function. Thus, analogies to developmental stages rather than specific definitions might have been made and used to describe different conditions.

Status of children

For Classical Greece, two stages of development seem to have existed for children: those under the age of 2/3 were infants, and those roughly aged 3 through to puberty were children. The evidence for this status is fairly consistent across the sources of surviving information. In Greek archaeological remains, neonates, infants, and toddlers under the age of 3 are most often found interred in shafts and wells that had gone out of use and below building foundations, indicating that their age designated a standing different from adults and older children. At the age of 3, children were introduced to the family clan in a ceremony known as the *Choes*; although the child had been given a name and was considered worth rearing at an earlier stage, it still had to survive this part of its life before being fully integrated into the social structure, which corresponds to their places of burial (Beaumont 2000; Papadopoulos 2000, 111). At the same time, Lagia notes that there are regional and temporal differences in the representation of children in ancient Greece, pointing out that, during the Late Classical and Hellenistic periods, there are few skeletal remains of children in Athenian cemeteries, whereas the numbers of skeletal remains are higher in the Archaic, High Classical, and Roman periods. This possibly points to different burial practices for children, which in turn might be indicated a change in their status (Lagia 2007).

Further indications about the precarious status of neonates and infants are expressed through the existence of naming rituals. In the Roman tradition, the waiting period differed: girls were named on the seventh or eighth day of their life, and boys on the ninth day (Dixon 1992, 134; Suetonius *Life of Nero* 6.2). When the pollution that came with the birth had been lifted, a celebration was held; in Greece it was the *amphidromia*, and in Latin the *dies lustricus* (Dixon 1992, 134; Parker 1996, 51; Plato *Theaetetus* 160e). These rites may have been set to see if a child was strong enough to survive the first week of its life and to allow time to consider whether an unhealthy infant should be exposed. The implication of the waiting period is that, during the stage between birth and acquiring a name, the infant was in some respects a liminal figure without any real status; in a manner of speaking, it was not perceived as wholly human (or wholly worth rearing) until it had demonstrated that it could survive its earliest days. This phase of existence might account for the unusual burials of infants in wells, under the eaves of houses, and in foundations, places where adults and older children are rarely found (Scott 1991, 116–9).

Children over the age of 2/3 were usually buried in different areas of cemeteries from adults. It is evident that, from about the seventh into the fifth century BC, child burials in Athens were placed alongside roads that seem to have been associated with stages of childhood development. For example, Houby-Nielsen (2000, 151–66) argues that the Plattenbau and Smeall-Dear areas of the Kerameikos led to the sanctuary of Demeter and Kore at Eleusis, and the Diochares Gate cemetery led to the sanctuary of Artemis at Brauron, both sanctuaries associated with girls. Furthermore, she states that, in association with male training, the cemetery near the Diplyon Gate led to the Academy. Archaeologists have found that children had specific places for interment that differed to those designated for adults in Iron Age, Archaic, and High Classical period sites throughout Greece (Snodgrass 1971; Whitley 2001). This difference is, therefore, a possible indication of their status in society and may be linked to the man found in the well on the slopes of the Acropolis.

Aristotle on the incomplete status of children

If the choice of burial location was dependent upon ancient definitions of the status of infants, children, and adults, then there is reason to argue that the males in the wells were identified as children on account of their physical and mental capacities. Aside from being found in social practices, ancient definitions of children are also found in philosophical discussions, particularly in Aristotle's works. In Aristotle, the child is deemed 'incomplete' because of its inability to fulfil the necessary duties required for life in the polis, its underdeveloped rational capacities, and its unstable physical nature on which these rational capacities depend. When commenting on the child's status as an incomplete citizen, Aristotle draws a comparison between the incomplete share in citizen rights held by the metic (a status he himself held) and the incomplete share in these rights held by a child (*Pol.* 1275a11–6). Of course, the metic's incomplete share in citizen rights is dependent on his status as a non-Athenian, whereas the child's incomplete status stems from its inability to behave in a rational fashion. This is a particularly important point to note because, for Aristotle, questions of rational capacity extend to matters of social status, and, in the *Politics*, he describes how the extent to which someone is capable of rational functioning marks their place in society.

Slaves, women, and children all had an incomplete share of a faculty for deliberation. The slave did not have it at all; the woman had it, but it is 'uncontrolled'; and the child had it, but it is incomplete (*atelês*; Arist. *Pol.* 1260a12–4). It is for this reason that each of these groups can only become 'whole' under the care of the free, adult, male Greek. This particular passage is part of Nussbaum's (1995) investigation into what Aristotle sees as sharing a fully human existence. She believes that Aristotle would not include the natural slave as he lacked the 'deliberative faculty' necessary for the good life, as qualified under Aristotle's function argument of *Nicomachean Ethics*. Those who lack this faculty, she presumes to be people 'who suffer some severe degree of mental retardation', and those who Aristotle classed as 'monstrous births' and those likely to have been exposed at birth should count among these. However, she does admit that some who lack incomplete rational autonomy may surpass 'mere human life' through associations such as their family (Nussbaum 1995, 117–8).

A child was a part of his/her father until a certain age, presumably when Aristotle deems full rational functioning should have developed (for the female child this was not full rational functioning but rather rationality appropriate to the female sex) and, until that time, was deemed a possession (*ktêma*) of the father (*EN* 1134b10). Hence, for Aristotle at least, the liminal status of children depended on their 'incomplete' rational capacity, a condition that excluded them from active participation in the adult world of the polis. This exclusion finds some parallel in the unusual burial of children seen in the well. In fact, if we consider the incomplete position of the child in Aristotle further, we may find some justification for the burials of the adults on the basis of his physical and subsequent possible mental state. The child's incomplete status was marked in Aristotle through his/her irrational behaviour, behaviour typified by a lack of rational decision and often impulsive actions. He says children manifest behaviour that is not fully rational: they pursue pleasure, their action is characterised by appetite, and, although their actions are voluntary, they are without rational choice (*EN* 1152b19–20; 1119b5–7; 1111a24–6; 1111b8–10). Much the same can be said for the young. The terms that Aristotle used for the young person (*neos*) and the child (*pais, teknon*, and *paidion* on occasion) in his ethical works are treated together here because they all fall short of complete rationality owing to their physical natures. The difference between the two stages of development appears to be one of increasing responsibility for the young agent; Aristotle used the child in discussions of basic appetite, friendship, and the overall experience of the young person (for experience, see *EN* 1095a3; 1142a12, 20, and friendship, *EN* 1155a12; 1156a26ff; 1158a5, 20).

We might consider then that the adult male interred in the well burial behaved in such a way that he shared the status of the child. Little and Papadopoulos suggested that the burial of the adult in the well may indicate that he was in some way excluded from society on the grounds of some crime or aberrant behaviour. However, although children are often seen to act incorrectly, they are not considered vicious (for Aristotle, vicious behaviour was deliberate behaviour, and deliberation was a condition that children do not share in), and as a result it is not clear why their status should in any way connect these two groups. It is not enough to say that the child and the unidentified males may have some share in incomplete rational function because, based on Aristotle's qualification of what constitutes 'complete' function, a direct correlation between Aristotelian theory and burial practice would mean that women and slaves would also be buried separately in ancient Greece. This was clearly not the case. Yet, what marks the child out from these other two groups is that they will, at some point, achieve rational function (appropriate to their sex), and that their current irrational behaviour depended on their unstable physical natures. It is this connection between unstable physical conditions and rational capacity that directly links the child to the mentally impaired individual in Aristotle's thought.

'Completion' for Aristotle was not merely marked by the transition to adulthood but also the physiological stability that normally accompanied adulthood, along with a process of habituation, which was the aspect of development for which an educator was responsible. Aristotle linked the incomplete nature of the child's rational capacity to their incomplete physical nature, which interferes with cognitive functioning and drives desires that overtake rational deliberation. According to Aristotle, the unstable physical nature of the youth caused behaviour based on desire, which was intense, but brief. The youth was compared to the sick in their sharp and powerful desires (*Rh.* 1389a4–9). This caused the young to be 'easily swayed', 'fickle', and have short but intense desire (*Rh.* 1389a6–7). These physical characteristics also impacted their temperaments (*Rh.* 1389a18–9; 24–5). This is peculiar not only to the child, but also to those who share some unstable state; for example, in the *Nicomachean Ethics*, certain types of people, such as the melancholic and the child, could not pursue rational pleasures because of their internal nature that caused them to pursue physical pleasures (*EN* 1154b5–15).

In *Parts of Animals*, Aristotle said that the 'dwarf-like' nature of the child prevented the 'movement' of the 'rational principle' contained within the child. He believed that pressure in the upper body could hamper the movement of the mind and the common sense (*koinê aisthesis*). Adults were more intelligent than animals because they stand upright and do not suffer from the burden of a heavy body pressing down upon them. In comparison, children are 'dwarf-like' and, therefore, they suffer from impaired movement of rational principle caused by the burden of a heavy body pressing downwards making the movement of the thought and central senses difficult (*PA* 686a24–b32; Coles 1997, 287–324).

This is also seen in *On Memory*, where the young human's difficulty in remembering is connected to his internal nature, a quality shared with people of restricted growth. Aristotle said that both the very young and the very old had difficulty remembering owing to being in a state of flux; in the young, this was from growth, and, in the old, decay (*Mem.* 450b5–7). Both the old and young had poor memories, as did people of restricted growth owing to the great weight bearing down on their central sense organ, which disrupted the movement of recollection. He added that young children experienced this not only owing to their internal flux, but also owing to being dwarfish, and thus they were doubly impaired (*Mem.* 453a31–b7). This unsettled physical state, and the subsequent effect it has on the ability of the individual to deliberate, is seen in melancholics as well as children, a condition that caused them to be described in the same passages. In essence, children showed a propensity to act on physical desires, and their characteristics were a direct result of this unstable physical state; more measured reactions only came with physical growth, internal stabilising, and associated rational development. It is not surprising that Aristotle should equate physical illness with lack of rational thought, because he believed that there needed to be some sort of internal physiological 'harmony' for rational function to take place. In the *Physics*, he discussed the effects that upset in the body has on psychic faculties; he stated that being drunk, asleep, and sick were examples of how psychic faculties were affected by restlessness, and, as such, people in these conditions only regained knowledge when they regained their stable physical state (247b1ff; 274b14). He also noted that knowledge was dependent on 'rest' in the psychic faculties, and this is the reason why children had inferior cognitive faculties, owing to the restless nature of their souls (*Ph.* 247b17–248a2). Dasen (2008, 50–2) also examines the ways Aristotle says children are intellectually and emotionally affected by their physical conditions.

In the *Nicomachean Ethics*, Aristotle also drew a comparison between the impulsive behaviour of the child and that of the melancholic, in that both were driven by internal unstable physiology to act in an irrational fashion (1154b5–15). In fact, unstable physiology is also seen to cause irrational behaviour in adults. Cognitive disturbance manifested itself in different ways in Aristotle, but clearly has a basis in the individual's physical condition. Aristotle used the term 'mania' to describe the condition itself, and the agent who manifests some sort of unbalanced condition is described as *mainomenos*. He also used the term 'paranoia' (*Athenian Constitution* 56, 6, 6; *PA* 653b5). In addition to mania and melancholia, epilepsy was also mentioned (Powell et al. 2005, 250–80), but it is not evident whether Aristotle considered this to be strictly an illness of the mind. Nonetheless, he clearly believed that mania and its various forms were the result of physical conditions; however, these conditions were not always illnesses, or symptoms of illnesses, as seen in the Hippocratic works, but in fact may be permanent, incurable conditions. When discussing the brain, Aristotle said that, if it became very fluid or solid, it would not perform its function properly and it would fail to cool the blood or set the blood, resulting in diseases, derangement (paranoia), and death (*PA* 653b3–5). Furthermore, owing to his hylomorphic theory, strong affections such as anger and sexual desire could change the state of the body, in some people causing mania (*EN* 1147a15–7). His 'diagnosis' of those who were incapable of rational functioning depended on an assessment of the agent with regards to normative cognitive processes such as decision-making. Those without the capacity for this had knowledge that they did not use, deliberated about things that nobody else would, were ignorant of their actions, or were compared to the 'insensible' types who fear nothing (*EN* 1147a12–4; 1112a19–21; 1111a6–7; 1115b26–7). The example of children is often used as a point of comparison with those who manifest irrational behaviour, such as in a notable passage where Aristotle, in describing pseudo-courage that arises from inexperience (*apeiria*) and ignorance (*agnoia*), gives the example of children and madmen (*mainomenoi*) who face that which rushes at them or who grab snakes (*EE* 1229a16–8).

Treating the madman like a child?

Aristotle clearly saw some parallel between the behaviour of the congenitally irrational adult and that of a child. Yet, would he go so far as to advocate treating the adult lacking in full capacity as a child? It seems much of this may depend on the nature of the condition. Furthermore, he was careful to distinguish between natural conditions and those caused by habituation (for example, failure to restrain strong emotions) and illness. He did make some distinction between curable and incurable incapacities and discussed the 'curability' of different types of uncontrolled behaviour (*EN* 1152a27–9). However, as far as those who would never achieve, or regain, full rational functioning were concerned, it seems that Aristotle was lenient towards adults who were incapable of achieving this status. He argued that we should not blame those who were incapacitated by nature or not through their own doing, and those whose actions were truly done in ignorance were to be pitied. When Aristotle was discussing states of character, he said if nature was the cause of these states, then these people were not liable to be blamed or called uncontrolled. He repeated this sentiment about bodily conditions, such as blindness, that may be natural or caused by one's own wrong behaviour (*EN* 1148b31–4; 1114a25; 1109b32; 1111a1).

Aristotle clearly held that the child, unable to exercise full rational functioning, was to remain a possession of his father until a time when he could function independently; thus, presumably, the incurable child would always remain a possession of his father. He was only considered 'whole' in his society by this relationship. In fact, it is clear that Athenian society considered those lacking in full rational capacity incapable of looking after their own affairs. It tends to be the case that evidence for how the mentally impaired were treated in Greek literature focused on medical treatment or punitive measures. Presumably, when the former of these two failed, or the family of the mentally impaired was not able to afford treatment, the latter became an issue. Greek law does appear to provide some support for drawing a parallel between children and those who are not considered by society to be fully rational. Plato described how, in Athens, prosecutors could call on the *dikê paranoias* to remove property and assets from a mentally incapacitated individual. This was usually a measure taken by a son against a senile father (a father suffering from paranoia), a measure that resulted in the parent taking the place of child (*pais*) in the household for the rest of his life (Plato *Leg.* 929d–e).

In Athenian law court speeches, this law is invoked against those who are no longer considered responsible for their actions. Plato tells us that, when a defendant was deemed to be suffering from insanity through being senile, sick, or in a childish state, he was given a lesser punishment (Plato *Leg.* 864d–e). It is difficult to see anything approaching 'compassion' in these accounts, although there is a clear notion that the family of the impaired individual should care for them (or, in cases of a slave, the owner), and, under these conditions, it does not seem surprising that the individual would return to the position of 'child' in the household. In the *Laws*, Plato noted that the mad person (*mainomenos*) must be kept indoors by his family, by any means possible, and that the person who failed to look after such a person in their charge (whether family or slave) should be fined (*Leg.* 934c–d). It may be that what we see in Aristotle is his intellectualisation of cultural phenomena, vestiges of which can be found in the burial record. It is also important to consider that, even if there was a tendency to treat the mentally impaired as if they were children, the attitudes of the ancients towards children, and any attitudes projected on to the mentally impaired as a result, are to be considered with caution.

Conclusion

Thus, to return the men in the well, although it is tempting to argue that an adult buried in an unusual manner is a sign of punishment that, therefore, identifies him as a social deviant, rather what we are seeing here is that the male was most likely identified as, in some ways, sharing the status of children. The reasons for this argument are as follows: first, the burial of a social deviant implies a careless disposal in unprotected ground, whereas here we have a person carefully placed in a well that is located between a settlement and a burial ground, rather than being cast away from both the living and the dead. Second, the choice of well burials seems to have been more closely associated with children. It is misleading to connect well burials with burials in pits used for criminals, such as the *barathon*; Herodotus's reference to a well burial, as mentioned above, seems to include a well in order to add a literary flourish. Third, the fact that they are buried in the manner of a child is more likely to be the significant factor in determining their status. It is clear from ancient legal and philosophical evidence that children were not considered complete in the way that adults were, either in their relation to the polis or in their own responsible behaviour, giving them a status that afforded them a different burial to adults. Furthermore, adults with mental incapacities were often referred to as children in that they shared, on the one hand, an underlying physical instability that caused their mental state and, on the other hand, that they needed to be cared for by family members.

References

Primary sources

Aristotle. *Art of Rhetoric.* Translated by John H. Freese (1926) Loeb Classical Library 193. Cambridge, MA: Harvard University Press.

Aristotle. *Athenian Constitution. Eudemian Ethics. Virtues and Vices.* Translated by Harris Rackham (1935) Loeb Classical Library 285. Cambridge, MA: Harvard University Press.

Aristotle. *Generation of Animals.* Translated by Arthur L. Peck (1942) Loeb Classical Library 366. Cambridge, MA: Harvard University Press.

Aristotle. *Nicomachean Ethics.* Translated by Harris Rackham (1926) Loeb Classical Library 73. Cambridge, MA: Harvard University Press.

Aristotle. *On the Soul. Parva Naturalia. On Breath, On Memory.* Translated by Walter S. Hett (1957) Loeb Classical Library 288. Cambridge, MA: Harvard University Press.

Aristotle. *Parts of Animals. Movement of Animals. Progression of Animals.* Translated by Arthur L. Peck and E.S. Forster (1937) Loeb Classical Library 323. Cambridge, MA: Harvard University Press.

Aristotle. *Physics, Volume I: Books 1–4*. Translated by Philip H. Wicksteed and Francis M. Cornford (1957) Loeb Classical Library 228. Cambridge, MA: Harvard University Press.

Aristotle. *Politics*. Translated by Harris Rackham (1932) Loeb Classical Library 264. Cambridge, MA: Harvard University Press.

Herodotus. *The Persian Wars, Volume III: Books 5–7*. Translated by Alfred D. Godley (1922) Loeb Classical Library 119. Cambridge, MA: Harvard University Press.

Livy. *History of Rome, Volume I: Books 1–2*. Translated by Benjamin O. Foster (1919) Loeb Classical Library 114. Cambridge, MA: Harvard University Press.

Plato. *Laws, Volume I: Books 1–6*. Translated by Robert G. Bury (1926) Loeb Classical Library 187. Cambridge, MA: Harvard University Press.

Plato. *Theaetetus. Sophist*. Translated by Harold N. Fowler (1921) Loeb Classical Library 123. Cambridge, MA: Harvard University Press.

Suetonius. *Lives of the Caesars, Volume II: Claudius. Nero. Galba, Otho, and Vitellius. Vespasian. Titus, Domitian. Lives of Illustrious Men: Grammarians and Rhetoricians. Poets (Terence. Virgil. Horace. Tibullus. Persius. Lucan). Lives of Pliny the Elder and Passienus Crispus*. Translated by John C. Rolfe (1914) Loeb Classical Library 38. Cambridge, MA: Harvard University Press.

Varro. *On the Latin Language, Volume II: Books 8–10. Fragments*. Translated by Roland G. Kent (1938) Loeb Classical Library 334. Cambridge, MA: Harvard University Press.

Xenophon. *Hellenica, Volume I: Books 1–4*. Translated by Carleton L. Brownson (1918) Loeb Classical Library 88. Cambridge, MA: Harvard University Press.

Secondary sources

Beaumont, Lesley (2000) 'The social status and artistic presentation of "adolescence" in fifth century Athens.' In Joanna Sofaer-Derevenski (ed.), *Children and Material Culture*. London and New York: Routledge, 39–50.

Carroll, Maureen (2018) *Infancy and Earliest Childhood in the Roman World*. Oxford: Oxford University Press.

Coles, Andrew (1997) 'Animal and childhood cognition in Aristotle's biology and the Scala Naturae.' In Wolfgang Kullmann and Sabine Föllinger (eds), *Aristotelische Biologie: Intentionen, Methoden, Ergebnisse*. Stuttgart: Franz Steiner, 287–324.

Cross, Morag (1999) 'Accessing the inaccessible: disability and archaeology.' *Archaeological Review from Cambridge* 15(2), 7–30.

Cross, Morag (2007) 'Accessing the inaccessible: disability and archaeology.' In Timothy Insoll (ed.), *The Archaeology of Identity: A Reader*. London and New York: Routledge, 179–4.

Dasen, Véronique (2008) 'All children are dwarfs: medical discourse and iconography of children's bodies.' *Oxford Journal of Archaeology* 27(1), 49–62.

Dixon, Suzanne (1992) *The Roman Family*. Baltimore: Johns Hopkins University Press.

Farwell, D.E. and Theya L. Molleson (1993) *Excavations at Poundbury 1966–80. Vol.* II *The Cemeteries*. Dorset Natural History Monograph Series. Dorchester: Dorset Natural History and Archaeological Society, 114.

Garland, Robert (1985) *The Greek Way of Death*. London: Duckworth.

Garland, Robert (1995) *The Eye of the Beholder: Deformity and Disability in the Graeco-Roman World*. London: Bloomsbury Academic.

González-del Angel, Ariadna (1999) 'Microtia: a clinical and genetic study at the National Institute of Pediatrics in Mexico City.' *Archives of Medical Research* 30(2), 120–4.

Hill, J.D. (1995) *Ritual and Rubbish in the Iron Age of Wessex*. British Series 242. Oxford: BAR.

Hodder, Ian (1982) *Symbols in Action*. Cambridge: Cambridge University Press.

Houby-Nielsen, Sanne (2000) 'Child burials in ancient Athens.' In Joanna Sofaer-Derevenski (ed.), *Children and Material Culture*. London and New York: Routledge, 151–66.

Hubert, Jane (2000) 'Introduction: the complexity of boundaries and exclusion.' In Jane Hubert (ed.), *Madness, Disability and Social Exclusion: The Archaeology and Anthropology of Difference*. London and New York: Routledge, 1–8.

Kurz, Donna C. and John Boardman (1971) *Greek Burial Customs*. New York: Cornell University Press.

Lagia, Anna (2007) 'Notions of childhood in the classical polis: evidence from the bioarchaeological record.' *Hesperia Supplements Constructions of Childhood in Ancient Greece and Italy* 41, 293–306.

Laubenheimer, Fanette (2004) 'La mort des tout petits dan l'Occident romain.' In Véronique Dasen (ed.), *Naissance et petite enfance dans l'Antiquité: Actes du colloque de Fribourg, 28 Nov.-1er Decembre 2001*. Fribourg: Academic Press, 293–315.

Liston, Maria A. and Susan I. Rotroff (2013) 'Babies in the well: archaeological evidence for newborn disposal in Hellenistic Greece.' In Judith Evans Grubs and Tim Parkin (eds), *The Oxford Handbook of Childhood and Education*. Oxford: Oxford University Press, 62–82.

Liston, Maria A., Susan I. Rotroff and Lynn M. Snyder (2018) *The Agora Bone Well. Hesperia*. Supplementary Series 50. Princeton: American School of Classical Studies.

Little, Lisa (1999) 'Abstract: Babies in Well G5:3: preliminary results and future analysis.' *American Journal of Archaeology* 103(1), 284.

Little, Lisa and John K. Papadopoulos (1998) 'A social outcast in Early Iron Age Athens.' *Hesperia* 67(4), 375–404.

Mays, Simon (2000) 'The archaeology and history of infanticide and its occurrence in earlier British populations.' In Joanna Sofaer-Derevenski (ed.), *Children and Material Culture*. London and New York: Routledge, 180–90.

Meskell, Lynn M. (1994) 'Dying young: the experience of death at Deir el Medina.' *Archaeological Review from Cambridge* 13, 35–45.

Molleson, Theya (1999) 'Archaeological evidence for attitudes towards disability in the past.' *Archaeological Review from Cambridge* 15(2), 69–77.

Moore, Henrietta L. (1982) 'The interpretation of spatial patterning in settlement residues.' In Ian Hodder (ed.) *Symbolic and Structural Archaeology*. Cambridge: Cambridge University Press, 74–9.

Nussbaum, Martha C. (1995) 'Aristotle on human nature and the foundation of ethics.' In James E.J. Altham and Ross Harrison (eds), *World, Mind and Ethics*. Cambridge: Cambridge University Press, 86–131.

Papadopoulos, John K. (2000) 'Skeletons in wells: towards an archaeology of social exclusions in the ancient Greek world.' In Jane Hubert (ed.), *Madness, Disability and Social Exclusion: The Archaeology and Anthropology of Difference*. London and New York: Routledge, 104–11.

Parker, Robert (1996) *Miasma: Pollution and Purification in Early Greek Religion*. Oxford: Clarendon Press.

Parker-Pearson, Michael (1999) *The Archaeology of Death*. Stroud: Tempus.

Powell, Andrew B., Michael J. Allen, James Chapman, Rachel Every, Rowena Gale, Phil Harding, Stephanie Knight, Jacqueline I. McKinley and Chris Stevens (2005) 'Excavations along the Old Sarum water pipeline, North Salisbury.' *Wiltshire Archaeological and Natural History Magazine* 98, 250–80.

Roberts, Charlotte and Keith Manchester (1995) *The Archaeology of Disease* (2nd edn). Stroud: Tempus.

Romm, James S. (1992) *The Edges of the Earth in Ancient Thought*. Princeton: Princeton University Press.

Rose, Martha Lynn (2003) *The Staff of Oedipus: Transforming Disability in Ancient Greece*. Ann Arbor: University of Michigan Press.

Rotroff, Susan I. (1999) 'The reanalysis of a well deposit from the second century BC in the Athenian Agora: animal sacrifice and infanticide in Late Hellenistic Athens.' *American Journal of Archaeology* 103(2), 284–5.

Scott, Eleanor (1991) 'Animal and infant burials in Romano-British villas: a revitalization movement.' In Paul Garwood, David Jennings, Robin Skeates and Judith Toms (eds), *Sacred and Profane: Proceedings of a Conference on Archaeology, Ritual and Religion, Oxford 1989*. Oxford: Oxford University Press, 116–9.

Snodgrass, Antony (1971) *The Dark Ages of Greece: An Archaeological Survey of the Eleventh to Eighth Centuries*. Edinburgh: Edinburgh University Press.

Snyder, Lynn M. (1999) 'The animal bones from Well G5:3: domestic debris, industrial debris and possible evidence for the sacrifice of domestic dogs in Late Hellenistic Athens.' *American Journal of Archaeology* 103(2), 284.

Sourvinou-Inwood, Christiane (1996) *Reading Greek Death to the End of the Classical Period*. Oxford: Clarendon Press.

Soren, David and Noelle Soren (1998) *A Roman Villa and Late Roman Infant Cemetery Excavation at Poggio Gramignano, Lugnano in Teverina*. Rome. L'Erma Di Bretschneider.

Whitley, James (2001) *The Archaeology of Ancient Greece*. Cambridge: Cambridge University Press.

Whittaker, Charles R. (1994) *Frontiers of the Roman Empire: A Social and Economic Study*. Baltimore: Johns Hopkins University Press.

Part 4

Classical reception as the gateway between Classics and disability studies

Ellen Adams

This volume began by exploring the voice of the forgotten othered, be it patient or person with impairment, and the challenges of articulating subjective experiences. Turning full circle, it returns to these themes, but with the added dimension of imagined stories and distorted dialogues between antiquity and modernity. These illusions, filters, and tensions generate a cognitive dissonance, whereby accounts of myriad and occasionally contradictory experiences present themselves simultaneously. Reality and representation do not sit at opposing ends of a spectrum, but rather fold into each other to produce the messiness of perception – including, and perhaps especially, that of the human body.

Modern western societies have established clear boundaries between the categories of myth, religion, historic past, and increasingly secular present. But these were blurred in antiquity: Greek myths shaped religion, while the present was overseen by a squabble of interfering and unpredictable gods. Gods were real for the Greeks, as in any religion, but they were also reborn in representations – theatre, poetry, art. And classical reception plays a vital part here. For example, there is a certain irony in how the Enlightenment witnessed the development of the scientific classification that distances us from the classical world, while engaging very closely with ancient authorities in its education and culture, including its understanding of medical conditions and treatments and attitudes towards disabled people (see King, Chapter 10).

Both Hall and King consider how ancient Greece and Rome have been 'good to think with'. The ancient world is familiar from being filtered through the channels of classical reception, while also being exotic enough to whet curiosity. In Chapter 9, Hall explores Nicolas Poussin's landscape *Blind Orion Searching for the Rising Sun* (1658), depicting three disabled classical figures, Orion, Cedalion, and Hephaestus, united on a shared mission. King considers the nineteenth-century creation of Nydia, a blind flower girl at Pompeii, who stands as 'a way of enabling those with disabilities to make sense of their bodies and those without disability to empathise with others'. Empathy is the ultimate imagined reality and can work to positive and negative ends. The positive is obvious: a reaching out, understanding, and kindness. 'False empathy', however, comprises the hollow acknowledgement and appropriation of a condition or situation, in order to evade dealing with the implications. 'Oh, I know *exactly* what you mean', is not an uncommon response to learning that someone is struggling in a particular environment, with the subtext being that, 'yes, I know it's hard, but if I can manage, so can you'.[1] Some misplaced empathy harms more than helps – much of the history of education for disabled people involves able-bodied people making the wrong assumptions with a colonial confidence. This includes the common assertion is that being impaired is overwhelmingly negative.

Both chapters consider the potential gain of disability, or the unforeseen advantages that dealing with impairments can produce. Hall explores how cooperation and mutual support can achieve shared goals perfectly well – each of the three figures, including blind Orion, contributing to the endeavour in their own way. King's Nydia is able not only to walk through a pitch-black Pompeii as she is accustomed to navigating without sight, but she is also able to lead her sighted companions. Blind Gain has been explored as a phenomenon whereby the lack of sight enhances other senses or generates strategies that bear other advantages. From Helen Keller onwards, an assertive response to such impairments does not constitute denial, but a realistic acknowledgement of humankind's ability for short-term adaptation. In considering blindness, both chapters explore text and image, which shape representations and construct realities in different ways. Classics has long explored the intermodal translation between the visual and the verbal (as ekphrasis – see Adams, Chapter 6, this volume), but here they serve as different tools used to explore perceptions of disability. And how visible the impairment itself is will clearly impact on such perceptions.

Dwarfism and club foot, as Hall explores, are visible conditions (some would say 'deformities') that do not necessarily indicate an inability to perform everyday activities. She considers literary sources of real or imagined symposia to reconstruct Greek perceptions of dwarfism – which may in turn flesh out the fragmentary profile of mythical Cedalion. He is not only able to work, but also constitutes a positive persona, as a tutor and contributor. What about invisible conditions, which may or may not have disabling consequences? If an impairment is not seen, then is it more difficult to perceive and understand? King charts the narrative of medical improvements in treatments for asthma, a hidden condition unless one is having an attack. This is an area that has seen continued medical advances, although its label of 'practising how to die' took on a heightened meaning in the age of Covid-19. She discusses whether Hippocrates merely described the symptoms or named the condition, and a global pandemic reminds us that such distinctions can matter (did people die *with* or *of* Covid?): knowledge is power in medicine, as elsewhere. But who sets the parameters of such knowledge?

The influence that ancient authorities have had in medical treatises and disability debates is difficult to explain. Presumably, most medics of a certain age started life with a good, solid classical education, which could be worn as a badge of honour for evermore. Hall investigates how historical authors have shaped our understanding of club foot, and King explores how medics are pleased to note that Hippocrates was right, and perhaps ahead of his time. The authority of the medic, noted in Part 1 of this volume, extends to that of the ancient author, providing a pleasing balance to the volume. And, if that authority is unsympathetic to certain ailments, then the consequences can be dire – as the grim misogyny behind the history of treating endometriosis illustrates (King, Chapter 10).

Hall rethinks ancient myth through modern concerns, whereas King reframes modern medicine through its engagements with ancient representations. This tipsy-topsy juxtaposition highlights, and indeed celebrates, how varied and wide-ranging our engagement with the classical world can be. King suggests that the vivid portrayal of Nydia in art, opera, and song 'almost' renders her a real historical figure, and Hall exhorts that literature has the power to undermine and shape ideology by presenting a world 'more politically advanced than the societies that produced them'. Specific to disability, this presents the sphere of representation as a forceful agent for social progressiveness. As such, classical representations have the power to go far beyond 'being good to think with' and can be deployed to enact real social change.

Note

1 My most startling experience of this occurred in the Old Bailey, when presenting myself for jury service. The very heart and symbol of our legal system struggled with its obligations to enact reasonable adjustments (cf. 2010 Equality Act). As a result of the subsequent lively discussion, I suspect that I am now permanently excused from being called up.

Chapter 9

The immortal forgotten other gang

Dwarf Cedalion, Lame Hephaestus, and Blind Orion

Edith Hall

Abstract

This article explores an ancient mythological narrative in which three disabled immortals unite in a quest. Lucian's *On the Hall* (28–29) describes a painting in which Orion, who has been blinded, carries the dwarf Cedalion on his shoulders. Cedalion directs him towards the sunlight that will restore his sight. Hephaestus, who is lame, watches them from his home island of Lemnos. This description inspired one of Nicolas Poussin's most famous classical landscapes, *Blind Orion Searching for the Rising Sun.* The myth of the three supernatural friends, disabled in different ways but mutually supporting one another, might reflect some aspect of the reality of the lives of disabled individuals in antiquity, or of medical procedures associated with Lemnos, or both. Although not claiming that the mythical narrative encapsulated in Lucian's ecphrasis has ever been previously interpreted, either in antiquity or more recently, as providing a positive representation of mutual self-help among disabled communities, my own interpretation springs from the premise that classical material needs to be open to new readings. If it can be reinterpreted from feminist, anti-racist, postcolonial, pro-youth, and anti-classist perspectives, why not from the perspective of 'the forgotten other'?

Poussin's Lemnian Encounter

One of Nicolas Poussin's most famous classical landscapes is *Blind Orion Searching for the Rising Sun*, which he painted for his Parisian patron, Michel Passart, in 1658. Passart was a scholarly individual, fond of arcane allusions to little-known classical texts. He will have been delighted that the inspiration for the painting was an ancient picture described as one ecphrasis among several in Lucian's *On the Hall* (28–9), written in the second half of the second century CE and much read by seventeenth-century art collectors (Cropper 1984, 169–72):

> Orion, who is blind, is carrying Cedalion. Cedalion is showing him the way to the sunlight. The rising sun is healing the blindness of Orion, and Hephaestus views the incident from Lemnos.

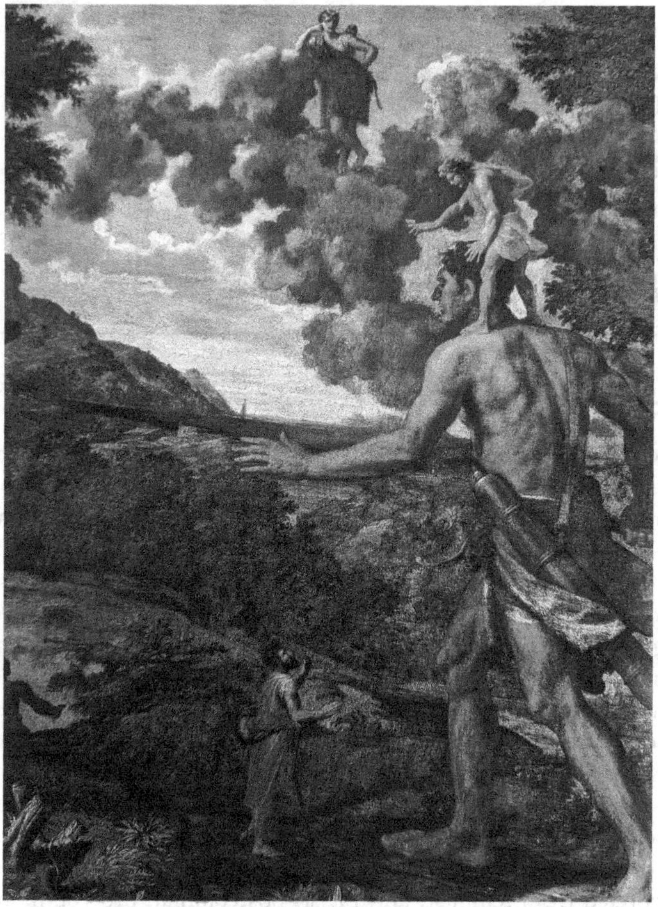

Figure 9.1 Nicolas Poussin (1658) *Blind Orion Searching for the Rising Sun* (Metropolitan Museum of Art, in public domain)

Now in the Metropolitan Museum of Art, New York, the imposing landscape across which Orion strides was once owned by Joshua Reynolds; it inspired a rhapsodically admiring essay, penned by William Hazlitt, after he saw it in 1821 on display at the British Institution (Burlington 1944). Hazlitt (1824, 34) states:

> He stalks along, a giant upon earth, and reels and falters in his gait, as if just awakened out of sleep, or uncertain of his way; – you see his blindness, though his back is turned. Mists rise around him, and veil the sides of the green forests; earth is dank and fresh with dews, the 'gray dawn and the Pleiades before him dance,' and in the distance are seen the blue hills and sullen ocean. Nothing was ever more finely conceived or done.[1]

The canonical reading of Poussin's picture these days, however, remains Ernst Gombrich's (1944). Noting that Poussin must have supplemented the Lucianic ecphrasis with details from an account of the myth in a compendium of mythology of 1567 by the arch-euhemerist Natalis Comes (1976 [1567], vol. II, Book 8, 895), Gombrich argued that the painting was an allegory for nature itself: Orion represents something produced by the elements of water and air, along with the sun, watched over by Diana, the moon. The painting portrays 'the drama of the circulation of water in nature', and the storm cloud is 'Orion himself in his "real" esoteric meaning'. His blindness is a 'transitory phase which will be over when he has passed the mist and approached the rising sun' (Gombrich 1944, 41).

Gombrich's allegorical interpretation is widely accepted. It informs, for example, the information given on the painting on the Metropolitan Museum's website, which discusses its 'meteorological subtext'.[2] But, in a sensitive reappraisal, David Carrier (1990–1) points out that a central concern of Lucian's *On the Hall*, like so much ancient writing on ecphrasis, is the rivalry between visual and verbal art, which in turn entails the comparison of the faculties of sight and hearing.[3] The painting defies the constraints of visual reality by collapsing vast distances (note the remote figures visible over Orion's arm). Orion's hand is stretching towards the place he will reach where his sight will be restored. And, in identifying this detail, the implied spectator of Poussin's painting is created. We look from somewhere high up on the hillside which Orion is descending. Poussin's Orion, in fact, suggests that vision is superior to speech. Speech may connect figures close to one another, but vision brings together what is near and far and enables viewers to locate themselves within the much larger narrative. Moreover, the painting 'corrects' the standard disadvantage of visual art, when compared with speech or writing, by the inclusion of Diana. She represents episodes within Orion's career subsequent to the Lemnos episode – in most accounts (see Fontenrose 1981 for citations and discussion) she is responsible for his death and sometimes for his katasterism: 'Poussin demonstrates that visual art has a power that literature lacks: a painting can simultaneously present several different stories' (Carrier 1990–1, 36).

Carrier's perception that the painting makes the viewer think about the relative advantages of sight and hearing is particularly suggestive given that the protagonist, Orion, has recently lost his sight and must listen to advice both from Hephaestus (clothed in blue, to the left of Orion's knees) and, presumably, the tiny Cedalion, perched on his shoulders to guide him. The angles of their heads suggest that Cedalion is at this very minute receiving verbal directions towards the rising sun from Hephaestus. Neer (2006–7, 337) points out that the location of the sun is unclear, and that the landscape with Orion thus 'invites the beholder to seek vainly for the sun and thereby to make the giant's dilemma his or her own'. But another way of thinking about this painting is that it brings together three ancient divinities who happened to have an impairment and shows them actively cooperating for the benefit of one of them.

They happen to be doing so on the island of Lemnos, an island closely associated with certain medical practices and healing cults in antiquity. Theoris, the woman healer prosecuted for her use of drugs and incantations in fourth-century Athens, was a native of Lemnos (Dem. *Against Aristogeiton* 25.79–80). The red earth of Lemnos was a sought-after ingredient in medicines, collected by the local priestess of Artemis, mixed with goat's blood, made into small discs, and impressed with the seal of a goat (Pliny, *NH* 35.6; Galen, *de Antidotis* II, 1; Scribonius, *de Compositione medicamentorum liber* 120). This procedure may have been connected with the famous Lemnian purificatory fire festivals held in August (Burkert 1970, 10). The hill, Moschylos, on which the precious red soil was found, was an extinct volcano identified in cult with the fall of Hephaestus from Olympus. The earth was used as in antidotes to poison, emetics, and as a poultice for ulcers and the bites of venomous reptiles (see Hasluck 1909–10, 221). Some traditions held that Philoctetes, suffering from some gangrenous infection of his leg after a snake bite, was cured not at Troy, but on Lemnos, using the local earth (Philostratus, *Heroica* VI.2); in one version, the healer is Hephaestus's son Pylius (Photius's *Epitome* 190, summarising Ptolemy Chennus's *New History*).

It is certainly possible that the myth of the three supernatural friends, disabled in different ways but mutually supporting one another, may reflect some aspect of the reality of the lives of such individuals in antiquity, or of medical procedures associated with Lemnos, or both. This chapter explores the information ancient sources offer us about the three friends and their respective impairments; among them, only Hephaestus has received any serious attention from scholars interested in representations of disability.[4] On the other hand, the sole discussion of the myth from a philological perspective makes no comment whatsoever on the shared feature of disability (Yoshida 1969). But I make no claim that the mythical narrative encapsulated in Lucian's ecphrasis has ever been previously interpreted, either in antiquity or more recently, as providing a positive representation of mutual self-help among the disabled community. My own interpretation springs from the premise that classical material has always been, and always needs to be, open to new readings. If it can be reinterpreted from feminist, anti-racist, postcolonial, pro-youth, and anti-classist perspectives, why not, in the twenty-first century, from the perspective of 'the forgotten other'? I will return to this question in the conclusion.

Cedalion

Aggravatingly little is known about Cedalion, the smith of restricted growth, except that Sophocles wrote a satyr play, *Cedalion*, about him (*TgrF* vol. IV, 328–33). We do not know whether this drama featured Orion, but it is most unlikely that it did not feature Hephaestus, as Cedalion has no life in ancient sources separate from his Olympian pupil. And Hephaestus was certainly a popular figure in satyr drama, as the satyrs traditionally assisted superior beings performing technological feats (see Hall 2006, 145–6, 156–8). Achaeus, the dramatist from Eretria famous for his satyr plays, composed a *Hephaestus*. In another Sophoclean satyr play, the satyrs participated in the invention of womankind. In a fragment of his *Pandora*, one individual, perhaps Hephaestus, possibly attended by Cedalion, is instructed by another to 'begin to manipulate the clay in your two hands' (fr. 482 *TgrF*). This leaves little doubt that Pandora, the first woman, was visibly constructed in the Athenian theatre, as she had been in Hesiod's accounts (*Theog.* 578–89, *Op.* 60–82). Other evidence links the satyrs with Hephaestus in the role of his workmen, and Hephaestus was important in early comedy. Among the titles of the Sicilian Epicharmus, according to Aristotle, one of the inventors of comic plots (*Poetics* 5.1449b5) is a *Hephaestus or Komasts*. The comic poet named Alcaeus, of Mytilene, wrote a mythological burlesque comedy entitled *Ganymede*. It staged a comic version of the story of Ganymede; Zeus took Hephaestus to earth to help acquire Ganymede, rather than sending an eagle; the fragments suggest what now seems tasteless slapstick humour at the expense of Hephaestus's limp (see Hall 2018, 383 and Storey 2011, fr. 3 [probably Zeus speaking]: 'Lame one, hurry up, or you will be struck by lightning').

Cedalion may have featured in some of these Hephaestus-centred satyr plays and comedies. The meagre literary sources relate that Cedalion came from Naxos. Shortly after Hephaestus was born, Hera had handed him over to Cedalion to care for him (as the root of the proper name, related to the verb *kēdō*, 'care for', implies). Cedalion was also commissioned to instruct the lame child in the arts of metalwork (Scholion on *Iliad* XIV.296 and Eustathius on *Iliad* XIV.294; see Vollkommer 1990). The appearance of a very small anthropomorphic figure on an important example among the many Athenian vases depicting the 'Return of Hephaestus' to Olympus may well have been assumed by any ancient viewer to be Cedalion (see Fig. 9.2). He walks along underneath Hephaestus's donkey, holding the end of the donkey's phallus so that the jug of wine whose handle is looped around the phallus cannot fall off and land on the floor.[5] In another, red-figure example, the very short satyr just in front of Hephaestus's donkey in the procession may perhaps have been thought to be Cedalion.[6] In these two examples, if dwarfism is implied, it is 'proportionate short stature' (PSS), in which the body parts are in typical proportion to one another, rather than 'disproportionate short stature' (DSS), most cases of which are fundamentally caused by skeletal dysplasia.[7]

No ancient picture of Cedalion on Orion's shoulders of the kind described by Lucian exists. But there are two depictions of Cedalion with Hephaestus in Roman art, sharing a similar iconography, which may imply that they both imitate a lost Hellenistic painting. It, in turn, may have been inspired by the Sophoclean satyr drama *Cedalion* (Welcker 1851, 158). One is a Pompeii wall painting in the Naples Museum (no. 9529), dated to around 70 CE (*LIMC* no.1).[8] Inside his workshop, Hephaestus sits on the left of the picture, opposite Thetis, and shows her Achilles's shield. Cedalion sits beneath Hephaestus and hammers Achilles's helmet. He wears a white pileus and a greenish loincloth. He hunches

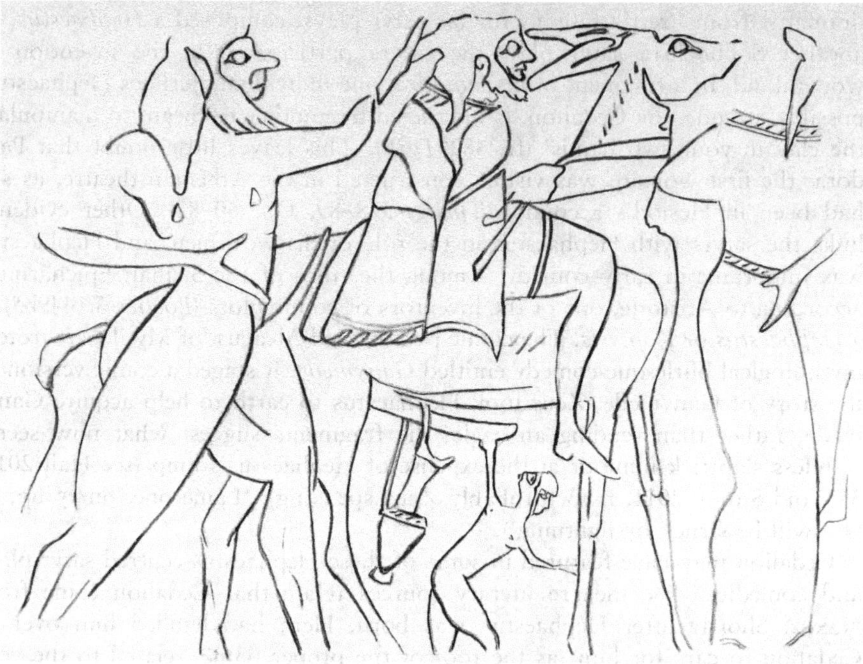

Figure 9.2 **Drawing reproduced by kind permission of Becky Brewis. Based on black-figure kantharosi in Dresden, Staatliche Kunstsammlungen ZV 1466 = *LIMC* 'Hephaestus' no. 142a**

over his work, showing developed muscles. He is bearded, has very tanned skin, darker even than Hephaestus, and is stockier and shorter in overall stature than the other figures – perhaps half their height, although the body position make it difficult to tell. Otherwise, there are no noticeable physical differences between them, and it is not clear whether his small stature entails relative disproportion between the parts of his body. The other image is a marble relief sculpture of the first or second centuries CE in the Louvre (see Fig. 9.3). There is no Thetis here: Hephaestus receives the shield, as yet unengraved, from a satyr. But Cedalion sits in a similar position, on the lower left, working on Achilles's helmet. He is depicted in a similar way, with beard and loincloth, although a playful touch is added with a young satyr trying to make off with the serious-minded and much older dwarf's pileus.

Dwarfs were staples of the nineteenth-century 'freak show' and continue to exert something of a fascination in popular culture; in fantasy fiction, they are often invested with a degree of authority and social status and special powers of intellect, divination, or magic (Backstrom 2012, 687–8; Adelson 2005, 5). The figure of Tyrion Lannister in the HBO television series *Game of Thrones*, played by Peter Hayden Dinklage, is the most famous example. Cedalion, as

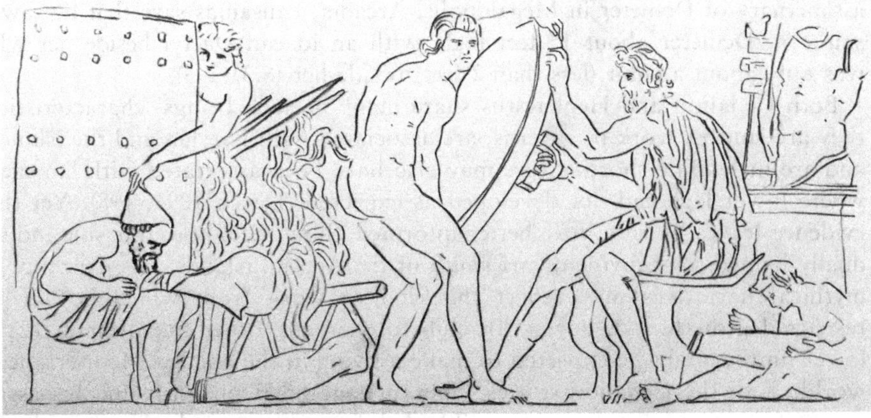

Figure 9.3 Drawing reproduced by kind permission of Becky Brewis. Based on marble relief sculpture in the Louvre, fr 109, *LIMC* no. 2

skilled craftsman, mentor, and companion to an Olympian god, seems to have been a forerunner of this type. In her 1993 study of dwarfs in ancient Egypt and Greece, Véronique Dasen sadly does not have an entry under 'Cedalion' in her index, although she has an interesting discussion of the Kerkopes, dwarfish and ape-like creatures who accosted travellers until Heracles captured them (Dasen 1993, 189–94). She shows that the terms *pugmaios* and *nanos* are usually used interchangeably and can mean both what we call 'pygmy' and what we call 'dwarf'. But Aristotle distinguished mythical pygmies from a real 'race of small people' to be found 'south of Egypt' who live in caves (*History of Animals* 8.12: Dasen 1993, 175–88).

Of more relevance to Cedalion are the beings Dasen (1993, 194–204) discusses in a section on Hephaestus and 'Small Demons'. Hephaestus is associated with several pairs or groups of (conventionally speaking) unattractive male supernatural beings who lived underground or in caves and shared his skills in metalwork. His sons, the Kabeiroi, lived in Lemnian caves and oversaw ecstatic mystery rites on Samothrace. Their small stature is at least implied by Herodotus's account of the Egyptian smith-god Ptah, who was identified with Hephaestus and depicted as a dwarf, as were the Egyptian equivalents of the Kabeiroi (2.37). Another term for the Kabeiroi, according to the *Suda*, was *Karkinoi*, or 'crabs', which may have had something to do with the identification of a crab's pincers with a smith's tongs (Detienne 1970; Detienne and Vernant 1978, 269–70); some of the terms used to describe Hephaestus's lameness (see below) are also found in association with a crab in *The Palatine Anthology*, 6.196.[9] The Kabeiroi were held by Diodorus Siculus (5.64.4) originally to have been Dactyls, another species of supernatural smiths, found in Phrygia, Rhodes, and Crete. They seem to have been imagined as very small. In a sanctuary of Demeter in Megalopolis, Arcadia, Pausanias says that he saw a statue of Demeter about 15 feet high, with an Idaean Dactyl beside her who was only about a cubit (less than 2 feet) beside her (8.31.2–3).

Both Cedalion and Hephaestus share many of such beings' characteristics: they are smiths, work in caverns, are associated with Phrygia and the islands, and are little. The short stature may also have been associated with lameness where lower legs had not developed as expected (Dasen 1993, 198). Yet this evidence leaves us very little better informed about Cedalion, our sole individually named semi-divine dwarf smith of the Aegean islands. His existence in mythical narratives may reflect the kind of work from which boys with restricted growth, like boys with club foot or any other impairment of the lower limbs, might be expected to make a living in the ancient Mediterranean world. Both the Cedalion stories – his tutelage of Hephaestus and his assistance of Orion – suggest a responsible, helpful, and avuncular figure of ready wits as well as advanced skills in metalwork. This may chime with some interpretations of the representations of dwarfs in ancient Egyptian art – for example, a group of five ivory figurines from Predynastic times in the Walters Art Museum in Baltimore, Maryland. Kozma (2010, 2556) has argued that these and representations of the Egyptian dwarf gods, Bes and Ptah, support 'the premise that dwarfs were accepted and integrated in the ancient Egyptian society, and with a few exceptions, their disorder was not depicted as a physical handicap [*sic*]'.

But, in the context of the less than sympathetic depictions of dwarfs in other Greek and Roman writing and iconography, the apparently positive persona and images of Cedalion as Hephaestus's tutor and Orion's benefactor seem exceptional and, therefore, surprising. As Nicole Kelley has shown, Greek vases depict dwarfs alongside hunchbacks and physically impaired individuals performing in entertainments intended to elicit derisive laughter. Augustus's granddaughter Julia kept a pet dwarf by the name of Cinopas (Pliny, *NH* 7.74–5). But it is not clear that dwarfs were regarded as freakishly monstrous: they are not included in Plutarch's list of the 'monsters' that could be purchased at special markets – people 'who have no calves, or are weasel-armed, or have three eyes, or ostrich-heads', at the sight of whom even the really curious person will soon 'have had enough and start to feel nauseous' (*de Curiositate*, ch. 10). Nor is dwarfism specified when Horace describes a banquet entertainment in which two deformed men traded abuse (*Satires* 1.5.50–70), or in Aelius Lampridius's account of the emperor Elagabalus's party, to which he invited groups of bald, one-eyed, gout-suffering or deaf men to dinner to arouse laughter (*Life of Heliogabalus* 29.3: Kelley 2007, 39–40; see further Stevenson 1975).

On the other hand, one 'miniature man' (*anthrōpiskos*) at another symposium, described by Lucian, was employed as a comic performer. The symposium is fictional, attended by various deceased intellectuals. Aristaenetus brings in the jester he either owns or has hired, by the name of Satyrion:

> a hideous fellow, his head shaven and only a few hairs standing up dead straight right on his crown. He danced in a disjointed and distorted way, which made him seem more ridiculous. He thought up some anapaests which he delivered in an Egyptian accent, and finished by cracking some jokes against the guests.
>
> *Symposium* (18)

One of them, Alcidamas, resented the witty, resourceful jester's success in capturing everyone's attention and challenged him to a bout of *pankration*, but conceded victory to his tougher – although much smaller – adversary (19).

Hephaestus

Satyrion's adeptness at producing laughter and holding his own against able-bodied antagonists is shared by Hephaestus, the dwarf Cedalion's ward and student, and the only disabled fully-fledged Olympian god.[10] As we shall see below, he is occasionally portrayed himself as of exceptionally diminutive stature, implying that he and his teacher were so closely identified as to be almost indistinguishable in some contexts. But his prominence in literature and cult, and the far greater interest in lameness than in dwarfism in ancient medical sources, mean that there is much more to say about him than about Cedalion.

What was Hephaestus's impairment? In archaic art, he is often portrayed with floppy lower legs, and feet and ankles incorrectly aligned with his shins and calves, riding a donkey – for example, on the colourful Caeretan hydria of about 525 BCE, now in the Vienna Kunsthistorisches Museum (3577).[11] One epithet used for him in Homer is *amphiguēeis* (e.g. *Iliad* 1.607 and *Od*. 8.300). But scholars are undecided as to its meaning. It is sometimes translated as 'ambidexterous', implying that he was unusually capable in both arms. But sometimes it was explained in antiquity as meaning 'lame in both legs' (see Deroy 1956). Neither explanation is helpful in terms of his precise condition. The only informative epithet is *kullopodiōn*, or 'with bent feet', as the stem *kull-* precisely corresponds with the technical terms used to describe club feet in the Hippocratic *de Articulis*, usually assumed to be a late fifth- or early fourth-century work.

Club foot, technically labelled congenital talipes equinovarus (CTEV), is a congenital musculoskeletal condition that occurs once in about a thousand live births. It makes the ankle look as though it has been bent inwards, so that the person appears to walk on their outside ankles or sides of their feet. It is not usually related to any other impairment. It occurs at double the rate in males as in females. In half of all cases it is bilateral, affecting both feet. There is believed to be an inheritable predisposition to club foot, although this is still the subject of intensive chromosomal research.

There are two passages in the Hippocratic *On Joints* that discuss club foot. In the first, it is treated as a sub-species of lameness, signified by the stem *chōl-*.

The adjective *chōlos* also occurs in Homer, being used of Thersites, who was 'lame in one leg' (*Il.* 2.217), and who is the butt of the laughter of the Achaean soldiers, as well as of the personified Prayers or *Litai* (*Il.* 9.503) and of Hephaestus himself (*Od.* 8.300). In the first passage, the Hippocratic writer has heard the story that the Amazons deliberately dislocate their sons' knees or hips when they are infants in order to make them lame and thus prevent any male conspiracy against their matriarchy: 'they used them as artisans to perform any sedentary work, such as that of a shoemaker or smith' (*On Joints* 53). The author then uses the verb *kulloein* to explain the consequences of such dislocations: 'The legs (*gounata*) are more bandied (*kulloutai*) when the dislocation is outward, but it is nevertheless easier for the possessor of outward-turning club foot to stand on his feet than if the legs are turned inwards'.

But the person with congenital club foot (the *kullos*), in whom the ankle is naturally present and the leg bones are not atrophied, is likely to be able to walk; the club-footed person is thus distinguished from someone who becomes acutely lame through injury. Later, in part 62, the author insists that:

> most cases of congenital club-foot are remediable, unless the declination is very great, or when the condition occurs at an advanced period of youth. The best plan, then, is to treat such cases at as early a period as possible, before the deficiency of the bones of the foot is very great, and before there is any great wasting of the flesh of the leg.

There is more than one variety of club foot, the author continues. Most of them are not complete dislocations, but impairments connected with the habitual maintenance of the limb in a certain position. Treatment consists of putting pressure on the bones of the legs and feet so they begin to grow or move into correct alignment, as a wax-worker moulds an object. Pressure is applied by plaster made from wax and resin, compresses, bandages and soles of soft leather or lead, which are stitched in place, and then an outer shoe or boot of lead. 'The most suitable are (those calf-length boots) which are called "mud-treaders" because they are used for travel on muddy ground; for this kind of shoe does not yield to the foot, but the foot yields to it.' Hephaestus's condition could have been treated by manipulation, orthotic bandaging, and stiff, structured footwear functioning as a splint.

One scene in Aristophanes makes fun of a man who I think was visually represented as club-footed – Cinesias, the dithyrambic poet in Aristophanes' *Birds*. Cinesias enters, and sings, 'On my light pinions I soar off to Olympus; in its capricious flight my Muse flutters along the thousand paths of poetry in turn', and most of his words consist of further ethereal poetry of this nature. But Peisetairos suggests that it would be difficult to get Cinesias off the ground at all (1375): 'This is a fellow will need a whole shipload of wings'. In his next retort he addresses Cinesias as the 'lime-wood man' and says that he is doing something circular with his club foot (1377–8):

> Welcome, Cinesias, you lime-wood man!
> Why have you come here twisting your club foot in circles?

He is chased from the stage. But the adjective *philurinos* is suggestive, given that Galen says that lime wood was used for medical splints (*Comm. On Hipp. Fractures* 18B.505k, *ek philirou*). I wonder whether *kullos*-legged Cinesias does not wear heavy splints, with which he draws dithyrambic circles in the soil of Cloudcuckooland.

The earliest mention of Hephaestus's impairment in the surviving literary tradition occurs during the Olympian council that closes the first book of the *Iliad*. Hephaestus is not explicitly said to be lame, but he reminds his mother, Hera, that resistance against Zeus is hopeless; once before he had tried to support her against Zeus, but Zeus had picked him up by the leg and hurled him down to Lemnos in retaliation. Now he serves the Olympians with their beverages (1.597–600): 'But he drew sweet nectar from the mixing-bowl and served it in cups to the other gods, moving left to right; and inextinguishable laughter arose amongst the blessed gods when they saw Hephaestus *poipnuonta* through the halls'. Hephaestus is an object of laughter not here specifically because he is lame, but because he is *poipnuonta*. This word is used of any kind of *servile* labour or effort, such as domestic cleaning; it is used of Hephaestus's own robotic metal maidservants when they help him move round his Olympian home (*Iliad* 18.421). It may well be that the reason the gods laugh is the contrast with the graceful service they are accustomed to from the beautiful Ganymede, as pointed out by a scholiast (scholion bT on line 584). But it is difficult to see how the audience does not think of Hephaestus's club foot, the image of which must have been insinuated by his own reference to how Zeus had picked him up by the leg a few lines previously.

Rinon argues that the presentation of Hephaestus in both Homeric epics is distinctively tragic. The reasons Rinon (2006, 18–9) gives are that he is portrayed in both epics as a god endowed with unusually human characteristics:

> Afflicted in body and limited in movement, suffering pain and humiliation, bound by human institutions such as marriage and divorce, and laughing stock of the other gods, he is unique among the Olympians in his humanized characterization. His unique status is used for dramatic effect, for this humanized god serves as a figure whose tragic depth is otherwise unavailable to immortals, one of whose main characteristics is a 'lofty levity' that often enables them to deride and mock the agonies of mortals. In the *Iliad*, Hephaestus' tragic awareness finds its most brilliant expression in his creation of the shield of Achilles, where his engravings reveal his humane perspective on the human lot. In the *Odyssey*, his betrayal serves as an emblem of the miseries of mortals and as a reminder of the ineradicable chasm between humans and gods. Despite differences between the epics, the portrayal of this exceptional god serves the poet in both cases as a means to

> represent a tragic perception of the human condition which is marked by pain and suffering.

I fear that this is to impose a twenty-first-century liberal, humanist view of deformity and ugliness on these texts, where pathos and what seems to us cruel laughter at the expense of disability can surely exist side by side. Rinon's reading does not take into account the subsequent close relationship between Hephaestus and the comic in both art and literature (explored at length in Hall 2018).

In *Iliad* Book 18, we finally learn that Hephaestus was *born* lame and was, therefore, disabled long before Zeus's punitive assault. When Thetis arrives at Hephaestus's house, she is received by his wife, Charis. From his workshop, he calls out to them that Thetis saved him when he fell from Olympus because his mother wanted to hide him on account of his lameness. Thetis and the Oceanid Eurynome had looked after him in their cave for 9 years, and he had forged pieces of jewellery there. We then receive the fullest description of his appearance and gait, which twice uses the verb *chōleuein* ('limp' or 'hobble'; *Iliad* 18.410–21):

> He spoke and rose from the anvil, an enormous, panting figure, limping, but his slim legs moved deftly beneath him. He placed the bellows away from the fire, collected all the tools he had been working with in a silver chest, and wiped his face and both arms and his thick neck and hairy chest with a sponge. He put on a tunic, and clasped a thick staff, and went limping towards the door; and his maidservants, made in gold to resemble living maidens, sped to support their master. They have intelligent minds, and speech and strength and they understand what to do from the immortal gods. And they served their master by supporting him.

This scene does not mention any laughter in response to Hephaestus's appearance, although it does mention his mother's desire to conceal him because of his lameness. This is the version retold by Hera herself in the Homeric *Hymn to Apollo* (316–8), where she brutally declares that she had cast him into the sea because he was born ugly and with a shrivelled leg. Perhaps the ancient audiences of the *Iliad* found the image of his sweat, his powerful upper body on his spindly legs, and his robot assistants more amusing than have people in more recent times.[12]

Hephaestus, intellectually, is easily the equal of the other Olympians, however. He can maintain his position among them by use of skill, cunning, and his ability to engender laughter. In the *Odyssey*, the smith-god metamorphoses from object of ridicule to mastermind of a comic spectacle. Demodocus sings the 'Lay of Ares and Aphrodite', about the adulterous affair of the gods. Helios informs Hephaestus, who goes to his smithy, 'pondering evil deep in his heart' (273). He makes a trap of bonds to bind his wife and her lover, hangs the trap from his bed-posts and the roof above them, and pretends to leave for Lemnos. Ares and Aphrodite seize their apparent opportunity, but are soon held fast in Hephaestus's snare. He returns, again tipped off by Helios. Now, in fierce anger and a terrible voice (304–5), he calls on Zeus and the other gods to witness what has happened (306–12):

> Father Zeus, and you other blessed gods who are forever, come here to see something laughable and intolerable. Aphrodite, daughter of Zeus, scorns me because I am lame and loves destructive Ares because he is beautiful and strong-limbed, whereas I was born feeble. Yet nobody is to blame for this except my two parents. I wish they had never conceived me!

He says that he expects the return of all the gifts he gave to Aphrodite's father when he wooed her. The male gods come to his house – Poseidon and Hermes and Apollo. The goddesses do not come out of shame, but the other gods stand in his gateway, and unquenchable laughter (326) arises among them when they see the crafty trick of Hephaestus. They agree that Ares owes a penalty. Poseidon pleads with Hephaestus to release Ares, who, he says, will pay the right recompense in front of the gods; in any case, he, Poseidon, will personally see to it that Hephaestus receives his due compensation. Hephaestus now agrees and releases the two lovers, who depart to Thrace and Paphos, respectively.

Hephaestus, by coming out better in the incident through deploying cunning and skill rather than physical strength and beauty, provides (as so often in the poem) a parallel with its hero, Odysseus (Newton 1987). Hephaestus stages a comic spectacle. But this is not just gentle humour: Hephaestus is dishonoured, angry, and *using* laughter in order to gain respect, public recognition that he has been grievously wronged, and that he is entitled to compensation. Poseidon, at least, is aware that the incident is a major threat to the stability of Olympian society and guarantees that Hephaestus will be compensated. Hephaestus can never win in a competition based on beauty or physique. But he can use his technological skill plus humour to protect his status in the community and counter-attack when he is insulted. Hephaestus here uses aischrologic laughter as an instrument of social justice (Brown 1989, 292).

If we had more than mere fragments of those precious archaic texts that told of his other famous technological ruse – designing a chair in which to imprison his mother, Hera – we would know much more about how Hephaestus could use comic spectacle in order to wreak revenge against one who had abused and insulted him, and to effect his own reinstatement as a god who deserved the respect of the Olympians, however ugly, disabled, and banausic he may have been. These lost texts are the Homeric *Hymn* to Dionysus quoted by Diodorus 3.66.3 (fragments of which have been edited by West 2001), a hymn by Alcaeus, and a poem by Pindar (Alcaeus fr. 349a–e Voigt; Pindar fr. 283 Snell-Maehler). 'Hera Bound by Her Son' constituted a popular and well-known myth. This is clear from Plato's *Republic* 2.378d, where it earns special disapprobation, along with the other Hephaestus story in which it is Zeus who hurls him from Olympus. They are, says Socrates, the sorts of story that must not be told to children because they provide examples of conflict between the Olympians.

The story was retold in several later sources (e.g. Paus. 1.20.3; ps.-Libanius, *Narr.* 30. 1; Hyg. *Fab.* 166; Serv. *auct. Ecl.* 4.62) and depicted on an Apulian amphora now in Foggia (see Fig. 9.4). Hephaestus, intriguingly, is himself depicted as stocky and of dwarfish size and arguably disproportionate body parts, as if he shared his tutor Cedalion's dwarfism (although the vase-painting may imply that, in one version of the story, he sent his mentor to release Hera in his place: see also Dasen 1993, 198). The story's outlines, as summarised by West (2001, 3), are these: from Lemnos, where Hera had hurled him in disgust, Hephaestus:

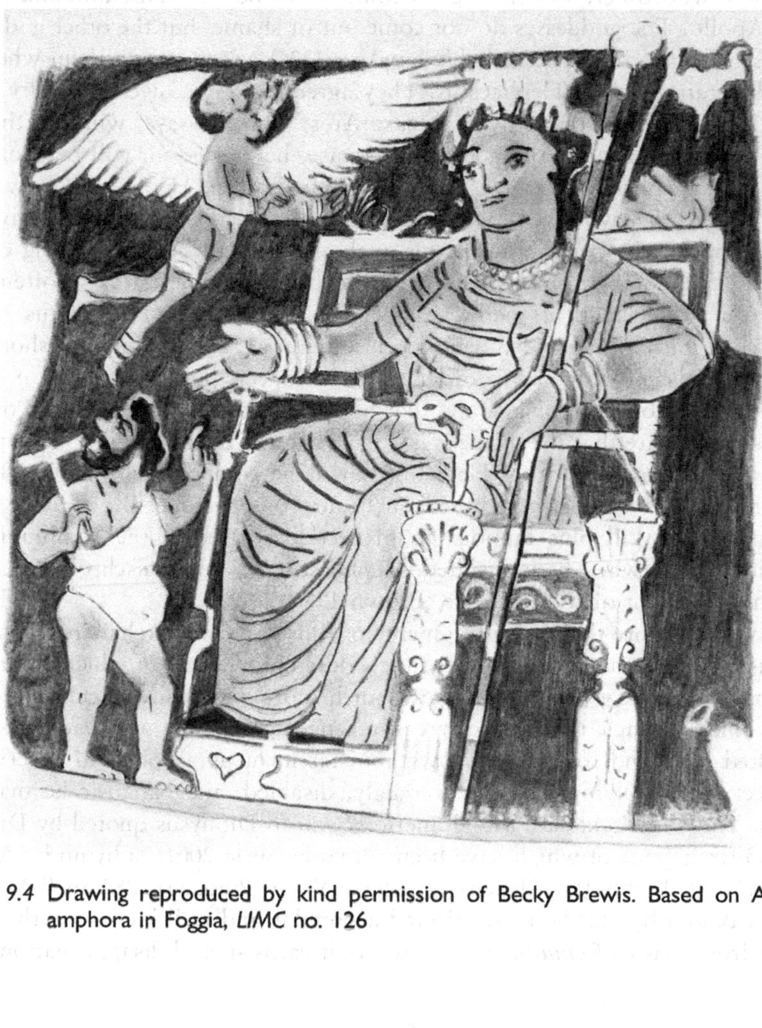

Figure 9.4 Drawing reproduced by kind permission of Becky Brewis. Based on Apulian amphora in Foggia, *LIMC* no. 126

> sent his mother a fine throne, in which he had incorporated a secret mechanism. When she sat down in it, she found herself trapped. None of the other gods was able to free her. It was clear that Hephaestus had to be induced to come back and undo what he had done. Ares undertook to go and fetch him by force. He went off, but failed to achieve his object, because Hephaestus defended himself with fire, which Ares could not face. Then Dionysus went equipped with wine, made Hephaestus drunk, and brought him back to Olympus in jolly mood, riding on a donkey or mule. He set Hera free, and she rewarded Dionysus by persuading the other Olympians to admit him to their number.

Hephaestus made a laughing-stock of Hera, and possibly of Ares, before joining Dionysus in the aboriginal divine *kōmos*, the first comic revel on Olympus.

The archaic evidence prompts further questions. First, had Hephaestus always been associated with the idea of obscene comic abuse, whether the satire of the archaic iambic poets or the insults delivered by members of the *kōmos* during Dionysiac festivals? There may be a special connection between aischrologic abuse and Hephaestus's club feet. In a tantalising line, the Hellenistic mimiambist Herodas claims Hipponax as his own poetic ancestor, and in doing so claims expertise in iambics and in the 'limping' or 'clubfooted' metre (8.75–9). He avers that he shares with Hipponax of old 'the ability to sing limping songs', and here uses the rare *kull-* stem of the choliambic metre (*ta kull' aeidein*), which reminds us of the *kull*-footed god of the *Iliad*. Hipponax, like Hephaestus, also used his technical skill, even if as a poet rather than as a smith, to extract revenge for public humiliation. According to a scholion on Horace's *Epodes*, there was a tradition that Hipponax wanted to marry the daughter of Bupalus, a painter of Clazomenae. He was despised because he was deformed, and Bupalus made a portrait of him looking hideous (in one version displaying the picture at the Panathenaea: Scholiast on Horace *Epodes* 6.11ff. (test. 9b Degani)) in order to make the viewer laugh. Hipponax got his revenge by attacking him so cruelly in his poetry that Bupalus hanged himself (Scholiast on Horace *Epodes* 6.11ff. (test. 9a Degani)).

The notion of limping or faltering gait also has something to do with the distinctive *skazon* or *choliambic* metre of invective poetry, which Hipponax had supposedly invented. This is an iambic senarius, but with a thumping spondee or trochee, two long syllables, replacing the final iambus. There is a suggestive description of what Hipponax achieved thereby in Demetrius of Phalerum's *de Elocutione* 301:

> In his desire to abuse his enemies he shattered the metre, making it lame instead of straightforward, and unrhythmical, i.e. suitable for vigorous abuse, since what is rhythmical and pleasing to the ear would be more suitable for words of praise than blame.

The very form of abuse poetry was, therefore, felt by the ancient Greeks to be somehow *de*-formed in a way that suggested the lopsided body and the distorted, uneven rhythm of the gait of a person with a limp. And the most instantly recognisable lame individual in their mythology was none other than club-footed Hephaestus.

The evidence in the archaic literary sources for Hephaestean laughter is here complicated by the visual depiction of lame carousers on many Corinthian black-figure pots, which some scholars have even argued represent a retinue of Hephaestus, or even a guild or ritual group of dancers all representing the smith-god, plural *Hephaistoi* (see e.g. Smith 2009). Another possibility, which I find more plausible, is that the club-footed god was drawn into a pre-existing tradition of deformed entertainers and bizarre phallic dances at Corinthian symposia. He first certainly joins the lame revels on a Middle Corinthian pot from the first quarter of the sixth century,[13] although the association might of course antedate this vase. But the wealth of visual evidence for lame dancers on archaic Corinthian pots has laid the playing field wide open for speculation here, like almost everything else to do with Greek entertainment in the sixth century BCE.

Orion

The scanty ancient sources on Orion tell us much less about the experience of being blind in antiquity than texts relating to other sightless figures – for example, Oedipus or Tiresias (well discussed in Bernidaki-Aldous 1990). But many more people may have identified with his experience than that of Cedalion or Hephaestus, as there were probably far more blind or partially sighted people in ancient populations than individuals with restricted growth or lameness. The cases where people had sought divine assistance for damaged eyesight among those recorded at the Athenian Asclepieion and in the Epidauros stelai are more numerous than cases of any other malady, although none of them was treated by looking directly into the rising sun (Horn 2013, 123–4).

Lisa Trentin points out, however, that certain aspects of ancient society, especially hand-to-hand combat without adequate helmet visors, in what were often semi-continuous wars, produced large numbers of men like Orion, blinded by injury in adulthood (Trentin 2013, 98–100). Gouging out of the eyes was also used as a punishment with some frequency, and so there will have been individuals in the ancient world who had experienced exactly the fate of Orion; rumours also circulate about miraculous restorations of vision parallel to the one he experienced (Trentin 2013, 100–4). Unlike Cedalion and Hephaestus, Orion is usually said to have been born a mortal, but an enormous one, with special powers as a hunter and the ability to wade through or walk on the deepest water. In the story of his blinding, almost certainly originating in Hesiod's *Ehoiai*, Orion had sexually assaulted Oenopion's daughter Merope on another eastern Aegean island, Chios. Consequently, Orion was blinded by Oenopion as a punishment before wandering on to Lemnos, where Hephaestus first pitied and then helped the blinded giant find a cure (Eratosthenes, *Catasterisms* 32; Hesiod Fr. 148a M.-W: Jackson 1997).

Blind people presumably often used slaves as guides, like the children who lead Tiresias onto the stage in Greek tragedy, but the exaggerated disparity in size between the gigantic Orion and dwarf Cedalion made possible the striking image of the guide perched on the blind man's shoulders, the dwarf's seeing eyes close to the giant's sightless ones, a perfect image of complementarity and cooperation.

Conclusion: repurposing antiquity

The incident on Lemnos described by Lucian and painted by Poussin seems to have been unique in ancient mythology in furnishing an imaginary instance of a divine disabled mutual support group. We shall probably never know whether anyone disabled in antiquity took comfort or inspiration from the story, or whether anyone able-bodied learned to respect the disabled more after hearing it. We can never be sure that Poussin recognised the potential importance of the theme of disability in the myth, although it is interesting that he painted this theme at the precise moment when he began to experience relentless tremors – perhaps Parkinson's disease – which seriously affected his ability to control his brush-strokes (Haggard and Rodgers 2000).

The unanswerable nature of these questions, however, hardly needs to prevent us from repurposing the story today. Poussin, after all, may himself have reinterpreted the myth of Orion as a nature allegory under the influence of the euhemeristic 'decoding' of classical mythology popular in his lifetime. In our time, the relentlessly patriarchal narratives of ancient myth and history have been systematically retold from the female viewpoint, by novelists and playwrights as well as scholars, since the 1970s, if not earlier (see Heilbrun 1990 [1985]; Hall 2008, 118–29). Anticolonial critiques and interpretations of ancient attitudes to ethnicity and slavery have fuelled intense creativity in anti-racist literature, art, and academic studies since the 1930s (see e.g. Greenwood 2010). Queer writing about and in response to antiquity is now abundant (see e.g. Clarke 2019). The lost voices of classical Athenian teenagers and young adults, destined for the battlefield or dangerously early childbirth, have been reclaimed (Shipton 2018). Even social class – long an 'ugly sister' within progressive Reception Studies – is beginning to be treated seriously by scholars, opening up possibilities for more class-conscious reworkings of ancient texts (Hall and Stead 2020). So why not adopt the meeting of Cedalion, Hephaestus, and Orion on Lemnos as an inspiration to scholars striving to use disability studies to deepen our understanding of ancient representations of the body?

Classical texts, such as Lucian's Lemnian ecphrasis, sometimes possess a transhistorical appeal that makes them seem eerily modern, and creative artists have adopted different metaphors to describe what they feel they are doing with the ancient material. The feminist poet Judith Kazantzis says that Homer's *Odyssey*, an epic of the high seas, 'is perennially open to plunder itself and I am a pirate' (Kazantzis 1999). The Marxist theatre director Peter Sellars, on the other hand, sees each classic text as an antique house that can be redecorated in the style of any era, while remaining essentially the same (quoted in Lahr 1993). The scholar Oliver Taplin (1989) proposes the more volatile image of Greek fire, a substance used as a weapon that burns under water. Greek culture, according to this analogy, is still present in invisible yet potentially incendiary forms. More ambivalent is Walcott's description, repeated in poems including *Omeros*, of 'All that Greek manure under the green bananas' (Walcott 1949, 15; see also Walcott 1990, 271); the Greek legacy is excrement, but has also fertilized his Caribbean imagination. This beautifully captures the paradoxical nature of ancient Mediterranean discourses to peoples colonized by Western powers, a paradox that must also affect disabled people, although for slightly different reasons and in different ways.

Various explanations have been proposed for the 'transhistorical' power of some ancient artefacts. Pierre Vidal-Naquet (1988, 361–80) argues that ancient literature transcends history because of its dialogic nature and unusual susceptibility to diverse interpretations. J.-P. Vernant (1988) further proposes that important artworks actively condition the shapes taken by future artworks, whether in imitation, adaptation, or reaction and rejection. Raymond Williams (1977, 120–7) would have suggested that this was in turn made possible by the ideological complexity of the original material, according to his notion that any moment in time contains three strands of ideology: old-fashioned ideas on their way out, dominant ideas that the majority of people hold, and emergent ideas developed only by avant-garde segments of the population that may not become mainstream for many centuries. On this argument, there are things in ancient culture – for example, the celebration of Penelope's intelligence in the *Odyssey*, the undermining of the cliched ethnocentric polarisation of Greek and barbarian in some Greek tragedies, or the positive light in which the dwarf Cedalion and the lame Hephaestus aiding the blind Orion are presented in Lucian – that might not become dominant ideology for millennia.

Williams's concept of 'emergent' ideology partially corresponds with the Russian formalist Mikhail Bakhtin's (1986) notion that literature holds 'prefigurative' meanings that can only be released by reassessments lying far away in what he calls 'great time' in the future. Another way of putting this, more mystically, is Erich Auerbach's concept of 'figura' or 'umbra', which draws on medieval allegorists to develop a metaphor of 'prefiguration' or 'foreshadowing' (see his essay 'Figura' (1944) as translated by Ralph Manheim in Auerbach 1959, 11–76). According to this argument, an element in an ancient text (e.g. Odysseus's wanderings) can in a mysterious but profound manner prefigure things that happen later (Columbus's voyages of exploration). The concept of literature's 'utopian bent' is also useful. From our twenty-first-century perspective, the patriarchal, slave-holding, beauty-obsessed ancient civilisations oppressed all their 'others'. But the fictional worlds created in myth and literature, with their juxtaposition of diverse voices and characters, had a licence to think, at least sometimes, in ways that were immeasurably more politically advanced than the societies that produced them. The human imagination has always been capable of creating egalitarian models of society, even when they are inconceivable in practice, such as the communistic utopias of 'golden age' myths (Hall 1997, 125–6 with further bibliography; Hall 2008, 148–55).

Might we see Lucian's ecphrasis as 'emergent' ideology, 'prefiguring', in a 'utopian' form of thinking, the drastic reconfiguration of attitudes to physical disability that has begun over the last few decades? If we do, we can read it, and view Poussin's masterpiece, in a progressive and humane spirit, alongside a few lines from the *Amenemope* (Chapter 25), an ancient Egyptian morality primer dating from between 1300 and 1075 BCE. These lines (Lichtheim 1997, 121; see also Walls 2007, 14) seem to me to be equally prefigurative, as well as to specify precisely the three forms of impairment that this chapter has discussed:

> Do not laugh at a blind man,
> Nor tease a dwarf,
> Nor cause hardship for the lame.
> Don't tease one who is in the hand of the god [i.e., ill or insane],
> Nor be angry with him for his failings.
> Man is clay and straw,
> The god is his builder.
> He tears down, he builds up daily.

Notes

1 Hazlitt has slightly adapted John Milton's *Paradise Lost* Book VII.373–4, 'the gray / Dawn, and the Pleiades, before him danc'd'.
2 www.metmuseum.org/art/collection/search/437326 (accessed 5 August 2020).
3 The way in which Lucian sets up this debate in *On the Hall* is well analysed by Newby (2002).
4 See e.g. Rose's influential *The Staff of Oedipus* (2003), which pays close attention to Hephaestus but never mentions Cedalion or Orion.
5 A black-figure kantharosi in Dresden, Staatliche Kunstsammlungen ZV 1466 = *LIMC* 'Hephaestus' no. 142a, where the figure is identified as 'un petit personnage'. Thanks to Dimitris Kanellakis for help on this image.
6 Metropolitan Museum of Art, New York. Attic Oinochoe c. 430 BCE, attributed to the Eretria Painter.
7 www.nhs.uk/conditions/restricted-growth/ (accessed 5 August 2020).
8 Conveniently viewable online at www.theoi.com/Gallery/F7.2.html (accessed 5 August 2020).
9 See also Aristophanes's *Peace* 781–91, a controversial passage where the sons of Carcinus are said to be dwarfish in size.
10 Hephaestus's own agency, wit, and success, as opposed to the mockery he suffers, are neglected in most studies of his disability; for example Garland (2010) 61–3; Kelley (2007) 35–9. Exceptions include Natale (2008) and Hall (2018).
11 Antikensammlung, IV 3577, an image conveniently viewable online at www.khm.at/en/objectdb/detail/56546/?offset=129&lv=list (accessed 5 August 2020).

12 See the dignity and pathos of the painting of Hephaestus, entreated by Thetis and supported by his handmaiden automata, by Henry Fuseli (1805), inspired by Pope's translation of the *Iliad*: number 1191 in Schiff (1975).

13 Athens, National Museum of Archaeology, no. 664; also noted by Dasen (1993) 199.

References

Adelson, Betty M. (2005) 'Dwarfs: the changing lives of archetypal "curiosities" – and echoes of the past.' *Disability Studies Quarterly* 25(3). Online at www.dsq-sds.org/article/view/576/753

Auerbach, Erich (1959) *Scenes from the Drama of European Literature: Six Essays* (= *Theory and History of Literature*, vol. 9). Manchester: Manchester University Press.

Backstrom, Laura (2012) 'From the freak show to the living room: cultural representations of dwarfism and obesity.' *Sociological Forum* 27, 682–707.

Bakhtin, Mikhail (1986) 'Response to a question from the *Novy Mir* editorial staff.' Trans. Vern W. McGee. In Caryl Emerson and Michael Holquist (eds), *Speech Genres and Other Late Essays*. Austin, TX: University of Texas Press, 1–7.

Bernidaki-Aldous, Eleftheria (1990) *Blindness in a Culture of Light*. New York: Peter Lang.

Brown, Christopher G. (1989) 'Ares, Aphrodite, and the laughter of the Gods.' *Phoenix* 43, 283–93.

Burkert, Walter (1970) 'Jason, Hypsipyle, and new fire at Lemnos: a study in myth and ritual.' *Classical Quarterly* 20, 1–16.

Burlington (1944) Anonymous editorial, 'The history of Poussin's Orion: a postscript.' *The Burlington Magazine for Connoisseurs* 84(491), 51.

Carrier, David (1990–1) 'Blindness and the representation of desire in Poussin's Paintings.' *RES: Anthropology and Aesthetics* 19/20, 31–52.

Clarke, Hannah (2019) 'Queer Classics: survey of LGBTQ+ Classicists reveals community and continuity.' *Eidolon*, 23 July. Online at https://eidolon.pub/queer-classics-b84819356f74

Comes, Natalis (1976 [1567]) *Mythologie*. Facsimile of the 1627 edition of the French translation by Jean Baudouin. 2 vols. New York and London: Garland.

Cropper, Elizabeth (1984) *The Ideal of Painting*. Princeton, NJ: Princeton University Press.

Dasen, Véronique (1993) *Dwarfs in Ancient Egypt and Greece*. Oxford: Clarendon Press.

Deroy, Louis (1956) 'À propos de l'épithète homérique d'Héphaistos ἀμφιγυήεις.' *RHR* 150, 129–35.

Detienne, Marcel (1970) 'Le Phoque, le crabe et le forgeron.' In Roland Crahay, Marcelle Derwa and Robert Joly (eds), *Hommages à Marie Delcourt* (Latomus Coll. 114). Brussels: Latomus, 219–33.

Detienne, Marcel and Jean-Pierre Vernant (1978) *Cunning Intelligence in Greek Culture and Society*. Trans. Janet Lloyd. Atlantic Highlands, NJ: Humanities.

Fontenrose, Joseph (1981) *Orion: The Myth of the Hunter and the Huntress* (= *UCPCS* vol. 23). Berkeley, Los Angeles and London: University of Chicago Press.

Garland, Robert (2010) *The Eye of the Beholder: Deformity and Disability in the Graeco-Roman World* (2nd edn). London: Bristol Classical Press.

Gombrich, Ernst H. (1944) 'The subject of Poussin's Orion.' *The Burlington Magazine for Connoisseurs* 84(491), 37–41. [Reprinted in his *Symbolic Images: Studies in the Art of the Renaissance*. London: Phaidon, 119–22.]

Greenwood, Emily (2010) *Afro-Greeks: Dialogues Between Anglophone Caribbean Literature and Classics in the Twentieth Century*. Oxford: Oxford University Press.

Haggard, Patrick and Sam Rodgers (2000) 'The movement disorder of Nicolas Poussin (1594–1665).' *Movement Disorders* 15(2), 328–34.

Hall, Edith (1997) 'The sociology of Athenian tragedy.' In Pat Easterling (ed.), *The Cambridge Companion to Greek Tragedy*. Cambridge: Cambridge University Press, 93–126.

Hall, Edith (2006) *The Theatrical Cast of Athens*. Oxford: Oxford University Press.

Hall, Edith (2008) *The Return of Ulysses*. London: IB Tauris.

Hall, Edith (2018) 'Hephaestus the hobbling humorist: the club-footed god in the history of early Greek comedy.' *Illinois Classical Studies* 43(2), 366–86.

Hall, Edith and Henry Stead (2020) *A People's History of Classics: Class and Greco-Roman Antiquity in Britain and Ireland 1689–1939*. London: Taylor & Francis.

Hasluck, Frederick W. (1909–10) 'Terra Lemnia.' *The Annual of the British School at Athens* 16, 220–31.

Hazlitt, William (1824) *'On a Landscape by Nicolas Poussin', in his Table-Talk: Original Essays on Men and Manners*, vol. II (2nd edn). London: Henry Colburn, 3–15.

Heilbrun, Carolyn (1990 [1985]) 'What was Penelope unweaving?', in her *Hamlet's Mother and Other Women*. New York: Columbia University, 103–11.

Horn, Cornelia B. (2013) 'A nexus of disabilities in ancient Greek miracle stories: a comparison of accounts of blindness from the Asklepieion in Epidauros and the shrine of Thecla in Seleucia.' In Christian Laes, Chris F. Goodey and M. Lynn Rose (eds), *Disabilities in Roman Antiquity*. Leiden and Boston: Brill, 115–43.

Jackson, Steven (1997) 'Callimachus, Istrus and two mortals' deaths.' *Quaderni Urbinati di Cultura Classica*, New Series 56, 105–18.

Kazantzis, Judith (1999) *The Odysseus Poems: Fictions on the Odyssey of Homer*. Tregarne, UK: Cargo Press.

Kelley, Nicole (2007) 'Deformity and disability in Greece and Rome.' In Hector Avalos, Sarah J. Melcher and Jeremy Schipper (eds), *This Abled Body: Rethinking Disabilities in Biblical Studies*. Leiden & Boston: Brill, 31–45.

Kozma, Chahira (2010) 'The ancient Egyptian dwarfs of the Walters Art Museum.' *American Journal of Medical Genetics. Part A.*, 152(10), 2556–62.

Lahr, John (1993) 'Inventing the enemy.' *New Yorker*, 18 October, 103–6.

Lichtheim, Miriam (1997) 'Instruction of Amenemope.' *COS* 1(47), 115–22.

Natale, Antonio (2008) *I riso di Hephaestus: all'origine del comico nella poesia e nell'arte dei greci*. Rome: L'Erma.

Neer, Richard T. (2006–7) 'Poussin and the ethics of imitation.' *Memoirs of the American Academy in Rome* 51(52), 297–344.

Newby, Zara (2002) 'Testing the boundaries of ekphrasis: Lucian's *On the Hall*.' *The Verbal and the Visual: Cultures of Ekphrasis in Antiquity* [Special Issue of *Ramus* 31(1–2), ed. Jaś Elsner]. Bentleigh, Victoria: Aureal, 126–35.

Newton, Rick M. (1987) 'Odysseus and Hephaestus in the *Odyssey*.' *Classical Journal* 83, 12–20.

Rinon, Yoav (2006) 'Tragic Hephaestus: the humanized God in the *Iliad* and the *Odyssey*.' *Phoenix* 60, 1–20.

Rose, Martha L. (2003) *The Staff of Oedipus: Transforming Disability in Ancient Greece*. Ann Arbor: University of Michigan Press.

Schiff, Gert (1975) *Henry Fuseli, 1741–1825*. Trans. S. Twohig. London: Tate.

Shipton, Matthew (2018) *The Politics of Youth in Greek Tragedy*. London: Bloomsbury.

Smith, Tyler Jo (2009) 'Komastai or "Hephaistoi"? Visions of comic parody in Archaic Greece.' *Bulletin of the Institute of Classical Studies* 52, 69–92.

Stevenson, William Edward (1975) 'The Pathological Grotesque Representation in Greek and Roman Art.' PhD thesis, University of Pennsylvania.

Storey, Ian C. (ed. and trans.) (2011) *Fragments of Old Comedy*, vol. 1. Cambridge, MA: Harvard University Press.

Taplin, Oliver (1989) *Greek Fire*. London: Cape.

Trentin, Lisa (2013) 'Exploring visual impairment in ancient Rome'. In Christian Laes, Chris F. Goodey and M. Lynn Rose (eds), *Disabilities in Roman Antiquity*. Leiden and Boston: Brill, 89–124.

Vernant, Jean-Pierre (1988) 'The tragic subject: historicity and transhistoricity.' In Jean-Pierre Vernant and Pierre Vidal-Naquet (eds), *Myth and Tragedy in Ancient Greece*. Trans. Janet Lloyd. New York: Zone Books, 237–47.

Vidal-Naquet, Pierre (1988) 'Oedipus in Vicenza and in Paris: two turning points in the history of Oedipus.' In Jean-Pierre Vernant and Pierre Vidal-Naquet (eds), *Myth and Tragedy in Ancient Greece*. Trans. Janet Lloyd. New York: Zone Books, 361–80.

Vollkommer, Rainer (1990) 'Kedalion.' *Lexicon Iconographicum Mythologiae Classicae* vol. 1. Zurich and Munich: Artemis, 978–9.

Walcott, Derek (1949) *Epitaph for the Young*. Bridgetown: Barbados Advocate.

Walcott, Derek (1990) *Omeros*. London: Faber & Faber.

Walls, Neal H. (2007) 'The origins of the disabled body: disability in ancient Mesopotamia.' In Hector Avalos, Sarah J. Melcher and Jeremy Schipper (eds) *This Abled Body: Rethinking Disabilities in Biblical Studies*. Leiden & Boston: Brill, 13–30.

Welcker, Friedrich G. (1851) *Alte Denkmäler*, vol. II. Göttingen: Dieterichschen Buchhandlung.

West, Martin L. (2001) 'The Fragmentary Homeric Hymn to Dionysus', *Zeitschrift für Papyrologie und Epigraphik* 134, 1–11.

Williams, Raymond (1977) *Marxism and Literature*. Oxford: Oxford University Press.

Yoshida, Atsuhiko (1969) 'Mythe d'Orion et de Cédalion.' In Jacqueline Bibauw (ed.), *Hommages à Marcel Renard* vol. II (= Collection Latomus 102). Brussels: Latomus, 828–44.

Chapter 10

A history of our own?

Using Classics in disability histories

Helen King

Abstract

This chapter discusses the uses of the classical world in constructing histories of disability and in considering what disability is. It investigates a range of conditions, including asthma, endometriosis, and conditions of hearing and sight. Some histories focus on key authorities from antiquity, such as Hippocrates, Aristotle, or Plato, while others look at inspiring individuals such as Quintus Pedius. The emphasis may be on continuity, or on change and progress. Modern literature and art can also use the classical world as a way of representing disability. In the case of Nydia, the blind flower girl of Bulwer-Lytton's *Last Days of Pompeii* who leads her companions to safety, nineteenth-century audiences found her so sympathetic that Randolph Rogers produced a sculpture of her, copies of which are still displayed across the world today. The response to her from more recent blind activists is less sympathetic.

Introduction

How do disability histories use the classical world, and in what other ways has the classical legacy been called on for help in constructing responses to disability? In this chapter I want to consider two approaches to these questions: the first using formal histories of particular conditions defined as disabilities, and the second based on more creative literary or artistic responses in which the ancient world is the subject of various types of reception.

Histories of disability may be created by awareness and support groups, or by medical specialists: in the former case, these are currently found in blogs and official sites online, whereas specialists tend to publish in medical journals. The material used in these histories comes from readings of ancient medicine and philosophy. The focus is often on the achievements of individuals with whichever condition is being discussed, although some such histories provide a less personalised timeline of key contributions (e.g. Bottrell n.d.).

The authors of such histories, like other writers of history, need to decide where to start: a decision that can be very significant for the message the history is intended to convey. A history of a disability can be presented as one that extends as far back as possible, thus stressing continuity and a shared experience between us and the past and invoking the key names of the Western tradition such as Hippocrates, Plato, or Aristotle; or, instead, it can concentrate on change, telling the story of a recent moment of breakthrough or enlightenment coming after millennia of darkness. If the first of these options is taken, then authors still need to decide where to position themselves in relation to the ancient world. This entails determining whether classical examples remain 'good to think with', or whether they should be dismissed as merely cautionary tales of a less enlightened time.

But it is not only ancient medicine and philosophy that are used in understanding disability. In the reception of the ancient world, classical myth can also be drawn on to represent disability and responses to it. Here, too, in artistic and literary works that engage with the Classics, considerations of whether to concentrate on similarity or on difference are brought into play. In the second part of this chapter, I shall look at some works of fiction created in the modern era that have contributed to views of ancient Greek and Roman approaches to disability as well as helping people to think about disability in their own contexts.

Creating genealogies of disability

Asthma

Histories of asthma provide excellent illustrations of the options available in using history to understand a disability. For example, a section of the *Journal of Asthma* takes the 'achievements of individuals' approach, with accounts of 'the experience of asthma in the life of outstanding persons' such as Seneca the Younger (Panzani 1988); in one of his letters, Seneca strikingly described an acute attack of 'shortness of breath' (Lat. *suspirium*), adding that he saw no reason to use the Greek name for it – *asthma* – and observed that doctors called it 'practising how to die' (*Ep.* 54.2; Jackson 2009, 17–9). This long history and the focus on achievements, with the personal touch of the voice of someone who apparently had the condition, clearly resonate with contemporary people with asthma who note that it was 'as though I had a special connection with this guy who lived more than 2,000 years before me' (Bottrell 2015a, n.p.)[1] and who also find it reassuring to remember that there was a time 'when there was no cure and no remedy that really provided any relief. It must have been pure hell to live like that' (Frea 2011, n.p.). Another journal, *Allergy and Asthma Proceedings*, includes a parallel series started by Sheldon Cohen on 'Asthma among the famous', with the classical individuals featured including Seneca, Pliny the Elder, and 'Augustus Caesar (63 B.C.–A.D. 14) first emperor of Rome' (King and Cohen 2001).

The respiratory therapist and freelance writer John Bottrell (who had asthma) included Seneca in his 'Asthma history' blog, set up in 2013 to 'provide a history of lung diseases from the beginning of time to today' (Bottrell 2015b). Over the blog as a whole, however, his focus is more on providing a long narrative account of the condition by providing brief biographies alongside summaries of texts. In his first post for this blog, he traced, 'The oldest description of asthma (sort of)' to 2697 BCE, to Chinese medicine and specifically to the *Yellow Emperor's Classic on Internal Medicine*; the 'sort of' is because the description referenced here is to difficulty in breathing rather than to a named disease (Bottrell 2013a; Jackson 2009, 40–1). Bottrell considers that the person 'who made asthma a household name' was Hippocrates, and, after medicine took a brief detour into considering that the condition was a nervous disorder, 'It wouldn't be until the early 19th century that it was proved that Hippocrates was right all along, at least about asthma being spasmodic in nature' (Bottrell 2013b).

Because the names of Hippocrates, Aristotle, and Galen continue to hold power, writers of disability histories are keen to include them. In most medical narratives that invoke the classical past, the key name remains that of Hippocrates, and, in my book *Hippocrates Now: The 'Father of Medicine' in the Internet Age* (King 2019), I demonstrated how Hippocrates today is almost always regarded as being 'right'. We meet him in many places where the body is under discussion, from Wikipedia to 'quotes', and from news outlets to social media. In contexts ranging from the validity of the Hippocratic Oath to the ideal diet, he is claimed as the father not just of medicine, but of health, of food science, and of holism. Histories of disability and of various medical conditions that are aimed at medical practitioners rather than at those with the condition may include Hippocrates not just to create a picture of continuity, but also to provide a sense of progress, as in Edmund Keeney's presidential address to the 1964 annual meeting of the American Society of Allergy, entitled 'The history of asthma from Hippocrates to Meltzer' (1964). Keeney's comments on the ancient world repeated what was then the standard textbook picture of movement from darkness to light and from superstition to 'rationality', a shift in which Hippocrates was thought to be crucial. Where the focus is on therapy rather than description or identification of a condition, however, Hippocrates may be considered less relevant. In 'A brief history of asthma and its mechanisms to modern concepts of disease pathogenesis', for a journal focusing on allergy, asthma, and immunology, Stephen Holgate highlighted the changes in understanding of the condition that led to a shift in therapy from bronchodilators to corticosteroids; for this particular story, only a single sentence on the Greek origin of the word 'asthma' was considered necessary, with the historical narrative beginning only in the late nineteenth century (Holgate 2010, 165).

Much hinges on how significant the use of the word *asthma* in the Hippocratic corpus is considered to be. It is certainly used there, as it is just a word meaning 'panting' or simply 'breath', but this can be blown up out of all proportion. There is no awareness in these histories that, in all instances in which the word features in Hippocratic treatises, it is used in the plural, *asthmata*, rather than as a disease label. Although some such histories at least recognise that Hippocratic usage concerns a symptom rather than a named condition, many do not make this distinction. A web page on 'Who discovered asthma?' currently offers, 'The history of the discovery of asthma as an acute respiratory disorder came to light in 400 BC. The term "Asthma" was first used by Hippocrates in his book *Corpus Hippocraticum*, where he also provided a definition for the medical term' (How to Use Inhalers 2012). Although the 'light' in this story of enlightenment is here firmly associated with Hippocrates, the date of 400 BCE is entirely arbitrary, probably based on taking the traditional dates for Hippocrates – 460–370 BCE – and then picking a round number in between.

Although Hippocrates is often credited with making *asthma* into a 'medical term', there is a variant that splits the roles of recognition of a symptom and describing a condition. In this version of the history, Hippocrates was aware of it simply as a symptom, and it was only with Aretaeus that it became something more, so that the credit for 'the first accurate *description* of asthma, as we know it today' (Karamanou and Androutsos 2011, n.p.; my italics) goes instead to Aretaeus (Sakula 1988, 35).

The search for medical wisdom in the past is by no means only a modern phenomenon, and other names from ancient medicine may also feature in histories of asthma. In his *Observations on the History and Cure of the Asthma* (1793), Michael Ryan claimed that he had:

> read most of the modern writers, and hitherto had tried their methods, and hot pectorals and cephalics in vain. I believed by my ill success in their way that they never understood this disease; and therefore turned over some of the old writers, Galen, Aegineta [Paul of Aegina], Aetius, &c. where I found more rational notions, and was directed by them to the use of that medicine which does very much relieve and prevent my fits.
>
> Ryan (1793, 65–6)

This picture of a turn towards history in order to help one's own condition feels very modern indeed. As this passage suggests, Ryan believed that the remedies used by classical authors were 'not only rational but successful' (Ryan 1793, 64). Hippocrates featured here too, as another hero of this story: whereas Hippocrates was 'intimately acquainted' with the nature of asthma (Ryan 1793, 57), Galen had 'pervert[ed] the intention and meaning of this illustrious writer' (Ryan 1793, 58). Ryan's favoured remedy was the cold bath; in the eighteenth century, the healing powers of both hot and cold baths were commonly traced back to Hippocrates (e.g. Floyer 1715, 47).

Not everyone agrees, or has agreed, that effective remedies can be taken from the past. One popular website observes that Aretaeus's 'suggested remedy of drinking a concoction of owl's blood and wine, however, is thankfully no longer a recommended intervention for asthma' (Felman 2018, n.p.). *Asthma: The Ultimate Teen Guide* attributes this remedy simply to 'The Romans' and contrasts it with Maimonides's 'more appetizing choice' of chicken soup (Paquette 2003, 1). The owl's blood remedy, part of the approach to ancient medicine that focuses on the 'curiosities' rather than making it into the ancestor of modern medicine, is variously attributed across histories of asthma. I have found no evidence that it derives from Aretaeus; although he does indeed describe asthma along with orthopnoea in his treatise *On Chronic Diseases* (1.1), this remedy does not feature in Aretaeus's *Cures for Chronic Diseases*. In histories of asthma produced for a general readership, it may be the better-known Galen, rather than Aretaeus, who is associated with owl's blood: for example, 'Galen the ancient Greek physician treated sufferers with the disgusting concoction of owl's blood in wine' (Thorpe 2015, n.p.). I have not so far managed to pin this story down, but it may originate in al-Rāzī's (Rhazes's) *al-Ḥāwī* (1955–68, Vol 4, 39), which records a remedy used in one of the medical treatises that, in the Middle Ages, was associated with the name of a ninth-century Christian physician, Yūḥannā ibn Māsawayh (known in the West as John Mesue).[2] According to Rhazes, Mesue:

> used for asthma and shortness of breath two drachmas of dried and powdered fox lung and decoction of figs added to a drink. In differing with Galen who reported many cured of asthma with owl's blood in a drink or giving owl's flesh with food and drinking its blood afterwards – owl's blood is not to be given in any case of asthma having seen it administrated and useless.
>
> Cserháti (2004, 258)[3]

In Mesue's reading, just because Galen reported the remedy – and the reference, in the treatise *De simplicium medicamentorum temperamentis ac facultatibus* 10.3 (Kühn 1965 12.257), is to the *noctua*, the night-owl – does not mean that anyone should use it now. In an odd twist on this story, an article on whether Hippocrates or Galen 'discovered' asthma states that Galen's treatment for it was 'owl's wine' (Cotto 2008, n.p.), the author adding that both authors 'described asthma correctly' in contrast to 'modern day physicians' who, until the 1980s, thought 'that asthma was purely a psychological condition'.

Other versions of the asthma origin story that focus on ancient Greece correctly note that the term *asthma* existed before the Hippocratic texts, so that the Hippocratic contribution is to transform it from an everyday word to a 'medical term' (e.g. Marketos and Ballas 1982). Such a claim raises the contentious issue of whether there was such a thing as a technical medical vocabulary in classical Greece. Does the terminology of the Hippocratic corpus simply repeat what was already in common use, or was the process the reverse, with non-medical writers picking up words from medical texts? For example, Thucydides, Euripides, and Aeschylus use terms that sound 'technical' to us, but does this mean that they took them from medical writing? These are important questions because of what they imply about the relationship between medicine and its wider cultural context. It is now nearly 70 years since Page (1953) noted what he considered to be 'technical' medical terminology in

Thucydides's description of the Plague of Athens, with Lichtenthaeler subsequently arguing that, 'il est donc établi comme une *certitude* que l'Historien athénien a écrit la peste à l'aide de la terminologie scientifique contemporaine' (1965, 33; author's italics). Another example would be Euripides's application to Philoctetes's disease of the word *phagedaina* (fr. 792 Nauck). This word is otherwise found only in the Hippocratic corpus, Democritus, Demosthenes, and in one of the Epidaurus *iamata* (Jouanna 2012a, 90–1, n. 22). As Jacques Jouanna has pointed out, in its use in Euripides, the word seems to be taken from Aeschylus's play on the same theme, and Aeschylus died at around the time Hippocrates was probably born. But is that enough to make it a 'technical term' borrowed by tragedy from medicine? Not necessarily; examples such as this one may instead preserve Ionian words that had gone out of usage except in medicine and drama (Jouanna 2012b, 74–5).

We can, therefore, see that the various versions of the history of asthma raise several questions applicable to disability history more widely. Is the story being told one of continuity, or of change and progress? Is a classical reference being used to provide a 'landmark in medical history', whether that is the origin of the name or the first clinically recognisable description? Is it reassuring to know that a condition which you have goes back a long way in time, and to encounter the 'achievements' of those who share it? Those who want to present a condition as having a long history often feel the need to include Hippocrates in this, even though they may find it difficult to go beyond stating that the word is used in the Hippocratic corpus. Where the diagnosis is presented as an old one, then the length of the history constructed for it becomes significant. If this is a long history, does it matter whether we go back to Hippocrates in the fifth and fourth centuries BCE, or only to Aretaeus in the second century CE, so long as there is a 'classic' somewhere in the story? Do we foreground the Greek and Roman Classics, or look to non-Western cultures – for example, to China in 2697 BCE? Is it age we want, or a Western classical pedigree? What about the Ebers Papyrus or the Code of Hammurabi (e.g. Sakula 1988; Cannizzaro 2017; Patel 2019)? Although ancient texts may be praised for recognising or describing a condition, or for finding a remedy that science subsequently forgot, there is also the tendency to dismiss older remedies for it as 'disgusting' or, in internet parlance, 'weird' (Saxena 2019). Perhaps what is most important is whether the story being told produces confidence in where we are now.

Endometriosis

These points can be illustrated further by looking briefly at the debilitating condition of endometriosis, a condition that, in the UK, is currently regarded as disabling but not a disability, not least because the pressure groups working to support those with it consider that it would increase discrimination against women in the workplace if it were to be so labelled. Nevertheless, women with endometriosis can apply for disability benefits (Endometriosis UK 2017).

Histories of endometriosis written for a general audience claim a Hippocratic origin that does not exist; for example:

> As with many medical conditions, there were a couple of blokes squabbling over who was the first to describe in [*sic*] around the 19th century, but there is even mention of the condition and its symptoms in the Hippocratic corpus which contains works from the 4th and 5th centuries BC.
>
> Mitra (2017, n.p.)

In an article published by three US medical doctors in 2012, 'Endometriosis, ancient disease, ancient treatments', endometriosis was identified with 'hysteria' – in itself, hardly a secure diagnosis (King 1993) – and a lengthy pedigree going back to the Hippocratic corpus was offered, along with the claim that the symptoms in the ancient Greek texts 'remarkably ... correspond nearly seamlessly to the set of symptoms identified today as emblems of endometriosis' (Nezhat et al. 2012, 3). Even leaving aside the many factual errors made in this 2012 article, which include attributing to the Hippocratic treatise *On Virgins* a passage that does not feature in it, presenting an image of the Delphic oracle as an example of the medical treatment of fumigation (Nezhat et al. 2012, 4 and Fig. 4), and colluding in the now-discredited myth of 'Trotula' as the name of 'one of the most celebrated female physicians of ancient times' (Nezhat et al. 2012, 13; ignoring, *inter alia*, Green 2001), this picture of continuity is remarkably strained. 'Nearly seamlessly'? On my own experience of severe endometriosis, I would certainly challenge identification with hysteria; it is nothing like the various symptoms from the 'hysteria' tradition that this article confidently presents, such as 'lying as if dead for seven days' (Nezhat et al. 2012, 6). This phrase, unattributed in Nezhat, comes from Pliny, *Natural History* (7.52.175), and is entirely serious about 'as if dead'; in the 'hysteria' tradition, this does not mean just feeling a bit rough, but suggests that there is a risk of premature burial (King 1993, 6 and 34).

The alternative to this 'longue durée' approach is to deny that any ancient references to endometriosis exist (e.g. Sutton 2006, 3) and instead to present this debilitating condition as having a far shorter history and as 'new' or 'modern', as for example in the title of an article arguing for its discovery only in the 1920s that was published in a medical journal in 2011, 'Endometriosis, a modern syndrome' (Brosens and Benagiano 2011). Like asthma, endometriosis has been linked to industrialisation, although even that claim is disputed (Jackson 2006, 148). But calling it 'a modern syndrome' and deciding that the length of its history is very short is also a political move because, from the 1940s, it was linked with women who were delaying having children because of their careers (Sanmiguel 2000). As late as 1991, US natural health magazine *Total Health* ran a story that included: 'It is called the "Career Woman's Disease" because it is predominantly found in women in their thirties, and occasionally twenties, who have not yet had children' (Binder 1991). This causation story, which suggests putting the blame on women for seeking fulfilment – or just an income – from something other than motherhood, is no longer as common as it was in the 1980s and 1990s (incidentally, the time when I was diagnosed). Although one may assume that the 'it's about career women' story militates against a search for a Hippocratic pedigree, that is not always the case; the 2012 'Ancient disease, ancient treatments' article bizarrely suggested that Hippocratic claims that pregnancy releases a woman from menstrual disorders – 'if she conceives, she is healthy' (King 2005) – are 'a near conceptual equivalent to the 20th-century notion of endometriosis as a "career woman's disease"' (Nezhat et al. 2012, 3).

Deafness

Asthma and endometriosis are very much hidden disabilities. Hearing impairments, while also being invisible, are more likely to become apparent in social interaction. In a culture such as that of the Greco-Roman world, a person who could not hear – whether this was permanent or temporary, total or partial – could follow practical instructions well enough to do many jobs (Adams 2020, 87–8), but this would not be the case for some elite roles based on orality, using persuasion and the skills of formal rhetoric. Christian Laes has already explored the complexities of classical terminology in *Disabilities and the Disabled in the Roman World: A Social and Cultural History* (2018), and I shall not revisit his arguments in any detail here. The link between hearing and speech does seem to be one recognised in antiquity. The Hippocratic *Fleshes* 18 mentions those who are deaf (*hoi kôloi*) from birth who can utter 'mere sounds' (*monophôna*) but cannot speak. The deaf-mute is, in Greek, *eneos* (Laes 2018, 122, citing Galen's definition of the term). The terminology can, however, sometimes make it difficult to distinguish those who are deaf-mutes from those who appear closer to our category of selective mutism, such as Pliny's Maecenas Melissus, who 'decided' to stay silent for three years after bringing up blood during a convulsion (Pliny, *NH* 28.62), or to autism (Laes 2018, 118–9). Are such modern diagnoses also appropriate to those healing miracles in which someone is unable to speak but then gives an answer in response to a question from the god, such as the mute boy who, during a sacrifice, spoke in answer to a slave who was helping with the firewood (IG IV^2 121.41–8; LiDonnici 1995, A5)?

As with asthma, and to a lesser extent endometriosis, Hippocrates features in the history of hearing and its disabilities. Here is a claim from 'A brief history of otorhinolaryngology' published in a Brazilian journal of the specialism in 2007: 'With merely empirical treatments, Hippocrates, was also interested in otology, however himself and his disciples were more concerned with the relations ear infections had with other organs, especially the brain and tonsils' (Nogueira et al. 2007, 694). So, even if Hippocrates is acknowledged as having little to contribute, he must at least be mentioned, even if only as 'interested in'. The wording here is taken almost verbatim from this article's stated source, an article by Joseph Hawkins, who co-wrote a series of 'historical sketches' of otohistory for the journal *Audiology and Neurotology* in 2004 and 2006, some of which were then published as a book (Hawkins and Schacht 2008). Hawkins mentioned:

> The acute observations of Hippocrates ... about the symptoms, diagnosis, course and treatment of diseases, including those of the ear ... His methods of treatment were almost entirely empirical, and he had scant knowledge of anatomy of the ear. He was mainly concerned with its infections and with their relations to other organs, including the tonsils and the brain.
>
> Hawkins (2004, 66)

The point about Hippocrates's main interest lying in the relationship between ear infections and the rest of the body is in turn based on a 1907 history of the discipline (Politzer 1907), widely repeated in medical literature on the 'giants of otology' (e.g. Traynor 2015), and is presumably what medical students were supposed to answer in response to a question in a Philadelphia 1941 exam on the history of otology: 'Write on the otological knowledge of Hippocrates' (Robinson 1941, 316). As for the tonsils, Hippocrates is also credited with the first tonsillectomy: 'The first operation on the tonsils has been attributed to Hippocrates (460–375 AD)' (Richardson 1999, 75; Vlayen et al. 2005, 49). The text that is the origin of this claim seems to be *On Glands* 7 and is a matter of 'interpreting' how to map the *paraisthmia* glands in the throat on to modern notions of anatomy; discussing this, the medical authors of a 2007 article – who, commendably, drew on the Loeb Hippocrates rather than relying on earlier pieces by their own peers – concluded that the author of *On Glands* 'should be recognized as a far-seeing pioneer in haematology and medical sciences' (Crivellato et al. 2007, 591–2).

This message that the pioneering Hippocrates 'was right' remains a strong one for many disabilities. For example, on the website for Epilepsy Canada, Hippocrates comes out as the hero, contrasted with the (alleged) Babylonian view that the condition was 'supernatural':

> Hippocrates believed that epilepsy was not sacred, but a disorder of the brain - a revolutionary view. He did not believe 'that a human could be invaded by a god, the basest by the most pure.' He recommended physical treatments and stated that if the disease became chronic, it was incurable.
>
> Epilepsy Canada (2016, n.p.)

The material here is taken from a World Health Organization publication (Reynolds 2005). Nor is this pattern unique to epilepsy. Along with statements about his empiricism, claims that Hippocrates moved perception of the condition being discussed from the result of divine intervention to having a natural cause are common on disability history sites; for example, on a history of developmental disabilities developed by a US group, 'For Hippocrates, care of the body was in the hands of man rather than the gods' (Minnesota Governor's Council on Developmental Disabilities 2019, n.p.). Other websites go rather further in their claims for Hippocrates's work on epilepsy – for example, a student project website arguing that 'Hippocrates also develops a diet for epileptics, possibly similar to the modern Ketogenic diet, which treats epilepsy' (Tuinstra 2001, n.p.). This appears to be assuming that the effects of fasting and of a ketogenic diet are the same.

Many histories are the product of disabled communities themselves, and because of this the history may be presented as that of a group rather than of a disability. The main example of this can be found in Deaf culture, which can present as a minority language group rather than as a disability group. In its histories, as elsewhere, the story can be created out of a series of individuals; significant here is Quintus Pedius, often described as 'the first deaf person in recorded history known by name'. 'Dumb from his birth', in the translation of John Bostock, this grandson of a former consul of the same name was taught to paint and 'made great progress in the art, but died … in his youth' (Pliny *NH*, 35.7; Bostock and Riley 1857, 231; Harrington 2006; Laes 2018, 118–9). Being non-verbal could, of course, point to conditions other than deafness (Adams 2020, 98).

Alternatively, in these histories, the focus can be on the development of sign language rather than on deaf people. To prove the antiquity of this mode of communication, the key text cited is Plato's *Cratylus*, and the key individual Socrates, although in this story he does not come off very well. On an Estonian website for the history of deaf people, based on a now-deleted page from Gallaudet University (which educates the Deaf and those with hearing disabilities), we read: '360 BC. Socrates mentions the use of signs by the deaf, Plato's Cratylus. Socrates discusses innate intelligence, and claims that Deaf people are incapable of language and ideas' (Estonian Association of the Deaf 2010, n.p.). This statement merges two ancient sources. First, in the *Cratylus* passage to which this refers, Socrates asks Hermogenes:

> Answer me this question: If we had no voice or tongue, and wished to make things clear to one another, should we not try, as dumb people actually do, to make signs with our hands and head and person generally?
> (422e–423b, tr. Harold N. Fowler 1921)

This passage, and this translation, is widely quoted, despite using the term 'dumb', which is no longer in current usage – for example, in a *History Today* article examining what the osteoarchaeological evidence of deafness can contribute to our knowledge of the past, although this glosses the translation to give 'as dumb [mute] people actually do' (Atkin 2015). Socrates goes on to describe how these people – the Greek is *hoi eneoi*, whatever that means here – use gestures, showing things that are light or higher up, or heavy or lower down, by raising or lowering their hands, or imitating the movement of a horse to say 'horse'. This passage may sound like a positive valuation of what non-verbal people do, but, in what he entitled 'a deaf reading' of *Cratylus*, Bauman noted the political implications of Socrates talking about gestures as preceding words (Bauman 2008, 134); the claim for 'preceding' is significant here, as it suggests that communicating by words is more 'advanced'. Drawing on the signs for 'heavy', 'light', and 'horse galloping' in American Sign Language, Bauman thus reads the key passage as denigrating sign languages, making signing into a primitive stage or an aberration rather than acknowledging that a fully grammatical language does not have to be based on speech, and can instead consist of gestures.

Second, that claim 'that Deaf people are incapable of language and ideas' is not a direct quotation from Plato, but seems to summarise Socrates saying, in a discussion of 'rational explanation', that anyone can make their thoughts clear by using speech; or, at least, anyone 'can show what he thinks about anything, unless he is deaf or dumb from the first' (*Theaetetus* 206d–e, tr. Harold N. Fowler 1921). But it also owes something to Aristotle, who is definitely not the hero of classical deaf history. Many online histories of the deaf repeat variations of: '355 BC. Aristotle says "Those who are born deaf all become senseless and incapable of reason"' (Estonian Association of the Deaf 2010, n.p.; Shaner 2013). This comes from a widely repeated sentence in the 1911 edition of the *Encyclopaedia Britannica* (Payne 1911) and, in the introduction to a history of deaf America by a deaf author, Jack Gannon, Mervin Garretson described it as 'The most *vicious* pronouncement' (Garretson 1981, p. xxi; my italics). Although, in *On Sense and Sensible Objects* (437a15–18), Aristotle claims that, 'of those who have been deprived of one sense or the other from birth, the blind are more intelligent than the deaf and the dumb' (tr. Walter Hett 1957), as Ellen Adams has noted: 'he does not explicitly state that the deaf were incapable of obtaining rational thought, as is often claimed in modern deaf studies' (Adams 2020, 89).

In these deaf histories that draw on the Classics, Hippocrates may come out relatively well, being seen as superior to Aristotle simply because he did not consider that those who were both deaf and mute were affected by any intellectual defect: in the 1911 *Encyclopaedia Britannica* article, for example, 'Hippocrates was in advance of Aristotle when he realized that deaf-mutes did not speak simply because they did not know how to' (Payne 2011, n.p.). But, in fact, there is very little in the Hippocratic corpus on those born deaf, let alone on their intellect. It is never clear whether those who do not speak are deaf, or have another condition that affects their ability to speak. The Hippocratic treatises are interested not in those who are born deaf, but in deafness as a stage of an acute disease (Adams 2020, 87, 93–4). For example, in *Prorrhetic* 1.29, suddenly becoming deaf is seen as a bad sign, which can be relieved by passing blood in the stools, but still presages death.

Nor is Hippocrates always presented as superior to Aristotle here. Giulio Ferreri, an oralist teacher of the Deaf – that is, not a supporter of sign language – noted in a paper translated into English in 1906 that the ancients handed down to us the error that being mute is about the tongue not being able to move properly, and, if it is released, then they can speak (hence our 'tongue-tied'), and argued that Aristotle had a better understanding of how speech happens than Hippocrates did. Ferreri also commented that, in contrast to the ancient habit of defining deaf-mutes by their inability to communicate in speech, the modern term 'deaf-mute' puts cause and effect in the correct order (Ferreri 1906). Here, then, it is Aristotle who is seen as having the knowledge.

In modern medical literature, there is also the view that Hippocrates was the source for Aristotle's alleged views on the intellectual capacity of deaf people. In a 2006 invited review for the *Mediterranean Journal of Otology*, an otologist, Anestis Psifidis (2006, 45–6), wrote:

> Hippocrates believed wrongly that, in deaf-mute patients, both the hearing and speech organs had been affected. His theory that deaf-mute children were developmentally challenged was adapted by such followers as Aristotle and Galen and influenced scientific knowledge and the progress of medicine for about 2000 years. Until the 16th century, deaf-mute children were treated as disabled, invalid, and demonized individuals and were rejected by society. In ancient Sparta, deaf-mute children were thrown down Keada, a precipitous ravine, to be killed.

This is, unfortunately, a typical example of what happens when someone writes the history of his own specialism using only previous work by people in exactly the same position. In this case, Psifidis is using a 1997 book by Panos Apostolides, *Ear, Nose and Throat Diseases in Hippocrates*. There is no evidence for this Spartan slaughter of the children, but the focus here fits another of the themes of disability history, the emphasis on past ill-treatment, which is part of the broader approach to the past as a bad place to be contrasted with modern enlightenment. For example, Omvig (2019, n.p.) states:

> It is reported that in many of the early great civilizations, blind babies were abandoned and left to die, either from exposure to the elements or to be eaten by wild animals. Later, some blind men were sold into galley slavery and some blind women were sold into prostitution. Others were used for amusement, but most lived their lives as beggars or were simply kept by families.

There is plenty of evidence for attitudes to disabled people that demean them. There is one reference in Plutarch to a dedicated market in Rome where they were sold as slaves:

> at Rome there are some who take no account of paintings or statues or even, by Heaven, of the beauty of the boys and women for sale, but haunt the monster-market, examining those who have no calves, or are weasel-

armed (i.e. short arms), or have three eyes, or ostrich-heads, and searching to learn whether there has been born some 'Commingled shape and misformed prodigy'.

On being a busybody (10, 520c, tr. William Helmbold 1939)

This is supported by, for example, Quintilian, who states that physically imperfect slaves cost more than attractive slaves (*Institutions* 2.5.10–12), but it is also clear that Plutarch, as Debbie Felton, observed, 'deplores' the existence of this market and those who use it (Felton 2012, 128–9). The 'bad emperors' are also associated with using individuals with disabilities for entertainment; although we find this disturbing, as Lisa Trentin (2011) points out, the idea that you do not treat people in this way is relatively recent.

It is clear that there are different valuations of ancient authorities in the medical and disability communities. In 1993, Edmund P. Fowler of the American Otological Society (founded 1868) wrote on its history, 'The second one hundred years: musings and dreams of things to come'. In discussing the number of developments in medical treatment over the first 100 years of the society, he referred to Hippocrates not as an otologist but in terms of 'primum non nocere', 'first do no harm'; the more new things there are on offer, the greater becomes the risk of accidentally doing harm (Fowler 1993, 88). Here, even where Hippocrates has nothing to say on a particular topic, his ethics at least still need to be referenced, because medicine needs Hippocrates. Fowler also observed that, although more information was needed on the history of the society:

> we cannot live on truth alone. The writers of history should use their *imagination* and so leave with us not just the words, nor just the tale, but a way of looking at things. They should record the myth as well as the facts.
>
> Fowler (1993, 88)

This is an interesting manifesto, not least because it suggests that there is some pure form of history in which the historian offers 'truth alone'.

Putting yourself in the story: myth and imagination

It is clear from this brief examination of disability histories that some play fast and loose with the available evidence in order to push home their point. In this final section, I want to examine two examples of a different use of the imagination, not to select and skew ancient evidence, but instead to provide both 'a way of looking at things' and also a way of enabling those with disabilities to make sense of their bodies, and those without disabilities to empathise with others. This involves using the ancient world – and its reception – in a different way. My first example picks up a condition already discussed here, endometriosis. Although, as I have shown, attempts have been made either to give this a history going back to Hippocrates or instead to deny that it has any history, ancient myths can also be brought into the endometriosis story. Enovid, originally sold as a treatment for endometriosis until 1960, used an advertisement showing Andromeda 'freed from her chains'; then, from 1960 it was marketed as a contraceptive (Enovid 1962; Junod and Marks 2002, 126). Here, the chains are 'the cyclic mechanism of her reproductive system', and Andromeda is labelled 'unfettered'. In his 2009 doctoral thesis, Ronald E. Batt went further, presenting Andromeda instead as 'the embodiment of every young woman with endometriosis', 'waiting to be rescued from torment' (Batt 2009, 9). He also offered the following unattributed lines:

> Look to the Sky and Imagine
> Beautiful Andromeda chained to her Rock
> Harried by the Twin Vultures of
> Pain and Infertility
> Now you have a Vivid Image
> Of every Young Woman
> Tormented by Endometriosis.

This image merges Andromeda with Prometheus, tied to a rock while a vulture comes to him each day to consume his liver (Fig. 10.1). As a former sufferer, I would question how helpful this is supposed to be to a woman with endometriosis, but the recognition of the severity of the pain with the suggestion of a cure may be encouraging.

I want to end by looking at a different aspect of constructing a history, this time not from a famous ancient medical writer, but from the point of view of a biography of an ancient person with a disability – in this case, blindness. Histories of the blind, like other disability histories, can focus on 'the blind as objects of charity rather than active agents in history', or on ill-treatment of those with disabilities, but may also construct their stories as 'a collection of biographies of "extraordinary" individuals, from Homer to Helen Keller', as the online *Encyclopaedia Britannica* puts it, pointing out that part of the reason for the focus on individuals is the absence of any 'sustained organized efforts by the blind to act in concert to achieve collective goals' (Miller 2014, n.p.).

One such extraordinary individual is Nydia, the blind flower girl of Pompeii. Although she is not a real historical figure, her life in art, opera, and song after she was created by Edward Bulwer-Lytton in *The Last Days of Pompeii* (1834) almost makes her one (Hunnings 2011, 181–2; Moormann 2015). Bulwer's novel was inspired by visits to Naples in 1833, including the sites of Pompeii itself – and the finds from there displayed in Naples Museum – and Florence, where he saw Karl Bruillov's painting *The Last Day of Pompeii* (1830–3). Drawing on an existing trope of the volcano disaster, and on a popular interest in staged volcanic eruptions from the 1770s onwards, his novel also reflects a growing tendency to focus on the individuals affected by such disasters rather than on the global picture (Daly 2011, 271). Earlier examples of this shift to the individual

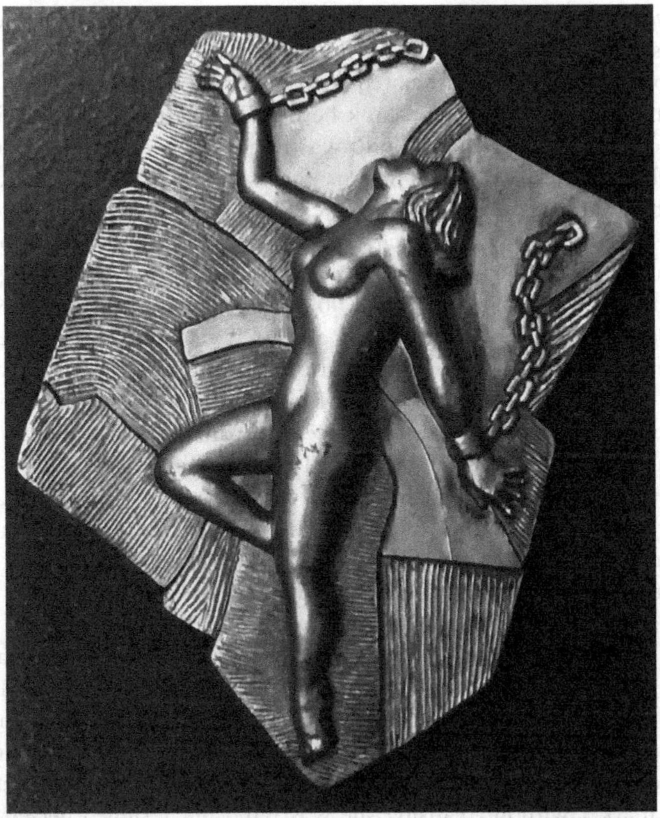

Figure 10.1 Enovid image of Andromeda supplied by Museum of Contraception and Abortion, Vienna (with permission)

included stories in which the earthquake saves a noble virgin from rape or a Christian from being attacked by a lion, as in Lincoln Fairfield's *The Last Night of Pompeii* (1832; Daly 2011, 268).

As a woman, a slave, and a blind person, Nydia is othered in more than one way. In the novel, she is treated badly by her owner Stratonice, then sold on to Glaucus, whom she loves, and then passed on by him to Ione, whom he loves. Her slave status is particularly significant when we consider that the novel was published one year after the abolition of slavery entered British law, and that Bulwer-Lytton was MP for Lincoln at publication. In 1838, he spoke in the House of Commons against the treatment of former slaves in the proposed Negro Apprenticeship Bill, under which those who had been freed were then expected to work for nothing as apprentices (Hunnings 2011, 185–6; Gross 1981). The only way in which Nydia could be further othered would be to make her of a different race; as Ato Quayson has observed, the language of disability and that of racial difference have been very close in the history of colonialism (Quayson 2007, 10).

One long-lasting trope associated with blindness is that it brings inner vision (Quayson 2007, 92–3); we may think here of Tiresias, blinded but given the gift of prophecy, or the idea that Homer was blind. Nydia's blindness does not give her insight or foresight, but it means that she can lead Glaucus and Ione to safety when darkness descends on the city after Vesuvius erupts. However, she then kills herself. Bulwer explicitly included among his inspirations the idea that the darkness after the eruption of Vesuvius would favour someone already blind (Daly 2011, 273; Schiller 1993, 40), and this remains a trope of fiction, as in the 1960s thriller (both a play and a film) *Wait Until Dark*, where darkness gives the trapped blind heroine her chance to turn the tables on the villains. The lead role in a stage production was not given to a blind actress until 2017, in a touring production in the UK; the actress, Karina Jones, said in an interview, 'I've totally got an advantage because I've got a lot of shorthand. I've got a head start because I have real insight into the character' (Finke 2017, n.p.). As blind heroine, Nydia has her own 'head start' in the darkness; Jessica L. Langworthy mentions a real example of blind girls leading their sighted teachers to safety through the smoke of a fire (Langworthy 1930, 276).

Nydia is very much an idealized nineteenth-century blind person, who, in the words of Leanne Hunnings, 'sits on the boundary between passivity and activity, objectivity and subjectivity, victimhood and agency' (Hunnings 2011, 182). The visual, in many forms, plays an important role in the book – witnessing a murder, witnessing the crucifixion – but Nydia is by definition always the Viewed, never the Viewer (Hunnings 2011, 199). Her previous owner, Stratonice, bought her at the slave market without realising she was blind but resigned herself to the purchase, especially when she found out that Nydia could sing (although her songs are always sad ones). In her ability to perform, Nydia reflects the nineteenth-century attitude that it is better to be blind than deaf, as described in this 1846 article in the *Westminster Review* (cited in Sharman 1996, n.p.):

> One of the most striking differences between the blind and the deaf is the tendency shown by the blind, in all ages, to poetry and poetical composition, – a taste which the deaf have never exhibited. The great command of language acquired by the blind, the excellence of their ear, and the absence of excitement and distraction from the sensations of sight, will go far to account for this peculiarity … The deaf, on the contrary, have no command of language, no ear, and a sad deficiency of ideas and emotions, while their possession of that admirable organ, the eye, tends to overpower their inner feelings, and to throw them upon visual sensations for a great part of their enjoyment.

Throughout, she is presented as someone to be pitied, but, as Stratonice found, there is an economic advantage to pity because people will pay more for the flowers she picks than they will to any other flower girl.

> 'I am often ailing,' said the blind girl, touchingly; 'and as I grow up I grieve more that I am blind. But now to the flowers!' So saying, she made a slight reverence with her head, and passing into the viridarium, busied herself with watering the flowers. 'Poor Nydia,' thought Glaucus, gazing on her; 'thine is a hard doom!'
>
> Bulwer-Lytton (1834, 42)

The switch to the upbeat 'Now to the flowers!' may reflect a nineteenth-century view that the blind were 'the most habitually cheerful of humankind' (Holmes 2004, 105).

I have found it useful to compare Nydia with the characterisation of another blind flower girl in the 1868 novel *Elsie, the Blind Flower Girl; A story of the Sheltering Arms*. This was one of several improving novels written to support an Episcopal foundation, The Sheltering Arms, in New York City, which from 1864 took in young children, including orphans, and those with disabilities (Higginbotham, n.d.). There is no evidence of direct influence of the Nydia story on this one, and the many similarities are likely simply to echo prevailing notions. We are told that God gave Elsie 'cheerfulness of spirit ... seemingly in compensation for her loss' (Anon. 1868, 57) and that, 'We only know that the blind from birth seem gifted with a particular serenity of spirit and cheerful sense of enjoyment' (Anon. 1868, 61). When we first meet Elsie, it is when Sister Phebe has gone out to buy some flowers to decorate the church for Easter; before she can enter the shop on Broadway, 'an engaging-looking child, between eleven and twelve years of age, carrying in her hand a basket of small, tastefully arranged bouquets' (Anon. 1868, 11) gains her attention. She has 'a strange vagueness of expression' in her eyes and uses a small dog, Gyp, as her guide. She is currently looked after by Margaret, but Sister Phebe is sure that the Sheltering Arms will be better for her. Blind from birth, like Nydia, she too not only has a way with flowers, but can also sing beautifully, 'a melody fresh and clear as a young bird's' (Anon. 1868, 21). An enhanced sense of touch helps her to learn to knit (Anon. 1868, 58–9). The modern reader may be desperate for a fire from which Elsie can save the nuns, but the novel instead goes through the stages of the liturgical and secular year, outlining how those at the Sheltering Arms occupy their time. Like Nydia, Elsie dies at the end of her story, but of consumption and not – of course – until she has been confirmed.

Nobody has to my knowledge suggested that *Elsie, the Blind Flower Girl* has any literary merit, but the immediate reception of Nydia was highly positive. The reviewer of *Last Days* for a women's magazine, *The Court Magazine and Belle assemblée* (November 1834, 217), wrote that she 'is a beautiful conception, and quite original. She wins our love by her artlessness and her generosity'. For *The Athenaeum*'s reviewer, she was 'the sweet blind girl', 'beautifully conceived' (362, Sept 1834, 707). In an appreciation of Bulwer's novels in *The Quarterly Review* (134, issue 268, April 1873, 487–515) it was observed that, 'Schoolboys read it with avidity, and German scholars quote it' (496). As for

Nydia, she 'stands out in bold relief' and 'her blindness gives her an individuality of her own', even if sometimes 'the sentiment is too refined, too modern' (497).

Nydia's most famous afterlife is in a statue by American sculptor Randolph Rogers (Fig. 10.2). The original model is from 1855, the eve of the Civil War, and there are both near-life-size 55-inch versions and smaller, 36-inch ones (Harris 2007, 197; Kovacs 2013, 37–8). It was a very popular sculpture; Rogers made around 100 copies, and a block on lower Fifth Avenue apparently had seven of the 55-inch statues (Kovacs 2013, 38–9). The rendition of the story 'as' ancient sculpture may confuse viewers who assume that there is a classical origin for it.

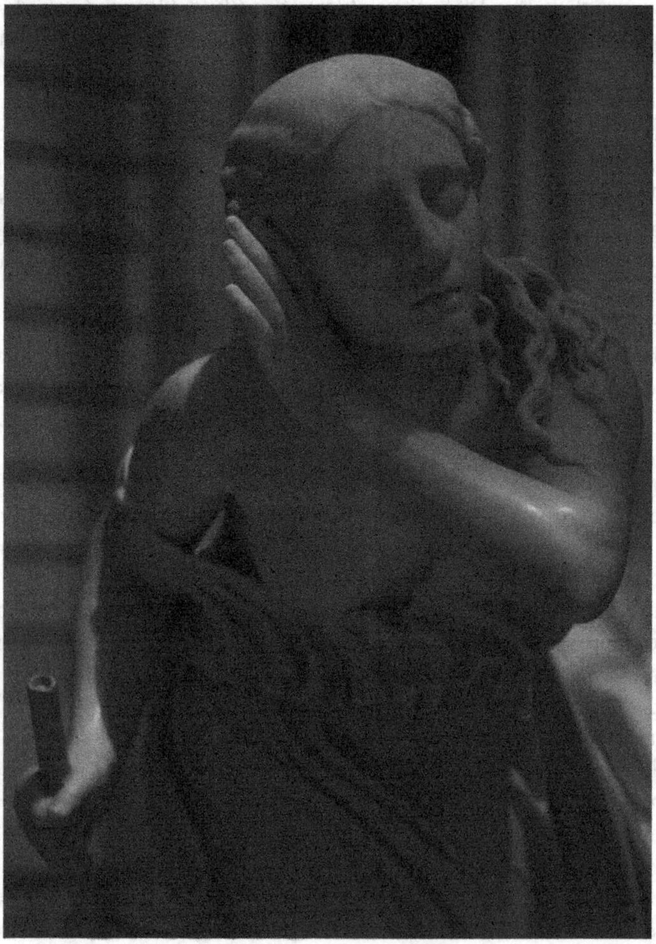

Figure 10.2 *Nydia*, by Randolph Rogers. 'Nydia, the blind flower girl of Pompeii, Metropolitan Museum of Art' by cphoffman42, licensed under CC BY-SA 2.0

Nydia's eyes are closed, and her hand is to her ear: she is listening, but the posture also emphasises that she cannot see. She has a cane to help her move about. It is left open here whether she is separated from Glaucus and Ione or is leading them to safety; her isolation as a figure may suggest the former. The broken piece of a Corinthian column stands in for the destruction of Pompeii.

Elsie dies young, but Nydia's more mature sexuality is clear from her right breast escaping from her dress, and Jon Seydl has suggested that we should also see her clothing in terms of what he calls 'the labial folds of the clinging drapery' (Seydl 2011, 219). Displayed at the 1876 Centennial Exhibition in Philadelphia alongside Rogers's *Ruth Gleaning* (1853), according to one critic 'The Ruth ... did not attract a tithe of the attention that the Nydia did, and did not awaken a tithe of the admiration' (Lessing 2011, 44, citing Clark 1978, 75). In 1865, however, when the rich plantation owner Adelicia Acklen was selecting sculptures for her home, she took Rogers's Ruth rather than his Nydia; Lauren Lessing suggest that perhaps this was because Nydia is presented as having too much of an active role here, rather than offering 'a pleasing, passive, feminine ideal' that fitted with cultural ideas of what a woman should be like and that would, thus, help Acklen's own reputation (Lessing 2011, 4).

It is clear even from the websites of the various museums that house a copy of this statue that it can be read in different ways. The Chicago Art Institute website states that, 'Randolph Rogers captured Nydia as she gropes her way through the burning city' (Art Institute Chicago, n.d.). That 'gropes her way', implying blindness as disability, contrasts strongly with Bulwer-Lytton's text in which she uses her staff 'with great dexterity' (Bulwer-Lytton 1834, 44) and also misses the whole point of the story: in the destruction of Pompeii, she is no longer at a disadvantage – the reverse, in fact, as her sense of hearing is superior to that of her companions. Bulwer-Lytton described her 'incredible dexterity' as she moved through the streets, 'so blessed now was that accustomed darkness, so afflicting in ordinary life' (Bulwer-Lytton 1834, 404). If we are supposed to imagine her separated from Glaucus and Ione, and listening for their voices, then her isolation is not a sign of her weakness, as she remains the one on whom they must rely for their safety. This point is made in the online description from another American university holding one of the sculptures, the University of Michigan: although the city is darkened by the ash blocking out the sun, 'Since Nydia is blind, she is still able to navigate the streets' (University of Michigan Museum of Art 2018, n.p.).

Not everyone loved Nydia, especially in the later twentieth century. In 1974, as Leanne Hunnings noted:

> Kenneth Jernigan of The National Federation of the Blind ... railed against this portrayal of the sightless Nydia as a literary character. He argues that she contributes to the perpetuation of the myth of the blind as 'dehumanized', and the manipulation of blindness for an aesthetic and commercialized aim.
>
> Hunnings (2011, 201)

Jernigan, a blind activist, gave addresses to the 1973 and 1974 Annual Conventions of the US National Federation of the Blind on the themes of history and literature, respectively, attacking 'the image of blindness as dehumanization, a kind of banishment from the world of normal life and relationships'. He held up for particular attention 'the saccharine sweet that has robbed us of humanity and made the legend and hurt our cause' (Jernigan 1974, n.p.). He referred to a range of characters including 'Caleb, the "little blind seer" of James Ludlow's awful novel, "Deborah". There is Bertha, Dickens's ineffably sweet and noble blind heroine of "The Cricket on the Hearth", who comes off almost as an imbecile.' And there he named 'the self-sacrificing Nydia, in "The Last Days of Pompeii"' calling such characters 'sweetness without light, and literature without enlightment'. Blindness in literature, for Jernigan, is:

> dehumanization, a kind of banishment from the world of normal life and relationships. Neither Dickens' blind Bertha, nor Bulwer-Lytton's Nydia, when they find themselves in love, have the slightest idea that anybody could ever love them back – nor does the reader.

It is true that Nydia, despite her depth of emotion, is unable to believe in herself as the object of love. A more recent analysis by Martha Stoddard Holmes suggests instead that Nydia is 'too feeling, too expressive and potentially too sexual for matrimony' (Holmes 2004, 39).

Leanne Hunnings noted that, from the Victorian period onwards, some women were turning Nydia's passivity into their own action. Nydia's song 'The Wind and the Beam loved the Rose' (Bulwer-Lytton 1834, 159) formed the basis of various musical compositions to be 'performed by young women in drawing-rooms', and 'classroom plays for educating the young' were also created from Bulwer-Lytton's novel (Hunnings 2011, 181–2). An even more active Nydia appears in an exercise designed by museum educator Anne Kindseth for the Art Institute of Chicago (Kindseth 2006). Describing the sculpture in a short piece for a journal aimed at teachers involved with art education, Kindseth produces an active Nydia who searches for her lost companions: 'Her body strains forward and her hand cups her ear as she desperately, and daringly, tries to listen for her lost friends'. Kindseth set an activity for those interacting with the sculpture:

> Activity
>
> *How do you think this woman feels? What makes you think that? Pose your body like Nydia. How do you feel standing this way? Think of a story that you would like to tell about an event in your life. Become a living sculpture by posing your body to convey the emotion of your story. Be sure to include props to help tell your story.*

Conclusion

In both formal histories and in imaginative engagement with the Classics, the stories we tell are forms of classical reception. Disability histories use the classical world in a number of ways, depending to some extent on whether they are written by those with the disability or by medical professionals. Greek and Roman history may feature as one source of stories of inspirational individuals, and, although the acknowledged 'great names' of the canon will often feature as 'discoverers', there is often little concern with the details of ancient vocabulary. Here, as elsewhere in histories of medicine and the body, Hippocrates is often seen as 'right', even if the medicine of the past did not realise this. The emphasis tends to be placed on continuity, giving the reassurance that what is being experienced now was also experienced then and offering a 'special connection' to the past, although it may also be suggested that the outcomes are far better today. The sense of continuity can also extend to myth, with characters from Greek and Roman myth being used to represent conditions or those who have them. In the case of Nydia, an imagined figure from the ancient world can be someone to pity, or to admire, with the enthusiasm for her literary and artistic representations varying over time. Although mythical or fictional stories may offer images of disability that are unhelpful to those who live with that condition, they have the potential to be used to foreground those with disability or to allow imaginative identification with a condition that the viewer or user does not share.

Notes

1 A revised version of this blog post appears as Bottrell 2015b. The connections between Bottrell's multiple blogs can be difficult to unravel, but see http://hardluckasthma.blogspot.com/2016/06/new-asthma-history-blog.html (accessed 18 April 2020) for some explanation.

2 Most of the pharmacy treatises associated with the name 'Mesue' were probably written in the eleventh century or later, perhaps in thirteenth-century Bologna, and were based on the Arabic pharmacological tradition (De Vos 2013, 683, 685). The earliest manuscripts of 'the divine Mesue' date to 1281 (De Vos 2013, 671).

3 The author cites Dols, *Medieval Islamic Medicine* (1984), here, but I have not found this passage in that book.

References

Adams, Ellen (2020) 'Deafness: sensory impairment as communication disability, past and present.' In Christian Laes (ed.), *A Cultural History of Disability in Antiquity*. London: Bloomsbury, 85–100.

Al-Rāzī (Rhazes) (1955–68) *Kitāb al-Hāwī fī l-ṭibb*, 23 vols, Hyderabad: Osmania Oriental Publications Bureau.

Anon. (1868) *Elsie, the Blind Flower Girl; A story of the Sheltering Arms*. New York: General Protestant Episcopal Sunday School Union and Church Book Society.

Apostolides, Panos (1997) *Ear, Nose and Throat Diseases in Hippocrates*. Athens: UCB Pharma.

Art Institute Chicago (n.d.) 'Nydia, the blind flower girl of Pompeii', www.artic.edu/artworks/2446/nydia-the-blind-flower-girl-of-pompeii (accessed 18 April 2020).

Atkin, Alison (2015) 'No longer deaf to the past.' *History Today* 3 December 2015, www.historytoday.com/no-longer-deaf-past (accessed 18 April 2020).

Batt, Ronald E. (2009) 'Emergence of endometriosis in North America: a study in the history of ideas.' PhD thesis, State University of New York at Buffalo.

Bauman, H-Dirksen L. (2008) 'On the disconstruction of (sign) language in the Western tradition: a deaf reading of Plato's Cratylus.' In H-Dirksen L. Bauman (ed.), *Open Your Eyes: Deaf Studies Talking*. Minneapolis: University of Minnesota Press, 127–45.

Binder, S. (1991) 'Endometriosis: the "career woman's disease".' *Total Health Magazine* 13(2), 37.

Bostock, John and Henry T. Riley (1857) *The Natural History of Pliny, Book VI*. London: Henry G. Bohn.

Bottrell, John (2013a) '2697 B.C.: The oldest description of asthma (sort of).' http://asthmahistory.blogspot.com/2013/10/2697-bc-oldest-description-of-asthma.html (accessed 18 April 2020).

Bottrell, John (2013b) '460–370 B.C.: What did Hippocrates think about asthma?' http://asthmahistory.blogspot.com/2014/05/460-370-bc-what-did-hippocrates-think.html (accessed 18 April 2020).

Bottrell, John (2015a) '4 B.C. to 65 A.D.: Seneca learns to cope with asthma.' http://respiratorytherapycave.blogspot.com/2015/05/4-bc-to-65-ad-seneca-learns-to-cope.html (accessed 18 April 2020).

Bottrell, John (2015b) '62 B.C.: Seneca the asthma philosopher.' http://asthmahistory.blogspot.com/2015/07/62-bc-seneca-asthma-philosopher.html (accessed 18 April 2020).

Bottrell, John (n.d.) 'Asthma timeline.' http://asthmahistory.blogspot.com/p/asthma.html (accessed 18 April 2020).

Brosens, Ivo and Giuseppe Benagiano (2011) 'Endometriosis, a modern syndrome.' *Indian Journal of Medical Research* 133(6), 581–593.

Bulwer-Lytton, Edward (1834) *The Last Days of Pompeii*. Paris: Baudry's European Library.

Cannizzaro, Theresa (2017) 'History of asthma (part one) – In the beginning.' https://asthma.net/living/history-of-asthma-part-one-in-the-beginning/ (accessed 18 April 2020).

Clark, William J.Jr (1978) *Great American Sculptors*. Philadelphia: Gebbie & Barrie.

Cotto, Bob (2008) 'Who discovered asthma Hippocrates or Galen?' https://ezinearticles.com/?Who-Discovered-Asthma-Hippocrates-Or-Galen?&id=1381520 (accessed 18 April 2020).

Crivellato, Enrico, Luciana Traban and Domenico Ribatti (2007) 'The Hippocratic treatise "On glands": the first document on lymphoid tissue and lymph nodes.' *Leukemia* 21, 591–592. www.nature.com/articles/2404618 (accessed 18 April 2020).

Cserháti, Endre (2004) 'The history of bronchial asthma from the ancient times till the Middle Ages.' *Acta Physiologica Hungarica* 91(3–4), 243–261. https://pubmed.ncbi.nlm.nih.gov/16438118/ (accessed 18 April 2020).

Daly, Nicholas (2011) 'The volcanic disaster narrative: from pleasure garden to canvas, page, and stage.' *Victorian Studies* 53(2), 255–85.

De Vos, Paula (2013) 'The "Prince of Medicine". Yūḥannā ibn Māsawayh and the foundations of the western pharmaceutical tradition.' *Isis* 104(4), 667–712.

Endometriosis UK (2017) 'Endometriosis – is it a disability?' https://endometriosis-uk.org/news/endometriosis-it-disability-37511 (accessed 18 April 2020).

Enovid (1962) 'Enovid: the first complete physiologic regulator of female cyclic function.' [advertisement]. *Canadian Medical Association Journal* 86, 1183. www.ncbi.nlm.nih.gov/pmc/articles/PMC1849248/pdf/canmedaj00949-0052.pdf (accessed 18 April 2020).

Epilepsy Canada (2016) 'History of epilepsy.' www.epilepsy.ca/history-of-epilepsy.html (accessed 18 April 2020).

Estonian Association of the Deaf (2010) 'Foreign deaf history.' http://www.ead.ee/foreign_deaf_history (accessed 18 April 2020).

Felman, Adam (2018) 'A brief history of asthma.' https://www.medicalnewstoday.com/articles/323526 (accessed 18 April 2020).

Felton, Debbie (2012) 'Rejecting and embracing the monstrous in ancient Greece and Rome.' In Asa S. Mittman and Peter Dendle (eds), *The Ashgate Research Companion to Monsters and the Monstrous*. Farnham and Burlington: Ashgate Press, 103–31.

Ferreri, Giulio (1906) 'The deaf in antiquity.' Translated into English for *American Annals of the Deaf* 51, 460–73.

Finke, Beth (2017) '50 years after its debut, a blind actor is cast in "Wait Until Dark".' https://blog.easterseals.com/50-years-after-its-debut-a-blind-actor-is-cast-in-wait-until-dark/ (accessed 18 April 2020).

Floyer, John (1715) *Psychrolousia, or, the History of Cold Bathing: Both Ancient and Modern. Part 1* (4th edn). London: printed for William Innys.

Fowler, Edmund P. (1993) 'The second one hundred years, musings and dreams of things to come.' In *History of the American Otological Society, Inc, 1868–1993: Six Score and Five Years of Progress* (printed by the Society), 88–90.

Fowler, Harold N. (1921) *Plato: Cratylus, Parmenides, Greater Hippias, Lesser Hippias*. Cambridge, MA: Harvard University Press.

Frea, Rick (2011) '62 B.C.: Seneca the asthma philosopherx [*sic*].' http://hardluckasthma.blogspot.com/2011/12/62-bc-seneca-asthma-philosopher.html (accessed 18 April 2020).

Garretson, Mervin D. (1981) 'Introduction.' In Jack R. Gannon, *Deaf Heritage: A Narrative History of Deaf America*. Washington, DC: Gallaudet University Press, xxi. http://gupress.gallaudet.edu/excerpts/DHintro.html (accessed 18 April 2020).

Green, Monica H. (2001) *The Trotula: A Medieval Compendium of Women's Medicine*. Philadelphia: University of Pennsylvania Press.

Gross, Izhak (1981) 'Parliament and the abolition of negro apprenticeship 1835–1838.' *English Historical Review* 96, 560–76.

Harrington, Thomas (2006) 'Earliest known deaf people (to 1700 AD).' https://web.archive.org/web/20071012084125/http://library.gallaudet.edu/deaf-faq-earliest-deaf.shtml (accessed 18 April 2020).

Harris, Judith (2007) *Pompeii Awakened: A Story of Rediscovery*. London and New York: I.B. Tauris.

Hawkins, Joseph E. (2004) 'Sketches of otohistory: Part 1 – otoprehistory: how it all began.' *Audiology and Neurotology* 9, 66–71.

Hawkins, Joseph E. and Jochen Schacht (2008) *Sketches of Otohistory*. Basle: Karger.

Helmbold, William C. (1939) *Plutarch, Moralia*. Vol. 6. Cambridge, MA: Harvard University Press.

Hett, Walter S. (1957) *Aristotle: On the soul, Parva naturalia, On breath*. Cambridge, MA: Harvard University Press.

Higginbotham, Peter (n.d.) 'Children's homes and institutions in New York, USA.' www.childrenshomes.org.uk/list/NewYork.shtml?LMCL=mo8hwf&LMCL=NLFA8_ (accessed 18 April 2020).

Holgate, Stephen T. (2010) 'A brief history of asthma and its mechanisms to modern concepts of disease pathogenesis.' *Allergy Asthma & Immunology Research* 2(3), 165–171. https://e-aair.org/DOIx.php?id=10.4168/aair.2010.2.3.165

Holmes, Martha S. (2004) *Fictions of Affliction: Physical Disability in Victorian Culture*. Ann Arbor, MI: University of Michigan Press.

How to Use Inhalers (2012) 'Who discovered asthma?' https://use-inhalers.com/who-discovered-asthma (accessed 18 April 2020).

Hunnings, Leanne (2011) 'Between victimhood and agency: Nydia the slave in Bulwer's The Last Days of Pompeii.' In Edith Hall, Richard Alston and Justine McConnell (eds), *Ancient Slavery and Abolition: From Hobbes to Hollywood*. Oxford: Oxford University Press, 181–207.

Jackson, Mark (2006) *Allergy: The History of a Modern Malady*. London: Reaktion Books.

Jackson, Mark (2009) *Asthma: The Biography*. Oxford: Oxford University Press.

Jernigan, Kenneth (1974) 'Blindness: is literature against us?' Address delivered at the National Federation of the Blind Banquet, July 3 1974. www.nfb.org/images/nfb/publications/convent/banque74.htm (accessed 18 April 2020).

Jouanna, Jacques (2012a) 'Disease as aggression in the Hippocratic Corpus and Greek tragedy: wild and devouring disease.' In Jacques Jouanna, *Greek Medicine from Hippocrates to Galen: Selected Papers*. Leiden: Brill, 81–96.

Jouanna, Jacques (2012b) 'Hippocratic medicine and Greek tragedy.' In Jacques Jouanna, *Greek Medicine from Hippocrates to Galen: Selected Papers*. Leiden: Brill, 55–80.

Junod, Suzanne W. and Lara Marks (2002) 'Women's trials: the approval of the first oral contraceptive pill in the United States and Great Britain.' *Journal of the History of Medicine and Allied Sciences* 57(2), 117–60.

Karamanou, Marianna and George Androutsos (2011) 'Aretaeus of Cappadocia and the first clinical description of asthma.' *American Journal of Respiratory and Critical Care Medicine* 184(12). https://doi.org/10.1164/ajrccm.184.12.1420b (accessed 18 April 2020).

Keeney, Edmund L. (1964) 'The history of asthma from Hippocrates to Meltzer.' *Journal of Allergy* 35, 215–26.

Kindseth, Anne (2006) 'Randolph Rogers. Nydia, the blind flower girl of Pompeii.' *School Arts* 105(7). https://go.gale.com/ps/i.do?p=AONE&u=tou&id=GALE%7CA142870861&v=2.1&it=r&sid=AONE&asid=e0670c2d (accessed 18 April 2020).

King, Helen (1993) 'Once upon a text: the Hippocratic origins of hysteria.' In Sander Gilman, Helen King, Roy Porter, G.S. Rousseau and Elaine Showalter (eds), *Hysteria Beyond Freud*. Berkeley, Los Angeles and Oxford: University of California Press, 3–90.

King, Helen (2005) 'Women's health and recovery in the Hippocratic corpus.' In Helen King (ed.), *Health in Antiquity*. London: Routledge, 150–61.

King, Helen (2019) *Hippocrates Now: The 'Father of Medicine' in the Internet Age*. London: Bloomsbury.

King, Jean R. and Sheldon G. Cohen (2001) 'Asthma among the famous. Augustus Caesar (63 B.C.–A.D. 14) first emperor of Rome.' *Allergy and Asthma Proceedings* 22(2), 101–9.

Kovacs, Claire L. (2013) 'Pompeii and its material reproductions: the rise of a tourist site in the nineteenth century.' *Journal of Tourism History* 5(1), 25–49.

Kühn, Karl G. (1965) *Claudii Galeni Opera omnia*. Vol. 12. Hildesheim: G. Olms.

Laes, Christian (2018) *Disabilities and the Disabled in the Roman World: A Social and Cultural History*. Cambridge: Cambridge University Press.

Langworthy, Jessica L. (1930) 'Blindness in fiction: a study of the attitude of authors towards their blind characters.' *Journal of Applied Psychology* 14, 269–86.

Lessing, Lauren (2011) 'Angels in the home: Adelicia Acklen's sculpture collection at Belmont Mansion, Nashville, Tennessee.' *Winterthur Portfolio* 45(1), 29–60.

Lichtenthaeler, Charles (1965) *Thucydide et Hippocrate vus par un historien-médecin*. Geneva: Librairie Droz.

LiDonnici, Lynn R. (1995) *The Epidaurian Miracle Inscriptions: Text, Translation and Commentary*. Texts and Translations 36; Graeco-Roman Religion Series I I. Atlanta: Scholars Press.

Marketos, Spyros G. and Constantine N. Ballas (1982) 'Bronchial asthma in the medical literature of Greek antiquity.' *Journal of Asthma* 19, 263–9.

Miller, Brian R. (2014) 'History of the blind.' Encyclopaedia Britannica online, www.britannica.com/topic/history-of-the-blind-1996241 (accessed 18 April 2020).

Minnesota Governor's Council on Developmental Disabilities (2019) 'Parallels in Time: A history of developmental disabilities.' http://mn.gov/mnddc/parallels/one/2.html (accessed 18 April 2020).

Mitra, Anita (2017) 'What is endometriosis?' www.gynaegeek.com/the-blog/2017/9/6/what-is-endometriosis (accessed 18 April 2020).

Moormann, Eric (2015) *Pompeii's Ashes: The Reception of the Cities Buried by Vesuvius in literature, music, and drama*. Berlin: De Gruyter.

Nezhat, Camran, Farr Nezhat and Ceana Nezhat. (2012) 'Endometriosis: ancient disease, ancient treatments.' *Fertility and Sterility* 98(65), 1–62.

Nogueira, João F. Júnior, Diego Rodrigo Hermann, Ronaldo dos Reis Américo, Iulo Sérgio Barauna Filho, Aldo Eden Cassol Stamm, and Shirley Shizuo Nagata Pignatari (2007) 'A brief history of otorhinolaryngolgy: otology, laryngology and rhinology.' *Revista Brasileira de Otorrinolaringologia* 73(5), 693–703. www.scielo.br/scielo.php?pid=s0034-72992007000500017&script=sci_arttext&tlng=en (accessed 18 April 2020).

Omvig, Jim (2019) 'History of blindness: summary of the history of the education and rehabilitation of the blind.' https://www.facebook.com/openoureyescommunity/posts/summary-of-the-history-of-the-education-and-rehabilitation-of-the-blindby-james-/10155124121210740/ (accessed 18 April 2020).

Page, Denys L. (1953) 'Thucydides' description of the Great Plague at Athens.' *Classical Quarterly* 3, 97–119.

Panzani, Raphael C. (1988) 'Seneca and his asthma: the illnesses, life and death of a Roman stoic philosopher.' *Journal of Asthma* 25, 163–74.

Paquette, Penny (2003) *Asthma: The Ultimate Teen Guide*. Oxford: Scarecrow Press.

Patel, H.H. (2019) 'Asthma history.' www.news-medical.net/health/Asthma-History.aspx (accessed 18 April 2020).

Payne, Arnold H. (1911) 'Deaf and dumb.' https://en.wikisource.org/wiki/1911_Encyclopædia_Britannica/Deaf_and_Dumb (accessed 18 April 2020).

Politzer, Adam (1907) *Geschichte der Ohrenheilkunde*. Vol. I. Stuttgart: Ferdinand Enke.

Psifidis, Anestis (2006) 'The prehistory of audiology and otology.' *Mediterranean Journal of Otology* 2, 41–6.

Quayson, Ato (2007) *Aesthetic Nervousness: Disability and the Crisis of Representation.* New York: Columbia University Press.

Reynolds, Edward H. (2005) 'Milestones in the history of epilepsy.' *WHO Epilepsy Atlas.* Geneva: WHO, 16–19. www.who.int/mental_health/neurology/Epilepsy_atlas_r1.pdf (accessed 18 April 2020).

Richardson, Mark A. (1999) 'Sore throat, tonsillitis, and adenoiditis.' *Medical Clinics of North America* 83(1), 75–83. https://doi.org/10.1016/S0025-7125(05)70088-2 (accessed 18 April 2020).

Robinson, Victor (1941) 'Examination in the history of otology.' *The Laryngoscope* 51(4), 315–6.

Ryan, Michael (1793) *Observations on the History and Cure of the Asthma; In which the Propriety of using the Cold Bath in that Disorder is Fully Considered.* London: printed for G.G.J. & J. Robinson.

Sakula, Alex (1988) 'A history of asthma.' *Journal of the Royal College of Physicians* 22, 35–44.

Sanmiguel, Lisa M. (2000) 'From "career woman's" disease to "an epidemic ignored": endometriosis in United States culture since 1948.' PhD thesis, University of Illinois at Urbana-Champaign.

Saxena, Surabhi (2019) 'Weird asthma cures you didn't know about!' https://cashkaro.com/blog/weird-asthma-cures-you-didnt-know-about/108240 (accessed 18 April 2020).

Schiller, Joyce K. (1993) 'Nydia: a forgotten icon of the nineteenth century.' *Bulletin of the Detroit Institute of Arts* 67(4), 36–45.

Seydl, Jon L. (2011) 'Experiencing the last days of Pompeii in late nineteenth-century Philadelphia.' In Shelley Hales and Joanna Paul (eds), *Pompeii in the Public Imagination from Its Rediscovery to Today.* Oxford: Oxford University Press, 215–31.

Shaner, Wendy (2013) 'Deaf culture timeline.' https://signlanguageco.com/deaf-culture-timeline/ (accessed 18 April 2020).

Sharman, Caroline (1996) 'Nineteenth-century views of blindness and deafness and Jane Eyre.' www.victorianweb.org/authors/bronte/cbronte/sharman10.html (accessed 18 April 2020).

Sutton, Christopher (2006) 'The history of endometriosis.' In Christopher Sutton, Kevin Jones and G. David Adamson (eds), *Modern Management of Endometriosis.* London and New York: Taylor & Francis, 3–16.

Thorpe, J.R. (2015) 'Science may have found a cure for asthma attacks.' www.bustle.com/articles/93817-a-cure-for-asthma-might-be-closer-than-youd-think-new-study-finds (accessed 18 April 2020).

Traynor, Robert (2015) 'International giants of otology: the earliest years.' http://hearinghealthmatters.org/hearinginternational/2015/international-giants-of-otology-the-pioneers (accessed 18 April 2020).

Trentin, Lisa (2011) 'Deformity in the Roman imperial court.' *Greece & Rome* 58(2), 195–208.

Tuinstra, Stephanie (2001) 'Disability timeline.' www.d.umn.edu/cla/faculty/tbacig/studproj/is3099/pplfrst/Untitled1.html (accessed 18 April 2020).

University of Michigan Museum of Art (2018) 'Nydia, the blind flower girl of Pompeii.' https://exchange.umma.umich.edu/resources/9627/view (accessed 18 April 2020).

Vlayen, Joan, Leentje De Bleser, Stephan Devriese and Walter Sermeus (2005) 'The use of clinical pathways in Belgium', KCE Reports 18A, *Prospectief bepalen van de honoraria van ziekenhuisartsen op basis van klinische paden en guidelines: makkelijker gezegd dan gedaan*, 34–56. https://kce.fgov.be/sites/default/files/atoms/files/d20051027319_0.pdf (accessed 18 April 2020).

Index

Page numbers in italics refer to figures. Page numbers in bold refer to tables. Page numbers followed by 'n' refer to notes.

9780367221959